Diversifying Food and Diets

Currently 868 million people are undernourished and 195 million children under five years of age are stunted. At the same time, over 1 billion people are overweight and obese in both the developed and developing world. Diseases previously associated with affluence, such as cancer, diabetes and cardio-vascular disease, are on the rise. Food system-based approaches to addressing these problems that could enhance food availability and diet quality through local production and agricultural biodiversity often fall outside the traditional scope of nutrition, and have been under-researched. As a consequence, there remains insufficient evidence to support well-defined, scalable agricultural biodiversity interventions that can be linked to improvements in nutrition outcomes.

Agricultural biodiversity is important for food and nutritional security, as a safeguard against hunger, a source of nutrients for improved dietary diversity and quality, and strengthening local food systems and environmental sustainability. This book explores the current state of knowledge on the role of agricultural biodiversity in improving nutrition and food security. Using examples and case studies from around the globe, the book explores current strategies for improving nutrition and diets and identifies key research and implementation gaps that need to be addressed to successfully promote the better use of agricultural biodiversity for rural and urban populations, and societies in transition.

Jessica Fanzo was formerly a Senior Scientist with Bioversity International and is now an Associate Professor of Nutrition at Columbia University in New York.

Danny Hunter is the Global Project Coordinator at Bioversity International for the UNEP/FAO/GEF project 'Mainstreaming biodiversity conservation and sustainable use for improved human nutrition and wellbeing' and Adjunct Associate Professor, School of Agriculture and Wine Sciences, Charles Sturt University, Australia.

Teresa Borelli is a Programme Specialist at Bioversity International working for the UNEP/FAO/GEF project 'Mainstreaming biodiversity conservation and sustainable use for improved human nutrition and wellbeing'.

Federico Mattei was formerly a Programme Specialist in the Nutrition and Marketing division at Bioversity International in Rome.

Issues in Agricultural Biodiversity

Series editors: Michael Halewood and Danny Hunter

This series of books is published by Earthscan in association with Bioversity International. The aim of the series is to review the current state of knowledge in topical issues associated with agricultural biodiversity, to identify gaps in our knowledge base, to synthesize lessons learned and to propose future research and development actions. The overall objective is to increase the sustainable use of biodiversity in improving people's well-being and food and nutrition security. The series' scope is all aspects of agricultural biodiversity, ranging from conservation biology of genetic resources through social sciences to policy and legal aspects. It also covers the fields of research, education, communication and coordination, information management and knowledge sharing.

Diversifying Food and Diets

Using agricultural biodiversity to improve nutrition and health

Edited by Jessica Fanzo, Danny Hunter, Teresa Borelli and Federico Mattei

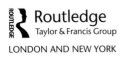

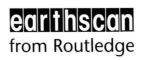

LONDON AND NEW YORK

from Routledge

This first edition published 2013
by Routledge
2 Park Square, Milton Park, Abingdon, Oxon, OX14 4RN

Simultaneously published in the USA and Canada
by Routledge
711 Third Avenue, New York, NY 10017

Routledge is an imprint of the Taylor & Francis Group, an informa business

British Library Cataloguing in Publication Data
A catalogue record for this book is available from the British Library

Library of Congress Cataloging-in-Publication Data
Diversifying food and diets : using agricultural biodiversity to improve
nutrition and health / edited by Jessica Fanzo, Danny Hunter, Teresa
Borelli, and Federico Mattei. – First edition.
     pages cm. – (Issues in agricultural biodiversity)
  Includes bibliographical references and index.
  1. Agrobiodiversity. 2. Nutrition – Environmental aspects.
  I. Fanzo, Jessica, editor of compilation. II. Hunter, Danny, editor of
  compilation. III. Borelli, Teresa, editor of compilation. IV. Mattei,
  Federico, editor of compilation.
  S494.5.A43D58 2013
  333.95–dc23   2012037893

ISBN: 978-0-415-63823-4 (hbk)
ISBN: 978-0-415-63824-1 (pbk)
ISBN: 978-0-203-08413-7 (ebk)

Typeset in Bembo
by HWA Text and Data Management, London

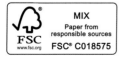

Printed and bound in Great Britain by MPG Printgroup

This book is dedicated to Lois Englberger, who passed away on the 29 September 2011 before she could see this book published. With our enormous gratitude and admiration for her work.

'At a time where fortification is widely promoted as the most effective solution to address micro-nutrient deficiencies, this book serves as an important reminder that nature provides an almost infinite variety of food species which are disregarded and therefore pushed into oblivion and extinction by the prevailing food production system. It is urgent to remind policy makers that agriculture is primarily about using natural resources to feed people. Sustainable development will only happen if we manage such resources in a sustainable way, building on local cultures, protecting and strengthening livelihoods, and ensuring good nutrition and health.' – *Florence Egal, Food Security, Nutrition and Livelihoods, Nutrition Division FAO*

'This book is important and deserves a wide readership. Only once governments are convinced of the importance of agricultural biodiversity shall they implement the policies that are urgently required to move away from the direction of agricultural development that is dominant today – one that favors uniformity over diversity, top-down research and development on new crops rather than bottom-up and participatory approaches, and monocropping over integrated farming systems.' – *From the foreword by Olivier De Schutter, United Nations Special Rapporteur on the right to food*

'I would like to take this opportunity to congratulate the authors and partner organizations on this milestone publication. Their work offers a comprehensive summary of contemporary information and good practices, identifies gaps in research and provides insight on potential opportunities for a variety of policy options. I look forward to more sustainable management of biodiversity in all ecosystems, but particularly in agricultural ecosystems, where we can truly achieve a healthy partnership between people and the planet.' – *From the foreword by Braulio Ferreira de Souza Dias, Convention on Biological Diversity*

Contents

Figures

Tables

Boxes

Contributors

Editors

Jessica Fanzo was formerly a Senior Scientist with Bioversity International, and is now an Associate Professor of Nutrition at Columbia University in New York.

Danny Hunter is the Global Project Coordinator at Bioversity International for the UNEP/FAO/GEF project 'Mainstreaming biodiversity conservation and sustainable use for improved human nutrition and wellbeing'.

Teresa Borelli is a Programme Specialist at Bioversity International working for the UNEP/FAO/GEF project 'Mainstreaming biodiversity conservation and sustainable use for improved human nutrition and wellbeing'.

Federico Mattei was formerly a Programme Specialist in the Nutrition and Marketing division at Bioversity International in Rome.

Contributors

Fabrice DeClerck, Bioversity International (Chapter 1)

Vernon H. Heywood, University of Reading (Chapter 2)

Irene Hoffmann and Roswitha Baumung, Food and Agriculture Organization of the United Nations (FAO) (Chapter 3)

Matthias Halwart, Food and Agriculture Organization of the United Nations (FAO) (Chapter 4)

Hervé B.D. Bisseleua and Amadou Ibra Niang, The MDG Centre, West and Central Africa (Chapter 5)

Ifeyironwa Francisca Smith, Lanrify Agriculture, Food and Nutrition Consulting Inc. (Chapter 6)

Roseline Remans, The Earth Institute at Columbia University and **Sean Smukler**, the University of British Columbia (Chapter 7)

Michael Hermann, Crops for the Future (Chapter 8)

Peter R. Berti, Healthbridge and **Andrew D. Jones**, Cornell University (Chapter 9)

Margaret McEwan and Gordon Prain, International Potato Center (CIP) and **Danny Hunter**, Bioversity International (Chapter 10)

Lois Englberger and Eminher Johnson, Island Food Community of Pohnpei (Case study 1)

Roshan Pudasaini, Sajal Sthapit and Rojee Suwal, LI-BIRD; and **Bhuwon Sthapit**, Bioversity International (Case study 2)

Katja Kehlenbeck, Ebenezar Asaah and Ramni Jamnadass, World Agroforestry Centre (ICRAF) (Case study 3)

Shakuntala Haraksingh Thilsted, WorldFish (Case study 4)

Jan Low, Ricardo Labarta, Maria Andrade and Sam Namanda, International Potato Center (CIP) and **Mary Arimond**, University California Davis (Case study 5)

C. Ojiewo, A. Tenkouano, J. d'A. Hughes and J.D.H. Keatinge, AVRDC – The World Vegetable Center (Case study 6)

Jennifer Nielsen, Nancy Haselow, Akoto Osei and Zaman Talukder, Helen Keller International (Case study 7)

Nadia Bergamini and Stefano Padulosi, Bioversity International, **S. Bala Ravi**, MSSRF, India and **Nirmala Yenagi**, University of Dharwad, India (Case study 8)

Kelly Donati, Christopher Taylor and Craig J. Pearson, University of Melbourne (Case study 9)

John Paull, University of Oxford (Case study 10)

Petra Bakewell-Stone, University of Kent (Case study 11)

Catia Grisa and Claudia Job Schmitt, Rural Federal University of Rio de Janeiro (CPDA/UFRRJ) (Case study 12)

About Bioversity

Bioversity International is one of 15 centres supported by the Consultative Group on International Agricultural Research (CGIAR). Bioversity is a world leading research-for-development non-profit organization, working towards a world in which smallholder farmers and rural communities in developing countries are thriving and sustainable. Bioversity's purpose is to investigate the use and conservation of agricultural and forest biodiversity in order to achieve better nutrition, improve livelihoods and enhance agricultural and forest sustainability. Bioversity International works with a global range of partners to maximize impact, to develop capacity and to ensure that all stakeholders have an effective voice.

> Bioversity International
> Via dei Tre Denari
> 00057 Maccarese,
> Rome, Italy
> www.bioversityinternational.org

About CTA

The Technical Centre for Agricultural and Rural Cooperation (CTA) is a joint international institution of the African, Caribbean and Pacific (ACP) Group of States and the European Union (EU). Its mission is to advance food and nutritional security, increase prosperity and encourage sound natural resource management in ACP countries. It provides access to information and knowledge, facilitates policy dialogue and strengthens the capacity of agricultural and rural development institutions and communities.

CTA operates under the framework of the Cotonou Agreement and is funded by the EU.

For more information on CTA, visit www.cta.int

Foreword

Olivier De Schutter

The first perspective

In international discussions, much less attention has been paid to agricultural biodiversity than to (non-agricultural) biodiversity. Yet, by domesticating and maintaining a variety of species, and by maintaining genetic diversity within each species, farmers and herders make a major contribution to the sustainability of our food systems. They contribute to the future resilience of food production in the face of climatic shocks and attacks from nature, which are by definition unpredictable and which require that we encourage diversity in farming systems (Swanson 1997: 52; Esquinas-Alcázar, 2005). They maintain the kind of diversity of crops or livestock that will allow us to support, in each specific agro-ecological environment, the reliance on the variety that will be best suited to that environment. And of course, they provide important nutritional benefits: while Green Revolution approaches in the past have primarily focused on increasing calorie availability by boosting cereal crops – particularly rice, wheat and maize – we have now come to realize that the shift from diversified cropping systems to simplified, cereal based systems has contributed to micronutrient malnutrition in many developing countries (Demment et al., 2003): of the over 80,000 plant species available to humans, only three (maize, wheat, rice) supply the bulk of our protein and energy needs (Frison et al., 2006), and nutritionists now increasingly insist on the need for more diverse agro-ecosystems, in order to ensure a more diversified nutrient output of the farming systems (Alloway, 2008; Burchi et al., 2011; DeClerck et al., 2011).

This message is not easy to get across. It runs against the tide. 'Green Revolution' approaches, in which farmers are supported by being given access to the main inputs (improved varieties of seeds, fertilizers and pesticides), are still dominant. This is understandable, since one of the reasons why small-scale farmers are poor and cannot move beyond subsistence farming is because of the high prices of inputs and the lack of access to credit. And input-intensive agriculture is still considered by many as the only realistic pathway towards its modernization, which we often equate to its industrialization.

But this form of support, it is increasingly recognized, can create its own problems. Commercial seed varieties may be less suited to the specific agro-ecological environments in which farmers work, and for which landraces (traditional farmers' varieties) may be more appropriate. Even where hybrid seed varieties (developed by professional plant breeders, in particular commercial seed companies) improve yields in the short term, their higher performance often has been a response to inputs (fertilizers) and to water availability, making it difficult for farmers unable to access such inputs and conditions to reap their benefits. Those who acquire inputs with their own means, often encouraged to do so during an initial period of subsidized inputs, may find themselves trapped in the vicious circle of debt as a result of a bad harvest and consequent impossibility to reimburse input loans. This may occur particularly when they have switched to mono-cropping, leading to revenues which may be higher in certain seasons but less stable across the years, and diminish resilience in the face of climate change: indeed, there exists a correlation between the switch to specialized and uniform varieties on the one hand and increased variability in productivity on the other (Duvick, 1989; Hazell, 1984, 1985).

The broader concern however, is that the expansion of agricultural areas cultivated with commercial seeds accelerates crop diversity erosion, as an increasing number of farmers grow the same crops, using the same, 'improved' varieties on their fields. It is this consequence that the authors of this book focus on, emphasizing in particular the links between the reduction of agricultural biodiversity linked to the spread of genetically uniform crops and the reduction in the range of species cultivated, on the one hand, and poorer nutrition for the rural communities concerned, on the other.

In order to redirect this trajectory, a number of measures should be taken. First, farming and herding practices that maintain and enhance diversity of species and genetic variability within species are more knowledge-intensive than practices that are based on uniformity and homogenization. Support for such practices therefore requires the development of both ecological literacy and decision-making skills in farmers' communities. Investments in agricultural extension and agricultural research are key in this regard. While agricultural spending is among the three top contributors to increasing rural welfare, along with public spending in education, health and roads, agricultural research in particular has the greatest overall impact on poverty and agricultural productivity in developing countries: it was found that it had 'the largest impact on agricultural production and second-largest impact on poverty reduction (after rural education) in China, and the second-largest impact on poverty reduction in rural India (after investment in roads)' (Fan, 2008). Research in agro-ecological practices in particular should be prioritized, because of the considerable, and largely untapped, potential of such practices. The role of the public sector here is particularly vital, since sound agricultural and herding practices that maintain and enhance agricultural biodiversity are generally not supported by the private sector, as the improvements in such practices are not rewarded by patents of plant breeders' rights (Vanloqueren and Baret, 2009).

Second, the social organization of farmers is also vital. Almost by definition, because of the localized nature of the knowledge that is to be mobilized, practices that support agricultural biodiversity and can help maintain and enhance it cannot be imposed top-down: they should be shared, rather, from farmer to farmer, in farmer field schools or through farmers' movements, as in the Campesino-a-Campesino movement in Central America and Cuba (Degrande et al., 2006: 6; Rosset et al., 2011). An improved dissemination of knowledge by horizontal means transforms the nature of knowledge itself, which becomes the product of a network (Warner and Kirschenmann, 2007). It should encourage farmers, particularly small-scale farmers living in the most remote areas and those on the most marginal soil, to identify innovative solutions, working with experts towards a co-construction of knowledge that ensures that advances will benefit them as a matter of priority – rather than only benefiting the better-off producers (Uphoff, 2002: 55).

Thirdly, farmers' seed systems must be supported (De Schutter, 2011; Santilli, 2012). In South Asia and sub-Saharan Africa, the overwhelming majority of farmers still rely on traditional farmers' seed systems in order to grow their crops. Reliance by farmers on farmers' seed systems, by the exchange and use of local 'landraces', allows them to limit the cost of production, and to preserve a certain degree of independence from the commercial seed sector. The system of unfettered exchange in farmers' seed systems ensures the free flow of genetic materials, thus contributing to the development of locally appropriate seeds and to the diversity of crops. In addition, these varieties are best suited to the difficult environments in which they grow. They result in reasonably good yields without having to be combined with other inputs such as chemical fertilizers. As already mentioned, because they are genetically diverse, such local varieties may be more resilient to weather-related events or to attacks by pests or diseases.

Allowing such farmers' seed systems to develop is not only in the interest of the poorest farmers. It is also in the long-term interest of professional plant breeders and seed companies themselves, who depend on the development of these plant resources for their own innovations. In order to achieve this, we must combine the discussion on intellectual property rights on seeds and the debate on access to genetic resources under the Convention on Biological Diversity and the International Treaty on Plant Genetic Resources for Food and Agriculture. By rewarding farmers for their contribution to the enhancement of agricultural biodiversity seen as a global public good, we also promote innovations through farmers' seed systems. The protection of farmers' rights, as stipulated under Article 9 of the International Treaty, and the gradual strengthening of the Benefit-Sharing Fund under the same instrument, have a key role to play in this transformation. And at local level, support for seed banks and seed fairs, and the adaptation of seed regulations in order to allow for an improved distribution of farmers' varieties, can also make an important contribution.

The implementation of such measures requires a serious commitment from states. This is why this book is important and deserves a wide readership. Only once governments are convinced of the importance of agricultural biodiversity, shall they implement the policies as outlined above, which are urgently required to move away from the direction of agricultural development that is dominant today – one that favors uniformity over diversity, top-down research and development on new crops rather than bottom-up and participatory approaches to plant breeding, and mono-cropping over integrated farming systems.

References

Alloway, B.J. (eds) (2008) *Micronutrient deficiencies in global crop production*, Springer Verlag, pp.354.

Burchi, F., Fanzo, J., and Frison, E. (2011) 'The role of food and nutrition system approaches in tackling hidden hunger,' *Int J Environ Res Public Health*, vol 8, no 2, pp.358–373.

DeClerck, F.A.J. et al. (2011) 'Ecological approaches to human nutrition,' *Food & Nutrition Bulletin*, 32(Suppl.1), pp.41S–50S.

Degrande, A. et al. (2006) *Mechanisms for scaling-up tree domestication: how grassroots organizations become agents of change*, ICRAF, Nairobi, Kenya.

Demment, M.W. et al. (2003) 'Providing micronutrients through food based solutions: a key to human and national development,' *J. Nutrition*, vol. 133, pp.3879–3885.

De Schutter, O. (2011) 'The right of everyone to enjoy the benefits of scientific progress and the right to food: from conflict to complementarity,' *Human Rights Quarterly*, vol. 33, pp.304–350.

Duvick, D. (1989) 'Variability in U.S. Maize Yields,' in J. Anderson and P. Hazell (eds), *Variability in Grain Yields*, Washington DC, World Bank.

Esquinas-Alcázar, J. (2005) 'Protecting crop genetic diversity for food security: political, ethical and technical challenges,' *Nature*, vol. 6, pp.946–953.

Fan, S. (2008) 'Public expenditures, growth, and poverty. Lessons from developing countries,' *IFPRI Issue Brief* 51, Washington DC.

Frison, E., Smith, I.F., Johns, T., Cherfas, J., and Eyzaguirre, P.B. (2006) 'Agricultural biodiversity, nutrition and health: making a difference to hunger and nutrition in the developing world,' *Food Nutr. Bull.*, vol 27, no 2, pp.167–179.

Hazell, P. (1984) 'Sources of increased variability in Indian and U.S. cereal production,' *American Journal of Agricultural Economics*, vol 66, pp.302–311.

Hazell, P. (1985) 'Sources of increased variability in world cereal production since the 1960s,' *American Journal of Agricultural Economics*, vol 36, no 2, pp.145–159.

Rosset, P. et al. (2011) 'The Campesino to Campesino agroecology movement of ANAP in Cuba: social process methodology in the construction of sustainable peasant agriculture and food sovereignty,' *Journal of Peasant Studies*, vol 38, no 1, pp.1–33.

Santilli, J. (2012) *Agrobiodiversity and the Law*, Earthscan, London.

Swanson, T. (2005) *Global Action for Biodiversity*, James & James Science Publishers, (originally published in Earthscan Publications, London, 1997).

Uphoff, N. (2002) 'Institutional change and policy reforms,' in Uphoff (eds), *Agroecological innovations. Increasing food production with participatory development*, Earthscan Publications, London.

Vanloqueren, G., and Baret, P.V. (2009) 'How agricultural research systems shape a technological regime that develops genetic engineering but locks out agroecological innovations,' *Research Policy*, vol 38, pp.971–983.

Warner, K.D., and Kirschenmann, F. (2007) *Agroecology in Action: Extending Alternative Agriculture through Social Networks*, MIT Press, Cambridge.

Foreword

Braulio Ferreira de Souza Dias

The second perspective

Biodiversity underpins ecosystem functioning and is essential to many aspects of our health and well-being, including nutrition. It is also the basis for future advances in food production through improved yields and nutritional quality and provides options for adaptation to climate change.

Globally, both food production and food security have increased over recent decades. This progress has been achieved through agricultural intensification but at significant environmental cost, illustrated by our overuse of land, water and chemicals. Alongside this, we have seen a trend towards a simplification of diets and accompanying nutritional degradation. To meet the challenge of achieving food security and healthy nutrition, we need to focus on ecologically sustainable intensification of farming systems that will also contribute to improved diets. This is a major challenge of our time, but the better management and use of biodiversity offer us solutions. For example, sustaining and restoring soil biodiversity, and thereby soil functions, offer significant opportunities to make better use of land and water in order to grow crops more efficiently. Biodiversity also offers options for crop diversification; including growing more locally appropriate crops and varieties better suited to different and changing conditions and consumer preferences. Another critical asset is the traditional knowledge associated with biodiversity, maintained by farmers and pastoralists.

Agricultural biodiversity was first addressed in a comprehensive manner by the Convention on Biological Diversity (CBD) in 1996. The CBD programme of work on agricultural biodiversity was detailed in 2000, and three related initiatives have since been launched: on soil biodiversity; on pollinators; and on biodiversity for food and nutrition. I welcome the growing international efforts to implement actions to support these policy instruments. Commitments to more sustainable food production and other policies that promote biodiversity-friendly practices will also support the implementation of the Strategic Plan for Biodiversity 2011–2020 and the Aichi Biodiversity Targets.

Major shifts in policies and approaches are required to achieve food security in all its dimensions: *availability* of sufficient food, *access* to it by all, good nutritional *quality*, and *stability* of supply. The conservation and sustainable use of biodiversity is essential to all four dimensions. The growing impacts of climate change will submit food production everywhere to unseen levels of stress and the most cost-effective solution to promote adaptation lies in biodiversity. Successful approaches will be founded on interdisciplinary collaboration and multi-scale partnerships. Consumers are a major driver of food production, so a shift in consumer preferences to choices that are both more sustainable and healthier will be critical.

Acknowledgements

I would like to take this opportunity to congratulate the authors and partner organizations on this milestone publication. Their work offers a comprehensive summary of contemporary information and good practices, identifies gaps in research and provides insight on potential opportunities for a variety of policy options. I look forward to more sustainable management of biodiversity in all ecosystems, but particularly in agricultural ecosystems, where we can truly achieve a healthy partnership between people and the planet.

Preface

This book is part of a larger series, *Issues in Agricultural Biodiversity*, published by Earthscan/Routledge in association with Bioversity International. It addresses the biodiversity dimensions of one of the greatest challenges our generation faces: to eradicate hunger and malnutrition from the planet. With the alarming pace of biodiversity loss and ecosystem degradation and their negative impact on poverty and health, this book makes a compelling case for re-examining food systems and diets. We hope this book serves to foster a deeper understanding and appreciation of the role of biodiversity in improving diets and nutrition security, particularly in the developing world which is home to the richest repository of biodiversity, and yet is also home to the world's poorest people. The book is also intended to be used as a tool and a guide to promote the use of biodiversity within food production systems, and to demonstrate that by providing local solutions for diversifying diets, nutritional status can be improved, effectively and sustainably.

The first half of the book outlines some of the challenges, and identifies potential solutions and opportunities to conserve, measure, and utilize biodiversity for improved diets and nutrition security. The second half provides twelve unique case studies on the links between agricultural biodiversity and diets and nutrition. The case studies are taken from diverse settings around the globe. This book builds on the work that Bioversity International and the UN FAO are doing on developing the concept of sustainable diets. Sustainable diets are those diets with low environmental impacts which contribute to food and nutrition security and to healthy life for present and future generations. Sustainable diets are protective and respectful of biodiversity and ecosystems; culturally acceptable, accessible, economically fair and affordable; nutritionally adequate, safe and healthy; while optimizing natural and human resources. Sustainable diets are therefore an important element for sustainable development and a green economy, providing a platform to promote strategies that emphasize the positive role of food biodiversity in human nutrition and poverty alleviation.

The book represents an important milestone in sharing our work on agricultural biodiversity, sustainable diets and nutrition, and their contribution to sustainable development and healthy food systems. It is also very timely, as it addresses several aspects of the Zero Hunger Challenge launched at the Rio+20 Conference by the Secretary General of the United Nations.

Sustainable food systems need better impact assessments and relevant policies based on the best evidence from agricultural landscapes. We hope the different chapters of the book demonstrate some of this impact and provide convincing arguments for engaging and strengthening policies and programmes. At the very least, the book and its authors have positioned nutrition, biodiversity and sustainable diets as important contributions to the post-2015 development agenda.

Emile Frison
Director General
Bioversity International

Barbara Burlingame
Principal Officer
Nutrition and Consumer
Protection Division
UN FAO

Acknowledgements

The editors would like to thank the many authors who contributed to the chapters and case studies included in this book. We would also like to thank Braulio Dias, Executive Secretary, Convention on Biological Diversity and Olivier De Schutter, United Nations Special Rapporteur on the right to food for the contributed forewords and Emile Frison, Director General, Bioversity International and Barbara Burlingame, Principal Officer, Nutrition and Consumer Protection Division, FAO for contributing the preface to the book. We extend our sincere thanks to Tim Hardwick, Ashley Irons and other staff at Earthscan. We also sincerely thank Sarah Fischer and Maria Merzouk at Bioversity International, both of whom provided support in the production of this book. A number of additional individuals generously contributed their expertise and time to the development of this book. We are grateful for their constructive review comments and valuable feedback and would like to thank the following: Deborah Markowicz Bastos, Mauricio Bellon, Bruce Cogill, Marie-Claude Dop, Adam Drucker, Carlo Fadda, Luigi Guarino, Timothy Johns, Judy Loo, Roseline Remans, and Adriana Zarrelli.

The development and publication of this book was made possible through support from the Global Environment Facility (GEF), the United Nations Environment Programme (UNEP) and the Food and Agriculture Organization of the United Nations (FAO) within the framework of the global project 'Mainstreaming biodiversity conservation and sustainable use for improved human nutrition and wellbeing'. We would also like to thank Dr Emile Frison, Director General of Bioversity International, and Jenessi Matturi, Co-publishing Programme, Technical Centre for Agricultural and Rural Cooperation (CTA) (ACP-EU) for their help in facilitating additional support for the publication of the book. We would also like to express our sincere thanks to the various host organizations that supported the editors, authors and other contributors.

Materials in this book have been sourced and referenced to the best of our knowledge. Every effort has been made to ensure that the originality of the source of copyright material has been provided within the text.

The editors would also like to add their personal acknowledgements to all who provided special support during the preparation of this work.

Teresa would like to thank her fellow editors Jessica Fanzo and Federico Mattei for their comradeship and support, as well as Maria Merzouk for her unfailing assistance. Special thanks, however, are directed to Danny Hunter, supervisor and mentor, for his kindness and constant guidance.

Jessica would like to thank Danny, Teresa and Federico for their partnership, creativity and friendship.

Danny would like to thank close members of his family especially his two children, Imogen and Callum, for their support and patience during the preparation of this book. He would also like to extend a special thank you to Sarah for her kindness, encouragement and support, and for providing a desk and a haven in Dublin where much of this book took shape. Finally, in addition to thanking his fellow editors, he would like to highlight the support, encouragement and discussions provided over the last few years by other colleagues at Bioversity International, namely Jojo Baidu-Forson, Nadia Bergamini, Mauricio Bellon, Pablo Eyzaguirre, Toby Hodgkin, Sara Hutchinson, Patrick Maundu, Stefano Padulosi and Laura Vuerich.

Abbreviations and acronyms

AICR	American Institute for Cancer Research
AnGR	animal genetic resources
ASF	animal source food
AVRDC	World Vegetable Center (previously known as Asian Vegetable Research and Development Center)
BMI	body mass index
CARD	Council of Agricultural and Rural Development
CBD	Convention on Biological Diversity
CBO	community-based organizations
CBS	Central Bureau of Statistics
CED	chronic energy deficiency
CFF	Crops for the Future
CFFRC	Crops for the Future Research Centre
CFS	Committee on World Food Security
CGIAR	Consultative Group on International Agricultural Research
CIAT	International Center for Tropical Agriculture
CIFOR	Center for International Forestry Research
CINE	Centre for Indigenous Peoples' Nutrition and Environment
CIP	Country Investment Plan
CONSEA	National Food Security Council
COP	Conference of the Parties
CPF	Collaborative Partnership on Forests
CRC	Co-operative Research Centre
CRP4	CGIAR Research Program 4 (Agriculture for Improved Nutrition and Health)
CSIRO	Commonwealth Scientific and Industrial Research Organization
CWR	crop wild relatives
DADO	district agricultural development office
DAG	disadvantaged groups
DD	dietary diversity
DFID	Department for International Development
ECOWAS	Economic Community of West African States

ENA	essential nutrition actions
ESSAN	National Food and Nutritional Security Strategy II 2008–2015 (ESAN)
ETC Group	Action Group on Erosion, Technology and Concentration
FAO	Food and Agriculture Organization of the United Nations
FFQ	food frequency questionnaire
FFS	farmer field school
FOS	fructo-oligosaccharides
FSM	Federated States of Micronesia
GEF	Global Environment Facility
GHG	greenhouse gases
GIS	geographic information system
GM	genetically modified
HFP	homestead food production
HH	household
HKI	Helen Keller International
HLPE	High Level Panel of Experts on Food Security and Nutrition
IAASTD	International Assessment of Agricultural Knowledge, Science and Technology for Development
IAEA	International Atomic Energy Agency
IBPGR	International Board for Plant Genetic Resources
ICRAF	International Centre for Research in Agroforestry (World Agroforestry Centre)
IDA	iron deficiency anaemia
IDD	iodine deficiency disorders
IET	Incredible Edible Todmorden
IFAD	International Fund for Agricultural Development
IFCN	International Farm Comparison Network
IFCP	Island Food Community of Pohnpei
IFPRI	International Food Policy Research Institute
IFT	indigenous fruit trees
IIAM	Institute for Agrarian Research in Mozambique (formerly known as INIA)
IIED	International Institute for Environment and Development
INIA	Institute of Agronomic Research for Mozambique (now recognized as IIAM)
IPGRI	International Plant Genetic Resources Institute
IRC	International Rice Commission
IRRI	International Rice Research Institute
ITPGRFA	International Treaty on Plant Genetic Resources for Food and Agriculture
IUCN	International Union for Conservation of Nature
IWMI	International Water Management Institute
LI-BIRD	Local Initiatives for Biodiversity Research and Development
LIFDCs	low-income food-deficit countries

LRD	land resources division
LTFs	local and traditional foods
MACH	management of aquatic ecosystems through community husbandry
MDG	Millennium Development Goal
MEA	Millennium Ecosystem Assessment
MNM	micronutrient malnutrition
MNP	multi-sectoral nutrition planning
MPT	multi-purpose tree
MSSRF	M.S. Swaminathan Research Foundation
MVP	Millennium Villages Project
NARC	Nepal Agricultural Research Council
NARES	National Agriculture Research Institute and Extension Services
NCD	non-communicable diseases
NDU	nutritional development unit
NFD	nutritional functional diversity
NFR	novel food regulation
NGO	non-governmental organization
NHS	national health scheme
NPC	National Planning Commission
NUS	neglected and underutilized species
NWFP	non-wood forest products
OECD	Organization for Economic Co-operation and Development
OFSP	orange-fleshed sweet potato
PAA	Brazilian Food Acquisition Programme
PDS	public distribution systems
PEM	protein energy malnutrition
PEN	poverty and environment network
PNAE	Brazilian National Programme of School Meals
PRA	participatory rural appraisal
PROTA	Plant Resources of Topical Africa
PVS	participatory varietal selections
QPM	quality protein maize
RBTA	Rare Breed Trust of Australia
RDA	recommended dietary allowance
RESEWO	Regent Estate Senior Women's Organization
REU	researching end users
ROPPA	Réseau des organisations paysannes et des producteurs de l'Afrique de l'Ouest (Network of Farmers' and Agricultural Producers' Organizations of West Africa)
RRC	rural resources centre
R&D	research and development
SETSAN	Technical Secretariat for Food Security and Nutrition in Mozambique

SHG	self-help groups
SIS	small indigenous fish species
SOFIA	State of World Fisheries and Aquacultures
SPC	Secretariat of the Pacific Community
SSA	Sub-Saharan Africa
SSP	sweet potato support platform
SUN	Scaling Up Nutrition Movement
TSNI	Towards Sustained Nutrition Improvement (in rural Mozambique)
UFRJJ	Federal Rural University of Rio de Janeiro
UNCED	United Nations Conference on the Environment and Development
UNCTAD	United Nations Conference on Trade and Development
UNDP	United Nations Development Programme
UNEP	United Nations Environment Programme
UNEP-WCMC	United Nations Environment Programme-World Conservation Monitoring Centre
UNESCO	United Nations Educational, Scientific and Cultural Organization
UNICEF	United Nations Children's Fund
UNISDR	United Nations International Strategy for Disaster Reduction
UNSCN	United Nations Standing Committee on Nutrition
USAID	United States Agency for International Development
USDA	United States Department of Agriculture
VAD	vitamin A deficiency
VITAA	Vitamin A for Africa
VMF	village model farms
WAHO	West African Health Organization
WCRF	World Cancer Research Fund
WEHAB	Water, Energy, Health, Agriculture and Biodiversity
WFP	World Food Programme
WHO	World Health Organization
WSSD	World Summit on Sustainable Development

Introduction

Agricultural biodiversity, diverse diets and improving nutrition

Danny Hunter and Jessica Fanzo

The global malnutrition burden and addressing the challenge

One of the world's greatest challenges is to secure adequate food that is healthy, safe and of high quality for all, and to do so in an environmentally sustainable manner (Pinstrup-Andersen, 2009; Godfray et al., 2010). With the growing demand of an ever-increasing human population, it remains unclear how our current global food system will sustain itself. Compounded with climate change, ecosystems and biodiversity under stress, population growth and urbanization, social conflict and extreme poverty, there has never been a more urgent time for collective action to address food and nutrition security globally.

This burdened food system impacts the most vulnerable people, as statistics clearly show. There are currently an estimated 868 million people suffering food and nutrition insecurity (FAO, 2012). In addition to those who are hungry, there are also 171 million children under five years of age who are stunted in their growth (UNICEF, 2012) and of those children, 90 per cent live in just 36 countries (Black et al., 2008).

Malnutrition takes its toll; it is responsible for 35 per cent of all child deaths and 11 per cent of the global disease burden (Black et al., 2008). Micronutrient deficiencies, known as hidden hunger, undermine the growth and development, health and productivity of over 2 billion people (Micronutrient Initiative, 2009). At the same time, an estimated 1.4 billion adults are overweight, and 65 per cent of the world's population live in countries where overweight and obesity kills more people than underweight (WHO, 2012). This pandemic contributes to the risk of non-communicable diseases such as diabetes and heart disease. With over-nutrition, many countries and urban communities in the developing world are experiencing the nutrition transition – going from undernutrition to obesity related to insufficient exercise, sedentary lifestyles and unhealthy diets (Doak et al., 2005; Popkin, 2008).

The global community has responded to the malnutrition crisis by focusing on interventions that aim to impact 90 per cent of the global population burdened by stunting and that largely address inadequate dietary intake, disease burden and poor childcare practices (Bhutta et al., 2008). There has been a particular focus on a window of opportunity, specifically, the first 1,000 days of a child's life from the nine months *in utero* to two years of age (Barker 2007; Golden, 2009; Victora et al., 2008). This window is critically important because nutritional setbacks during this time can result in irreversible losses to growth and cognitive development and can reduce educational attainment and earning potential (Martorell et al., 1994; Shrimpton et al., 2001; Victora et al., 2008).

These core nutrition-specific interventions are critically important in addressing nutrition insecurity, particularly during the window of opportunity. However the design, testing and scaling of more holistic multi-sectoral packages that combine child and maternal care and disease control with nutrition sensitive programming from agriculture, education, social protection, and education, have been limited in their development and implementation. Practical operational strategies for localizing and applying sensitive interventions must be further clarified and defined as to how such interventions impact nutritional outcomes. What has become clear is that agriculture is and will continue to be part of the solution in improving the health and nutrition of all populations regardless of age, during their lifespan.

Our global food system

Redirecting the global agricultural system to ensure better nutrition is important as the supplier of the world's food. The global agricultural system is *currently* producing enough food, in aggregate, but access to enough food that is affordable and nutritious for all populations has been more challenging. Most agricultural systems are extremely efficient at producing a handful of staple grain crops, mainly maize, rice and wheat. In developing countries and particularly those in nutrition transition, people obtain most of their energy from these staple grains along with processed oils and fats and sugars, resulting in diets that often lack micronutrients and other necessary dietary and health components.

Agricultural systems vary across the world, spanning large-scale monocrop landscapes to smallholdings of farmers who typically live on less than two hectares of land. Taking into account the differing agro-ecosystems and landscapes, it is necessary to understand how our agricultural system can promote positive nutrition outcomes. A recent review showed that agriculture interventions have done little to impact undernutrition (Masset and Haddad, 2012), as measured by core nutrition indicators including growth indicators. However, more research needs to be done to better understand the role of value chains, biodiversity, and ecosystem services on nutritional and dietary outcomes, and what are the best ways to measure agriculture's impact on nutrition and dietary outcomes.

Big drivers of trends in food consumption globally are the private sector, markets, processed food and diet shifts. Research and development practitioners must start thinking about new and sustainable approaches to improving the quality and variety of food produced and consumed around the world and to develop innovative new roles that agriculture can play that will ensure value chains are more nutrition sensitive, and that will improve dietary diversity and nutrition outcomes at all stages of life. To do this, nutrition must be a central goal of agriculture and production systems, as well as value chains and marketplaces, and be recognized as a potential avenue to improving dietary diversity, quality and health as well as a means of restoring and preserving ecosystems. But one size does not fit all and this approach must ensure that agriculture – the backbone of food production – is tailored to respond adequately to the diverse conditions of major agro-ecological, socioeconomic and epidemiological situations.

Agricultural biodiversity as a potential tool for improving nutrition security

Productive terrestrial and marine ecosystems, both wild and managed, are the source of our food – a prerequisite for health and life (Millennium Ecosystem Assessment, 2008). It is well understood that the sustainability of the global ecosystem in general and of the agriculture in particular, is dependent on the conservation, enhancement and utilization of biological diversity, or biodiversity (Frison et al., 2011; Lockie and Carpenter, 2010). Biodiversity includes the variety of plants, terrestrial animals and marine and other aquatic resources (species diversity), along with the variety of genes contained in all individual organisms (genetic diversity), and the variety of habitats and biological communities (ecosystem diversity). Biodiversity is essential for humanity, providing food, fibre, fodder, fuel, and medicine in addition to other ecosystem services.

Biodiversity is the lifeblood of what we eat. Biodiversity – both wild and cultivated – underpins the sustainability of agricultural production by providing the genetic diversity and material needed to drive innovation and adaptation, as well as essential ecosystem services and processes. Far too often the human nutritional and health ecosystem services that biodiversity provides have been ignored (DeClerck et al., 2011, see Chapter 1 in this volume). When linked, biodiversity, agriculture and nutrition form a common path leading to food and nutrition security, and achievement of the Millennium Development Goals (Toledo and Burlingame, 2006).

Agricultural biodiversity (agrobiodiversity), that sub-component of biodiversity important for food and agriculture, plays an important role in productivity and the livelihoods of all farmers, regardless of resource endowment or geographical location. Agricultural biodiversity refers to the biological variety exhibited among crops, animals and other organisms used for food and agriculture, as well as the web of relationships that bind these forms of life at ecosystem, species, and genetic levels. It includes not only crops and livestock directly relevant to agriculture, but also many other organisms that have indirect effects on agriculture, such as soil fauna, weeds, pollinators, pests and predators. Agricultural biodiversity provides the basic resources farmers need to adapt to variable conditions in marginal environments and the resources required to increase productivity in more favourable settings. Agriculture is the bedrock of the food system and biodiversity is important to food and agricultural systems because it provides the variety of life (Tansey and Worsley, 1995).

FAO (2010) estimates that of a total of 300,000 plant species, 10,000 have been used for human food since the origin of agriculture. Out of these, only 150–200 species have been commercially cultivated of which only four – rice, wheat, maize and potatoes – supply 50 per cent of the world's energy needs, while 30 crops provide 90 per cent of the world's caloric intake. Intensification of agricultural systems has led to a substantial reduction in the genetic diversity of domesticated plants and animals. Some on-farm losses of genetic diversity have been partially offset by conservation in gene banks (Millennium Ecosystem Assessment, 2008). Even so, the implications of this loss of agricultural biodiversity (as well as loss of associated ecological knowledge) for the biodiversity and quality of the global food supply are scarcely understood, especially from the perspective of nutrition.

Agricultural biodiversity furthermore includes species with under-exploited potential for contributing to food security, health, income generation, and ecosystem services. Terms such as underutilized, neglected, orphan, minor, promising, niche, local and traditional are frequently used interchangeably to describe these potentially useful plant and animal species, which are not mainstream, but which have a significant local importance as well as a considerable global potential for improving food and nutrition security.

Even so the research reveals that the major causes of neglect and underuse of these important species (see Box 0.1) are often related to factors that include poor economic competitiveness with commodity cereal crops, a lack of crop improvement, poor cultivation practices, inefficiencies in processing and value addition, disorganized or non-existent market chains as well as a perception of these foods as being 'food of the poor' (Jaenicke et al., 2009).

As this book highlights, inter-species and intra-species variability represents a considerable wealth of local biodiversity and, with a better understanding of their contributions and use, could have potential for contributing to food security and nutrition. They also have considerable potential for enhancing adaptation to global climate change. Some of these species are highly nutritious and have multiple uses.

It is essential to understand how the global agricultural system and the benefits derived from agricultural biodiversity influence the drivers of global dietary consumption patterns, nutrition and health status, in particular in the developing world. The lack of diversity is shown to be a crucial issue, particularly in the developing world where diets consist mainly of starchy staples with less access to nutrient-rich sources of food such as animal proteins, fruits and vegetables. Dietary diversity is a vital element of diet quality and the consumption of a variety of foods across and within food groups and across different varieties of specific foods more or less guarantees adequate intake of essential nutrients and important non-nutrient factors. Research demonstrates that there is a strong association between dietary diversity and nutritional status, particularly micronutrient density of the diet (Arimond and Ruel, 2004; Hoddinott and Yohannes, 2002; Kennedy et al., 2007; Moursi et al., 2008; Rah et al., 2010; Ruel, 2003; Sawadogo et al., 2006; Thorne-Lyman et al., 2010; World Bank, 2006, 2007).

Box 0.1 Some barriers to the promotion and mainstreaming of agricultural biodiversity for improved diets and nutrition

- Disconnect between the biodiversity, agriculture and health sectors and other sectors (including education)
- Continued neglect by the international and national research and extension systems
- Biodiverse food-based approaches all too often fall outside the traditional scope of clinical nutrition and public health
- Lack of skills and institutional capacity necessary to promote multi-sector approaches to fully exploit biodiversity, agriculture and health linkages
- Lack of data linking biodiversity to dietary diversity and improved nutrition outcomes
- Poor information management and accessibility: relevant information is highly fragmented, scattered in various publications and reports or not easily accessible databases to policy makers and practitioners
- Lack of evidence demonstrating or comparing the most (cost-)effective methods and approaches for delivering or mobilizing biodiversity for dietary and nutrition outcomes
- Poorly developed infrastructure and markets for the majority of biodiversity for food and nutrition
- Reach and influence of the modern globalized food system and trade policies which impede or undermine promotion and consumption of biodiversity for food and nutrition and which favour the consumption of unhealthy processed foods
- Inadequate agricultural and food security policies and strategies that promote major cereal staples have often diminished the dietary role of more nutritious species such as millets, indigenous fruits and vegetables and roots and tubers
- Few practical examples on how to successfully mainstream biodiversity for nutrition objectives
- Negative perceptions and attitudes to local, nutritionally-rich traditional biodiverse foods
- Non-tariff barriers and strict food safety assessment regulations such as the European Union's Novel Foods Regulation (NFR) which places a considerable burden of proof on those attempting to bring traditional biodiverse foods and their products to markets
- The 'artificial' cheap cost of exotic or imported foods which externalize their health and environmental costs

Key research questions and potential solutions: What this book delivers

The current climate for the promotion of food-based approaches including a greater role for agricultural biodiversity to improving diets and nutrition is favourable with renewed global political interest in addressing nutrition issues through better multi-sectoral approaches. In particular, the Scaling Up Nutrition (SUN) movement (see Chapter 10) has taken up the initiative to rally political attention and action to address the problem of undernutrition through cross-sectoral action. In early 2011, IFPRI's 2020 conference on leveraging agriculture for improving nutrition and health, reiterated calls for greater synergies and partnerships among relevant sectors, and underlined the need for a new paradigm for agricultural development to be driven by nutrition goals (IFPRI, 2011; Fanzo and Pronyk, 2011).

At the global level, the Consultative Group on International Agricultural Research (CGIAR) reform process aims to develop improved research-for-development synergies with multiple actors and is prioritizing cross-sectoral collaboration. The new CGIAR Collaborative Research Programme 'Agriculture for improved nutrition and health' (CRP4) (IFPRI, 2011) is the main vehicle for achieving this and has two of four components (Value Chains for Enhanced Nutrition, and Integrated Agriculture, Nutrition and Health Programs and Policies) where agricultural biodiversity has been accorded significant recognition. This has been matched from the biodiversity community with representatives from the Convention on Biological Diversity (CBD), DIVERSITAS and IUCN calling for strengthened international cooperation for biodiversity and health (Campbell et al. 2011).

However, there remain important, yet unanswered, questions about agricultural and ecosystem biodiversity and its role in improving dietary diversity and quality, and which will help to ensure nutrition security and increased health benefits. We hope that through this book and its case studies, answers to key research questions will provide clarity for governments, development programmers, value chain and food sector actors, academic and research institutions, health and agriculture workers, farmers and communities.

Book structure

The book is divided into three parts. Part I (Chapters 1–4), describes novel and interdisciplinary approaches to nutrition, agriculture and biodiversity as well as providing an overview of agricultural biodiversity and its importance to nutrition and health. Chapter 1 makes the case for human nutrition as an ecosystem service and considers how ecology, as one element of any cross-disciplinary solution, with its focus on complex systems can make contributions to several global development challenges related to agriculture, environment and nutrition. The chapter offers refreshingly new interdisciplinary perspectives on the problem of food production, biodiversity and nutrition that offer hope for longer-term sustainable solutions to these problems. These perspectives fall under the three 'eco' concepts of eco-system services, eco-nutrition and eco-agriculture, all of which link agriculture, human well-being, and environmental sustainability. Despite the highlighted advantages of using diversity as a development tool, it is stressed that the concepts discussed still struggle to gain wide support in the face of more targeted and short-term interventions, in part because of the focus on complexity rather than simplification. The chapter suggests that as with the management of eco-agricultural landscapes, interventions must be multifunctional and offer solutions at the expense of other development problems.

Chapter 2 provides an in-depth overview of the multiple elements of agricultural biodiversity which impact most directly on nutrition and health and how this diversity has evolved over time and been nurtured by countless generations of farmers and local communities. It draws attention to the relatively recent diminishing diversity of agriculture including loss of agricultural biodiversity and subsequent ecological, social and nutritional impacts of this. The challenge of building production systems that deliver intensification without simplification is stressed, drawing attention to the need for new paradigms such as sustainable intensification which produce more output from the same area of land while reducing negative environmental impacts including improving biodiversity. However, the difficulty of convincing governments and policy makers of the need for agricultural production practices which embody a greater use of biodiversity for food and agriculture is highlighted. Reasons for this and possible solutions are suggested including a lack of knowledge about the species that are involved; much of the evidence on their nutritional or health benefits of particular species is partial or anecdotal and there is a need for critical scientific assessments.

Chapter 3 outlines the links between changes in human food consumption patterns and animal genetic resources for food and agriculture with a focus on domesticated avian and mammalian species genetic diversity. It introduces the concept of sustainable diets largely from an environmental perspective but also touches briefly on social and economic aspects. While significant increases in food production have occurred in recent decades, largely through intensive practices, this has come with a significant cost to animal genetic resources with estimates that around one-third of cattle, pig and chicken breeds are already extinct or currently at-risk. With expected growing demand for animal food products the prospect for animal genetic resources is not promising unless major transformations occur in the food system. However we know that animal source proteins are important in improving nutrition. With the exception of marginal areas and extensive grazing systems, it is related that we can expect at the breed level that local breeds and their multiple functions and benefits will increasingly be replaced by transboundary breeds. These losses may be exacerbated by future breeding programmes which focus on narrow breeding objectives and the application of new biotechnologies may add to this. The chapter concludes by suggesting solutions which have a focus on sustainable diets which favour the conservation and sustainable utilization of animal genetic resources.

Chapter 4 deals with the role of aquatic organisms in agricultural landscapes and their importance for food and nutrition security and livelihoods of the rural poor. It argues that the integration of fisheries, aquaculture and agriculture provides numerous options for sustainable exploitation of a wide diversity of food items that can address the nutritional needs of different members of the household and society at large which are particularly important for avoiding micronutrient-related nutritional disorders. The chapter relates studies on the availability and use of aquatic biodiversity from rice-based ecosystems in Cambodia, China, Laos and Vietnam which have documented 145 species of fish, 11 species of crustaceans, 15 species of molluscs, 13 species of reptiles, 11 species of amphibians, 11 species of insects and 37 species of plants which are directly caught or collected from the rice fields and utilized by rural people during a single season. A case study from Laos is presented to illustrate this diversity which demonstrates the critical importance of flooded rice fields for the availability and utilization of aquatic organisms. While the chapter highlights that data is scarce on the nutritional composition of much of this aquatic diversity, it argues that evidence suggests it has considerable potential as a cost-effective food-based strategy to enhance micronutrient intakes or as a complementary food for undernourished children. The chapter draws attention to the fact that aquatic biodiversity is a much undervalued and neglected 'safety net' rarely captured by national statistics or reports. It stresses the need for better awareness-raising and mainstreaming to make aquatic biodiversity more 'visible' as critical. It concludes that relevant international forums and conventions – the International Rice Commission (IRC) and the Conventions on Biological Diversity (CBD) and on Wetlands (Ramsar) – recognize the importance of aquatic ecosystems and the biodiversity for food and nutrition they provide and support this aim.

Part II (Chapters 5–10) examines approaches to mobilizing agricultural biodiversity including delivery mechanisms, cross-sectoral collaborations and partnerships and markets, as well as methodological approaches and challenges to measuring biodiversity's contribution to diets. Chapter 5 discusses how homestead food production (HFP) in Mali has contributed to improved food security for nearly 150,000 vulnerable people using a cross-cutting approach to promoting agricultural biodiversity for food and nutrition with examples taken from the Millennium Villages Project. While Africa continues to struggle with significant nutrition problems the chapter points out it does have access to a high diversity of under-utilized micronutrient-dense vegetables adapted to local conditions. However these have been much neglected by research and extension resulting in reduced consumption, loss of local knowledge and genetic diversity. In this context the chapter relates how initiatives of the Millennium Villages Project enhance the role of this under-utilized diversity in improving the nutritional status and livelihoods of vulnerable groups, particularly women and children. The initiative has reported significant achievements including increasing agricultural production and enhancing ecosystem function by restoring and maintaining soil productivity, improving crop diversification, developing community gene banks, capacity building and empowerment of women and strengthening farmer cooperatives. However, impacts on micronutrient status in target communities have yet to be published.

Chapter 6 continues the focus on Africa and examines the agro-ecology of the West Africa region and the role played by diversity within the local food systems in shaping the region's well-known but disappearing rich and healthy food culture, an often neglected topic in discussions of solving the malnutrition pandemic. The chapter reviews the changes that are taking place in the food culture and dietary habits influenced by globalization, urbanization and changes in food production practices, and the nutrition transition before outlining research and intervention programmes that have been put in place by organizations such as Bioversity International and FAO working with the West African Health Organization (WAHO), the Economic Community of West African States (ECOWAS), Réseau des organisations paysannes et des producteurs de l'Afrique de l'Ouest (Network of Farmers' and Agricultural Producers' Organizations of West Africa) (ROPPA), and national agencies and universities, to counteract these changes and which are expected to generate positive changes in the food choices of the population eventually leading to increased diversification in household diets.

Chapter 7 explores novel research methodologies employing tools used largely in ecology and agricultural sciences that might be applied to better integrate nutrition and which might help answer such questions as *how can we manage biodiversity and the ecosystem services it provides for human nutrition, while also managing other components of human well-being?* Or, *how do different plant species compositions differ in nutritional function?* Taking the latter question, and by using examples from rural villages in sub-Saharan Africa, the chapter illustrates how an ecological concept, the Functional Diversity (FD) metric, has potential to address this question by applying it to the nutritional traits of plants (and potentially animals) present in a farming system or landscape. The chapter also explores the importance of understanding possible synergies and trade-offs with other ecosystem services and components of human well-being as well as to identifying drivers of change before discussing some tools considered important for enhancing inter-disciplinary collaboration and communication among individuals and agencies working in relevant fields and sectors.

Chapter 8 focuses on three native domesticated plant species – maca, yacon and quinoa – common to South America and that have provided food to native Amerindian populations for countless generations and which have each seen in recent years quite a remarkable turnaround in terms of international profile which has contributed to considerable interest in commercial product development and research. Central to this turnaround in all three cases has been the discovery or substantiation, and growing consumer awareness, of particular nutritional attributes of each species. In particular, this chapter attempts to distil the critical factors that have shaped the re-emergence of these previously neglected crops and in doing so attempts to determine commonalities and derive broader lessons that might be important for the broader promotion and marketing of nutritionally relevant agricultural biodiversity.

Chapter 9 focuses on the role of biodiversity at the dietary level and stresses that while biodiversity has often been considered a prerequisite for dietary diversity and the health benefits that flow from having a diverse diet, the question of whether multiple varieties of single plant or animal species are required for a diverse diet is not something that is usually discussed in the biodiversity literature. Commencing with a review of what dietary diversity means and how it is measured, the chapter moves on to review the arguments made and the evidence for a relationship between biodiversity and dietary diversity. The chapter considers the magnitude of biodiversity from a nutrition perspective, and presents the case for how biodiversity and dietary diversity might be considered in nutrition programming in a rural Bolivian population. The chapter concludes by integrating information from across various sections to come up with a series of questions that should be considered prior to embarking on a biodiversity-based nutrition intervention.

Some of the chapters mentioned above have drawn attention to the multi-faceted nature of nutrition problems and provide examples of how agriculture and biodiversity can contribute to dietary diversity and quality. They have highlighted the need for improved cross-sectoral collaborations and partnerships, more effective inter-disciplinary working relations and improved integration across sectors and disciplines, all of which have parallels in renewed global calls for greater leveraging of agriculture and biodiversity for improving nutrition and health including greater synergies among the relevant sectors. The final chapter, Chapter 10, reviews how new findings from research on partnerships could contribute to more effective cross-sectoral partnerships in nutrition, agriculture and environment. The chapter explores some of the factors that have limited practical responses to previous calls for such cross-sectoral collaboration with a brief examination of pre-World War II efforts to implement multi-sectoral and collaborative approaches between agriculture and health in Malawi. This is followed by an overview of the evolution of disciplinary perspectives in the agriculture, environment and nutrition sectors which have occasionally demonstrated some meeting of concepts and approaches; yet this never seems to have been translated into practical, effective cross-sectoral and inter-disciplinary collaboration required to address current nutrition problems. The chapter concludes with an example of how a national model, Fome Zero in Brazil, has successfully linked strengthening agricultural biodiversity and improved nutrition; and an examination of what current reforms in the CGIAR and the UN Standing Committee on Nutrition might have to offer for greater mobilization of agricultural biodiversity. Finally the chapter poses the question as to what is different now that may make our future efforts more successful.

Part III comprises 12 case studies from Africa, Asia, Australia, Europe, the Pacific and South America which demonstrate practical examples where agricultural biodiversity has been deployed to enhance dietary diversity and nutrition. Case study authors were asked to provide a brief description of the context including a statement of the problem being addressed, how agricultural biodiversity was used as a solution or intervention, the mechanisms used to mobilize agricultural biodiversity; evidence to show the impact of the intervention using targeted agricultural biodiversity; efforts to scale-up interventions using agricultural biodiversity; how the work impacted in influencing relevant policies and the key lessons learned from the work described. Highlights include the example of a community-based, Go Local, approach to promote local yellow-fleshed varieties of banana, giant swamp taro, breadfruit and pandanus rich in beta-carotene and other carotenoids to alleviate vitamin A deficiency in the Federated States of Micronesia; efforts to promote nutrient-rich small indigenous fish species in Bangladesh; the participatory tree domestication approach used by ICRAF to select and promote indigenous fruit trees with high nutritional value in sub-Saharan Africa; the role of farmers markets and community gardens as localized food systems and their potential for improving dietary diversity and nutrition, supporting biological diversity and linking production to consumption in Australia; the efforts of the Incredible Edible Todmorden (IET) initiative to address the issue of food self-sufficiency and quality of diet in the town of Todmorden in the UK; and the role of a public policy, the Food Acquisition Programme (PAA), in promoting diversification and the sustainable management of biodiversity for food and agriculture and food and nutritional security in the overall Fome Zero (Zero Hunger) strategy in Brazil.

References

Arimond, M. and Ruel, M.T. (2004) Dietary diversity is associated with child nutritional status: evidence from 11 demographic and health surveys, *Journal of Nutrition*, vol 134, no 10, pp.2579–2585.

Barker, D.J.P. (2007) Introduction: The Window of Opportunity, *Journal of Nutrition*, vol 137, pp.1058–1059.

Bhutta, Z.A., Ahmed, T., Black, R.E., Cousens, S., Dewey, K., Giugliani, E., Haider, B.A., Kirkwood, B., Morris, S.S., Sachdev, H.P., Shekar, M., Maternal and Child Undernutrition Study Group (2008) What works? Interventions for maternal and child undernutrition and survival, *Lancet*, vol 371, pp.417–440.

Black, R.E., Allen, L.H., Bhutta, Z.A., Caulfield, L.E., de Onis, M., Ezzati, M., Mathers, C. and Rivera, J. (2008) Maternal and child undernutrition: global and regional exposures and health consequences, *Lancet*, vol 371, pp.243–260.

Campbell, K., Cooper, D., Dias, B., Prieur-Richard, A.H., Campbell-Lendrum, D., Karesh, W.B. and Dazak, P. (2011) Strengthening international cooperation for health and biodiversity, *EcoHealth*, vol 8, pp.407–409.

DeClerck, F., Fanzo, J., Palm, C. and Remans, R. (2011) Ecological approaches to human nutrition, *Food and Nutrition Bulletin*, vol 32, ppS41–S50.

Doak, C.M., Adair, L.S., Bentley, M., Monteiro, C. and Popkin, B.M. (2005) The dual burden household and the nutrition transition paradox, *Int J Obes*. Vol 29, no 1, pp.129–136.

Fanzo, J. and Pronyk, P. (2011) A review of global progress toward the Millennium Development Goal 1 Hunger Target, *Food and Nutrition Bulletin*, vol 32, no 2, pp.144–158(15).

Food and Agriculture Organization of the United Nations (FAO) (2010) *The State of Food Insecurity in the World*, FAO, Rome, Italy.

Food and Agriculture Organization of the United Nations (FAO) (2012) *The Commission on Genetic Resources for Food and Agriculture (CGRFA) Second Report on the State of the World's Plant Genetic Resources for Food and Agriculture (PGRFA)*, FAO, Rome, Italy.

Frison, E., Cherfas, J. and Hodgkin, T. (2011) Agricultural biodiversity is essential for a sustainable improvement in food and nutrition security, *Sustainability*, vol 3, pp.238–253.

Godfray, H.C.J., Crute, I.R., Haddad, L., Lawrence, D., Muir, J.F., Nisbett, N., Pretty, P., Robinson, S., Toulmin, C. and Whiteley, R. (2010) The future of the global food system, *Phil. Trans. R. Soc. B2010*, vol 365, pp.2769–2777.

Golden, M. (2009) Proposed nutrient requirements of moderately malnourished populations of children, *Food and Nutrition Bulletin*, vol 30, no 3, ppS267–S343.

Hoddinott, J. and Yohannes, Y. (2002) Dietary diversity as a food security indicator, Discussion paper 136, International Food Policy Research Institute (IFPRI), Washington DC.

IFPRI CGIAR Research Programme 4 (CRP4) (2011) *Linking Agriculture, Nutrition and Health* (CGIAR Multi Center Grant Proposal).

Jaenicke, H., J. Ganry, I. Hoeschle-Zeledon and R. Kahane (Eds) (2009) *Proceedings of the International Symposium on Underutilized Plants for Food Security, Nutrition, Income and Sustainable Development*, Acta Hort. ISHS. 806 (Vol I–II).

Kennedy, G.L., Pedro, M.R., Seghieri, C., Nantel, G. and Brouwer, I. (2007) Dietary diversity score is a useful indicator of micronutrient intake in non-breast-feeding Filipino children, *J Nutr* vol 137, pp.472–477.

Lockie, S. and Carpenter, D. (2010) *Agriculture, Biodiversity and Markets*, Earthscan.

Martorell, R., Khan, L.K. and Schroeder, D.G. (1994) Reversibility of stunting: epidemiological findings in children from developing countries, *Eur J. Clin Nutr* 48, Suppl 1: S45–57.

Masset and Haddad (2012) Effectiveness of agricultural interventions that aim to improve nutritional status of children: systematic review, *BMJ* 2012, p.344, doi: 10.1136/bmj.d8222.

Micronutrient Initiative (2009) *Investing in the Future: A united call to action on vitamin and mineral deficiencies* www.unitedcalltoaction.org, accessed December 2010.

Millennium Ecosystem Assessment (2008) *Ecosystems and Human Well-Being: Biodiversity Synthesis*, World Resources Institute, Washington DC.

Moursi, M.M., Arimond, M., Dewey, K.G., Trèche, S., Ruel, M.T. and Delpeuch, F. (2008) Dietary diversity is a good predictor of the micronutrient density of the diet of 6- to 23-month-old children in Madagascar, *J. Nutr.* 138(12): 2448–53.

Pinstrup-Andersen, P. (2009) Food security: definition and measurement, *Food Security*, vol 1, pp.5–7.

Popkin, B. (2008) *The World Is Fat: The Fads, Trends, Policies, and Products That Are Fattening the Human Race*, Penguin.

Rah, J.H., Akhter, N., Semba, R.D., de Pee, S., Bloem, M.W., Campbell, A.A., Moench-Pfanner, R., Sun, K., Badham, J. and Kraemer, K. (2010) Low dietary diversity is a predictor of child stunting in rural Bangladesh, *European Journal of Clinical Nutrition*, vol 64, pp.1393–1398.

Ruel, M.T. (2003) Operationalizing dietary diversity: a review of measurement issues and research priorities, *Journal of Nutrition*, vol 133 (11 Suppl 2), pp.3911S–26S.

Sawadogo, P.S., Martin-Prevel, Y., Savy, M., Kameli, Y., Traissac, P., Traore, A.S. and Delpeuch, F. (2006) An infant and child feeding index is associated with the nutritional status of 6- to 23-month-old children in rural Burkina Faso, *J Nutr*, vol 136, pp.656–663.

Shrimpton, R., Victora, C.G., de Onis, M., Lima, R.C., Blossner, M. and Clugston, G. (2001) Worldwide timing of growth faltering: implications for nutritional interventions, *Pediatrics* 107: E75.

Tansey, G. and Worsley, T. (1995) *The Food System*, Earthscan, London.

Thorne-Lyman, A.L., Valpiani, N., Sun, K., Semba, R.D., Klotz, C.L., Kraemer, K., et al. (2010) Household dietary diversity and food expenditures are closely linked in rural Bangladesh, increasing the risk of malnutrition due to the financial crisis, *J Nutr*, vol 140, pp.182S–188S.

Toledo, A. and Burlingame, B. (2006) Biodiversity and nutrition: a common path toward global food security and sustainable development, *Journal of Food Composition and Analysis,* vol 19, pp.477–483.

UNICEF (2012) Childinfo.org .

Victora, C.G., Adair, L., Fall, C., Hallal, P.C., Martorell, R., Richter, L. and Sachdev, H.S. (2008) Maternal and child undernutrition: consequences for adult health and human capital, *Lancet*, vol 371, no 9609 pp.340–357.

WHO (2012) *Obesity and Overweight*, WHO Fact Sheet No 311. WHO, Geneva.

World Bank (2006) *Repositioning Nutrition as Central for Development*, World Bank, Washington DC.

World Bank (2007) *From Agriculture to Nutrition: Pathways Synergies and Outcomes*, World Bank, Washington DC.

Part I

The state of agricultural biodiversity and nutrition

Overviews, models and themes

1   Harnessing biodiversity

From diets to landscapes

Fabrice DeClerck

Introduction

There is an increasing sense that we are at a global crossroads, at the peak of human potential while on the edge of global disaster. Several authors highlight critical planetary thresholds that have been largely surpassed (Rockstrom et al., 2009), particularly the loss of biodiversity, the failure to meet the 2010 Convention on Biological Diversity targets (Butchart et al., 2010), and the increasing scepticism that we will attain many of the Millennium Development Goals. Amongst these goals, halving the number of people who regularly go hungry is prominent. Novel solutions are urgently required to confront these issues.

There are also refreshingly new perspectives on these problems that offer both guidance and hope that solutions are within reach if we are committed. The most exciting of these solutions are those that are the product of interdisciplinary collaborations aimed at integrated solutions, rather than disciplinary band-aids that offer solutions at the expense of other development problems. These solutions often come from a combined process of divergent and convergent thinking (DeHaan, 2011). Divergent thinking is fostered by brainstorming freely on a problem using a defocused, intuitive approach, while maintaining a particular receptiveness to a broad range of associations (i.e. thinking across disciplinary boundaries). Convergent thinking is then used to synthesize these ideas and bring them back into focus. One way to foster this kind of thinking is by encouraging disciplinary scientists to consider how their specific skill set or knowledge base could be applied to tackle an issue or problem outside of their disciplines (DeClerck et al., 2011a).

This practice has become increasingly common with ecologists, amongst other fields, leading to novel interdisciplinary realms such as ecosystem services (Daily, 1997; Naeem et al., 2009), eco-nutrition (Deckelbaum et al., 2006), eco-health (Borer et al., 2012) and eco-agriculture (McNeely and Scherr, 2003) for example (Table 1.1). Ecosystem services blend the domains of ecology, economic and social sciences; eco-nutrition brings together the science of nutrition, agronomy and ecology; eco-agriculture calls on close collaboration with landscape planners, political leaders, farmers and community groups and a broad

Table 1.1 Definition of four interdisciplinary communities of practice, their core disciplines and groups involved, stated goals and key references regarding select examples of ecology's integration in other disciplines

Integrated efforts	Core disciplines/groups	Goals	Reference
Eco–nutrition	• nutrition • agronomy • ecology • economics	Integrate nutrition and human health, agriculture and food production, environmental health, and economic development to jointly reduce malnutrition, increase agricultural productivity, protect the environment, and promote economic development.	Deckelbaum et al., 2006
Eco-agriculture	• ecology • agriculture • economics • development practitioners • community groups	Rural communities jointly manage their resources to enhance rural livelihoods, conserve biodiversity and ecosystem services; and develop more sustainable and productive agricultural systems.	McNeely and Scherr, 2003
Ecosystem services	• ecology • countless other fields	To recognize the contribution of natural and managed ecosystems to human well-being and livelihood. In the broadest sense these include services such as clean water, clean air, agricultural productivity through pollination and pest control services for example.	Daily, 1997 MEA, 2005
Eco-health	• ecology • health sciences	To better understand the connections between nature, society, and health, and how drivers of social and ecosystem change ultimately will also influence human health and well-being.	Wilcox et al., 2004

range of professionals from ecology, agronomy, and economics amongst other disciplines within mixed-use landscapes. In each case, traditional disciplinary boundaries are broken and interaction between disciplines is fostered. The first step in fostering this interaction is 'semantic mediation', or creating a common language. More importantly it requires participants to focus on process and to hold off on considerations of specific contexts until a broader interdisciplinary perspective is developed. This chapter explores how integrating ecology and ecological thinking into nutrition and agricultural development can be used to develop novel solutions to development problems by particularly focusing on ecology, nutrition and agriculture.

A rapid review of the problem

Nutrition

Unfortunately, the first similarity between the fields of nutrition, agriculture and environment is the current gloomy outlook! It is often cited that more than one billion of the world's population lack access to food or are chronically malnourished. On the flip side, a 2006 World Health Report predicts that by 2015 there will be 2.3 billion overweight adults and more than 700 million obese. This 'double burden' suggests that nearly half (47 per cent) of the global population is suffering from some form of nutritional disorder. The poor are particularly hard hit with these two paradoxical problems, hunger and obesity. In many parts of the world, the poor are dependent on subsistence systems subject to the vagaries of rainfed agriculture where the primary challenge is a struggle to simply produce enough calories to survive. In contrast, many of the urban poor, including in the United States, are faced with levels of obesity tapering off at 35 per cent for adults. Again, in developed countries such as the United States, rates have risen to nearly 60 per cent among non-Hispanic black women and to nearly 45 per cent among Mexican American women since 2004. Among children and teens, about 21 per cent of Hispanics and 24 per cent of blacks are obese compared with 14 per cent of non-Hispanic whites (Ogden et al., 2012; Flegal et al., 2012). Several studies have suggested that the poor cannot afford to eat healthily, which at times is due to a lack of access to food (calories), or which can be driven by a lack of access to dietary diversity (Franco et al., 2009) leading to literal food deserts typically found in poor urban neighbourhoods (Gordon et al., 2011; though see recent articles discrediting this notion: An and Sturm, 2012). There is growing recognition however that the food we eat has a direct impact on our own health, as well as the health of the environment (Nugent, 2011).

Agriculture

Agriculture is faced with similar challenges. Recent reviews and analyses highlight the current twin challenges of feeding the 9 billion global inhabitants projected for 2050 while decreasing the growing environmental footprint of agriculture (Tilman et al., 2011; Foley et al., 2011; Rockstrom et al., 2009). While agriculture has met the challenge of producing for growing populations in the past, notably through the Green Revolution, this increase has come at tremendous environmental cost. Agricultural expansion is the primary driver of biodiversity loss with more than 70 per cent of global grasslands, 50 per cent of savannahs, 45 per cent of temperate deciduous forests, and 27 per cent of tropical forests converted to agriculture. Global fertilizer use has increased more than 500 per cent leading to significant impacts on global water and nitrogen cycles in particular. In terms of disruptions to the carbon cycle, agriculture has contributed to 30–35 per cent of global greenhouse gases (Foley et al., 2011) and is likely to be one of the industries most impacted by global climate change. The focus on agricultural intensification has also led to a singular focus on a handful of crop species, primarily in the grass family. Three crops, wheat, maize and rice, occupy approximately 40 per cent of the global agricultural landscape (Tilman, 1999a). Not only is tremendous crop diversity lost though agricultural intensification, the intraspecific, or genetic diversity of both major and minor crop species is lost, eroding the capacity of agricultural systems to weather shocks.

Agricultural systems are increasingly vulnerable to climate change, globalization, the increasing price of inputs such as water and fertilizer, and the degradation of the natural resource base. These problems are likely to be significant obstacles, particularly for small-scale farmers. The free pass that agriculture has enjoyed over the past decades regarding agricultural productivity at any cost is coming to a close with increasing public pressure for food production systems that contribute to environmental protection while supporting farming communities. The agriculture of the next three decades will need to continue its impressive yield increases while halting or reversing its negative impact on the environment. Agricultural landscapes must become net producers of ecosystem services rather than consumer services. This necessitates a movement towards multifunctional landscapes.

Environment

As with human nutrition and agriculture, global environmental concerns are rising. Butchart et al. (2010) highlight that most indicators of the state of biodiversity are declining with no significant reductions in rates observed. In contrast, indicators of pressures on biodiversity continue to increase. In many cases, the negative declines are tied to agriculture and include the direct impact of agricultural expansion on the loss of habitat for biodiversity. Although species extinctions are natural, never in the history of the earth has one species, our own, been the cause of the mass extinction of so many others. Current extinction rates are 1,000–10,000 times greater than background extinction rates (Rockstrom et al., 2009); a disaster that E.O. Wilson (1994) argues has far greater consequences than economic collapse or nuclear war. Rockstrom et al. (2009) evaluated nine critical planetary thresholds that require the effort of a global collective and which must not be surpassed in order to maintain a stable and resilient human society. Of the nine thresholds identified (phorphorus/nitrogen cycle, climate change, global freshwater use, change in land use, biodiversity loss, atmospheric aerosol loading, chemical pollution, stratospheric ozone depletion and ocean acidification), two have been significantly surpassed: the rate of biodiversity loss is more than ten times the proposed threshold value; and disruption to the nitrogen cycling is approximately 3.5 times the proposed threshold value. It is hard not to see the impact of agriculture in both of these out-of-bounds indicators in addition to the environmental impacts mentioned above.

Integrated approaches to solutions

Traditionally, issues of hunger have been the domain of nutrition, crop production, the domain of agronomy, and environmental conservation, the domain of ecology. The review of emergent global concerns above however demonstrates the important role of agriculture in all three issues. The majority of the foods that provide us with our nutrition come from agricultural fields that compete with biodiversity for space. There are deeper relationships that are not as obvious however. The nutritional value and the flavours of our foods are ultimately the result of complex interactions between crops and their environment. The protein content of beans is the result of a symbiotic relationship with bacteria inhabiting the roots of legumes; the pungent flavour of peppers is the result of an antagonistic interaction between the chilli pepper, a weevil and a fungus. Most of the flavours that spice our meals are the result of these negative interactions, or arms races, between plants and their pests and diseases. These are all interactions that have occurred on evolutionary timescales.

On shorter timescales, the production of many fruits such as almonds, apples and pears is wholly dependent on a host of bees and other insects that pollinate the flowers facilitating fruit production. The conversion of leaf litter to soil organic matter is the result of a host of invisible, and underappreciated communities of soil microflora and fauna (whose value we would quickly learn to appreciate if they disappeared). Whether the nutritional value of the foods we eat, or simply the production of many of these crops within farmers' fields, we quickly realize that food production and nutrition are tied to ecosystem services, and that human nutrition is a component of human well-being that is ultimately dependent on numerous ecosystem services that operate from microscopic to landscape scales (Figure 1.1; Table 1.2).

Ecosystem services

The late 1990s brought a fresh look at humans and their interactions with the environment starting with a renewed realization of society's dependence on nature's services. Daily's (1997) multi-authored volume *Nature's Services* and the more recent synthetic work of the Millennium Ecosystem Assessment (MEA, 2005) were key to highlighting this dependence. Ecosystem services

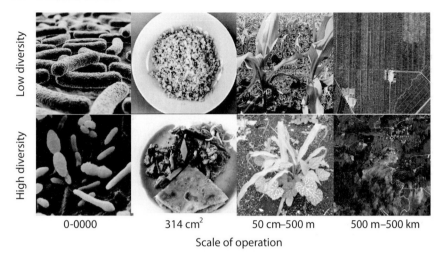

Low diversity

High diversity

| 0-0000 | 314 cm^2 | 50 cm–500 m | 500 m–500 km |

Scale of operation

Figure 1.1 Different levels of species richness contribute to nutritionally important ecosystem services at different scales, increasing from left to right in this figure. Species poor systems (top row) may be well suited for singular functions, but generally fail at maintaining the stability of the function, and at the provision of multiple functions where species rich communities (lower row) are better suited. From left to right: (1) the microbiome of the human gut with the obese gut (above), and the lean gut (below); (2) the species richness of the food we eat; (3) field scale monocultures (above) or polycultures such as the Mayan three-sister system (below); and (4) landscape scale land use diversity such as the simplified banana monoculture (above) and the diversified landscape of a biological corridor (below), both in Costa Rica.

are defined as the conditions and processes through which ecosystems and the species that comprise them sustain and contribute to human livelihoods (Table 1.1; Daily, 1997). The MEA (2005) further classifies these into four broad categories: provisioning, regulating, cultural, and support services (Table 1.2). The fundamental understanding here is that ecosystems, including agricultural ecosystems, or other managed ecosystems are comprised of a community of species (or biodiversity) interacting with each other, and with their environment. The product of these interactions, which include competition, predation, reproduction, and cooperation for example, can be considered ecosystem services when they benefit humanity (Table 1.1; nicely summarized in Loreau et al., 2002; Naeem et al., 2009, 2012). When the species composition of ecological communities is altered, the functions provided by those communities are likewise altered. As a general rule, though there are exceptions, increasing the number of species in a community will increase the number of functions provided by that community (Hector and Bagchi, 2007; Isbell et al., 2011), and will increase the stability of the provisioning of those functions.

A subset of these ecosystem functions are identified as essential to human well-being – and are called ecosystem services (Tables 1.1 and 1.2). In the simplest sense, ecosystem services are the ecosystem functions with human

Table 1.2 Adaptation of the Millennium Ecosystem Assessment classification of ecosystem services.

Those services that have ties to human nutrition are italicized and the scale at which the service operates is identified: human body (B), field (F), and landscape (L). Human nutrition is a function of provisioning services which provide us with the raw materials of our diets, the fuels and clean water with which it is often prepared. Regulating services ensure the stability of food production systems (on farm) and nutrient absorption (within the human body). The recipes and food traditions that are prevalent in most cultures are the result of long-term interactions between human societies, the ingredients of the agroecological landscapes of our ancestors, and trade systems. Supporting services in agricultural landscapes are often overlooked and include soil formation, pollination, nutrient cycling, and soil formation. The microbiome of the human gut also provides numerous supporting services, including transforming the food we consume into forms that can be taken up by our bodies and serving as a first line of defence against disease.

Provisioning services	*Regulating services*	*Cultural services*
Products obtained from Ecosystems	*Benefits obtained from regulation of ecosystem processes*	*Non-material benefits obtained from ecosystems*
Food (F, L)	Climate regulation (L)	Spiritual and religious
Freshwater (F, L)	Disease regulation (B, F, L)	Recreational and tourism
Fuelwood (F, L)	Water regulation (L)	Aesthetic
Fibre (F, L)	Water purification (F, L)	Inspirational
Biochemicals (B, F, L)	Pollination (F, L)	Educational
Genetic resources (F, L)		Sense of place (B)
		Cultural heritage (B)
		Traditional recipes and culinary heritages (B)

Supporting services

Services necessary for the production of all other ecosystem services

Soil formation (F)
Nutrient cycling (B, F)
Primary productivity (F)

value including non-economic values. Understanding the *concepts* and *processes* through which biodiversity provides ecosystem services, from human nutrition to landscape scale services (Figure 1.1), generates novel insights and promising solutions to global problems as we will see below.

Ecosystem services represent one of the most exciting examples of interdisciplinary integration. The initial idea with its focus on ecosystems falls squarely in the disciplinary realm of ecologists though the evolution of the concept was to communicate the benefits of conservation to non-ecologists (Daily, 1997). Considering the services that ecosystems provide brings social scientists and human interests to the table. The recent growth of programmes on payments for ecosystem services has involved economists and political scientists when the economic valuation of these services is warranted. Whereas ecosystem services that have received the most attention to date include carbon sequestration for climate mitigation, water quality, and regulation of hydrological cycles, there is a growing interest in ecosystem services in agricultural landscapes, including pollination and pest control services. Less evident from a contextual point of view, but clear from a process-based interpretation, human nutrition is dependent on several ecosystem services including provisioning, regulating, supporting and cultural services (Table 1.2), and alternatively may even be considered one of the most fundamental ecosystem services (DeClerck et al., 2011b). The capacity of ecosystems to provide us with the energy and nutrition needed to go about our daily lives fully depends on the foods that agriculture provides us. The means by which our internal ecosystems, or the bacterial communities that reside in the human gut, process and make nutrients and calories available (Turnbaugh et al., 2009; Jumpertz et al., 2011) is also very much an ecosystem service.

Eco-nutrition

In 2006, a paper was published introducing the concept of eco-nutrition (Deckelbaum et al., 2006; Deckelbaum, 2011). The fundamental goal of eco-nutrition was to show the linkages between agriculture, human well-being, and environmental sustainability. Eco-nutrition was defined as the interrelationships among nutrition and human health, agriculture and food production, environmental health, and economic development (Deckelbaum et al., 2006). It argued that individuals and families caught up in the poverty trap find themselves in a negative feedback loop, unable to practise productive agriculture because of lack of access to resources leading to environmental degradation through unsustainable agricultural practices; that environmental degradation leads to low yields which further provokes problems of malnutrition which leads to increased incidence of disease, or simply insufficient caloric intake to provide the human energy needed for labour-intensive sustainable field management. The cycle thus repeats itself. Central to the proposal of eco-nutrition is that reversing this negative feedback requires integrated and targeted solutions that simultaneously address the agricultural, nutritional and environmental dimensions of the problem; that is that human nutrition in subsistence communities cannot be resolved without addressing agricultural problems, which in turn cannot be resolved without addressing environmental degradation.

A classic example of eco-nutrition in subsistence systems is the indigenous 'American three-sisters' polyculture where farmers simultaneously sow maize, beans and squash not only in the same field, but in the same planting hole (Figure 1.1). The critical element of the system is not that it includes three distinct taxonomic species, but that it includes three species that are functionally distinct. A three-species system comprised of rice, maize and wheat for example, would not feature the same environmental or nutritional benefits. Focusing on processes from the agro-ecological point of view, the species represent three distinct functional groups. Maize is a C4 grass with highly efficient ability to convert sunlight to energy in tropical environments. Very few plant families outside the grass family have the C4 photosystem. Beans are C3 herbs, unique in their ability to convert abundant atmospheric nitrogen into plant useable forms. Very few plant families other than the bean, or legume family (Fabaceae to botanists) have the ability to capture and use atmospheric nitrogen. Bean cover crops are often used in agricultural systems as a nature source of nitrogen fertilizer. Squash in contrast, has a photosystem as with beans, but does not share its nitrogen fixing ability. When grown in combination, the maize provides the primary productive elements, but also provides the physical support structure, a trellis of sorts, for the climbing bean. Mayan farmers have suggested that the beans growing on the corn provide the additional benefit of hiding the ripe ears of corn from crop pests. The beans and the maize capture the majority of the sunlight, but not all; the remaining light that reaches the ground is captured by the third species, squash, which as a prostrate plant occupies the space remaining and whose less efficient C3 photosystem may be benefited by the shade and increased micro-environment humidity offered by the other species.

The combination of these three species harnesses several important ecological processes. Resources are partitioned between the niches of the three species, and complementary interactions are also favoured, particularly in the support provided by maize to the beans, the nitrogen provided to the maize and squash by the beans, and the more humid micro-environment provided to the squash. Nutrient flows are maintained and managed within the system, with little overflow into adjacent areas, or requirements for external inputs. The more efficient partitioning of resources and great occupation of niche space by the three species also benefits the provision of ecosystem services such as soil conservation and fertility.

There is also important nutritional complementarity between the three crop species of the three-sisters system. Carbohydrates and energy are primarily provided by the maize, protein by the beans, and vitamin A by the squash. The combination of these three crops is nearly nutritionally complete. One critical point however is that the protein provided by the system is derived from the unique ability of the bean family to convert atmospheric nitrogen to plant usable forms through a symbiotic relationship with a bacteria found in the plants' roots – the trait that makes beans ecologically unique is the same trait that makes the species agronomically unique as a source of biological nitrogen fertilizer, and the same trait that makes the family nutritionally unique as a source of plant-based protein. Mayan farmers, traditionally consume their meals with sauces (salsas) prepared with lime juice from citrus plants grown in their home gardens (DeClerck and Negreros-Castillo, 2000). The beans supply amino acids lacking in corn, while the addition of lime makes the niacin within the beans bio-available.

The important contribution of eco-nutrition to human nutrition is in defining the relationship between crop diversity, nutritional diversity and human health. DeClerck et al. (2011b) working with subsistence farmers of Western Kenya, found that farmers who had greater in-field crop nutritional diversity, where the unit of measure was not species diversity but the nutritional diversity of the crops, were less likely to suffer anaemia than farmers with lower field-based nutritional diversity. Other studies have also shown ties to agricultural diversity and human nutrition (Remans et al., 2011a; Penafiel et al., 2012). However, available crop nutritional diversity is not necessarily linked to improved nutrition (Termote et al., 2012) because it must pass through important social filters such as cultural preferences, social pressures, and other elements of human behaviour, highlighting the need for eco-nutrition to add social and behaviour scientists to the equation.

Eco-nutrition as an interdisciplinary field of study considers human nutrition to be a function of multiple ecosystem services. Considering the definition of ecosystem services, the benefits that humans receive from ecosystems, and the MEA (2005) distinction of four categories of services, multiple nutrition entry points become evident.

- The production of foods in agro-ecologically intensified systems is a primary provisioning service.
- Maintaining soil fertility or the inter-annual productivity of cropping systems are defined as regulating services.
- Soil microflora and fauna that convert soil organic matter into nutrients available to plants play important support services.
- Cultural services are central to nutrition – how you eat may be as important as what you eat (Pollan, 2009) as diets are the product of an evolutionary interaction between groups of people and the edible species found in our environments.

Most cultures can identify with a traditional dish, such as the Mayan meal of corn-based tortillas, with whole or fried beans, and tomato salsa prepared with citrus. Cultures that took corn from Latin America without the beans or the lime missed added value obtained from the combination of these species with important nutritional consequences such as pellagra. As with mixed cropping systems described earlier, traditional foods are more than the sum of their parts (Figure 1.1).

Eco-agriculture

The third 'eco' concept introduced earlier is that of eco-agriculture. Eco-agriculture is the management of landscapes for both the production of food and the conservation of ecosystem services and wild biodiversity (McNeely and Scherr, 2003). The concept explicitly recognizes the multifunctional role of agricultural landscapes arguing that they should contain space for nature (biodiversity), food (agricultural productivity), people (livelihoods), and that they should contain the institutions that support these multiple goals. Like eco-nutrition, it highlights the relationship between three elements and suggests that a focus on any single element in isolation deviates from the path of sustainable development.

Inherent in the notion of eco-agriculture is the recognition that productive agriculture is dependent on biodiversity through the provision of ecosystem services such as pollination, pest control services and healthy soils (also important elements of eco-nutrition); that human livelihoods are dependent on agricultural land uses, not only for the production of healthy foods, but also for the production of clean water and other ecosystem services; and that both the conservation and production goals of eco-agricultural landscapes are dependent on human communities. Eco-agriculture takes us away from the paradigm that conservation should only occur in natural reserves and protected areas, with agriculture parsed to designated production areas. Rather, eco-agriculture suggests that landscapes should provide both production and conservation functions, and that the additive value of this integration is greater than their segregation. Eco-agriculture values the contribution that agricultural landscapes can make to conservation (complementing reserves), and recognizes the contribution of conservation to agricultural production and sustainability.

Why diversity struggles as a strategy

Eco-nutrition, eco-agriculture, and ecosystem services all feature elements of managing diversity whether this be genetic diversity, species diversity, or landscape diversity (Figure 1.1). Managing for biodiversity can be complicated, particularly when attempting to understand the details of all possible interactions. Ecologists revel in complexity, describing ecosystems as 'complex adaptive systems' (Levin, 1999). Ecology is often hard-pressed to be predictive, with solutions that are often complex and context specific. Nutrition is similar, because as we shall see, the human body is in many ways its own complex adaptive system. As Pollan (2009) says, 'eating in our times has gotten complicated'. The diversity and often changing recommendations of nutritionists are enough to be mind-boggling, not unlike recommendations made by ecologists which frequently are so context specific and complex to be wholly unusable. Complexity should not lead to inaction however, by focusing on processes rather than contexts, and when managing for diversity we may find that the solution is simpler than we think, much in the same way that Pollan (2009) reduces nutrition to three simple rules: eat food, not too much, mostly plants.

Despite the advantages of using diversity as a development tool, the concept still struggles to find greater adoption in the face of more targeted interventions in part because of the focus on complexity rather than simplification and on context rather than process. The focus on complexity means that diversity-based strategies tend to be knowledge intensive. Two key ecological processes are focused on below, resource partitioning and resource acquisition. Both of these processes are comparable to concepts of harvest or yield in agronomy, and nutrient capture in nutrition.

Methods used by community ecologists often call for measuring the number of species, species composition, or the abundance of distinct species in an ecological community (or ecosystem). We then try to understand how changes in these community attributes affect ecosystem services. The positive effect of biodiversity in ecosystem services is most notably observed in those that relate resource acquisition and productivity (Hector et al., 1999; Hooper and Dukes, 2004). There are two primary mechanisms identified for the effects of diversity on the delivery of an ecosystem service, and one example of the effects of nutrient enrichment and impacts on biodiversity, which have parallels to human nutrition.

First, there are two mechanisms that relate biodiversity to the provision of ecosystem services. The first of these is the sampling effect (Tilman, 1999b), which notes that increasing species richness (the number of species in an ecological community), also increases the probability of including a species that is particularly good at providing a specific ecosystem service. The fundamental notion behind this concept is chance, and that increasing diversity is simply a matter of hedging one's bets. The maximum level of ecosystem service provision evidenced in the sampling effect is equal to the provisioning level of a monoculture of the dominant species. For example, under the rules of the sampling effect, the community productivity cannot exceed the productivity of the most productive species in the species pool. In other words, the total productivity is the sum of the parts.

The second mechanism is through species complementarity. Complementarity occurs when increasing species richness increases the number of niches that are filled, increasing resource use efficiency and productivity, as well as increasing the probability of positive interactions such as symbioses. This complementarity increases the efficiency of the system and yields a service provisioning that is greater than the sum of its parts. The quantity of ecosystem service provided in a diverse community is greater than the quantity provided by a monoculture of even the most productive species. There are numerous examples of both mechanisms in the ecological literature.

One problem with many of these studies is that they have focused on singular ecosystem services such as productivity, carbon sequestration, or pollination for example. It is often the case that when focusing on a single service, there is a single species that is best able to provide that service. A classic example is for carbon sequestration. If the land management objective is to store carbon, then a dense plantation of a fast growing, high wood density species such as eucalyptus is ideal. Bunker et al. (2005) demonstrated this with their study of carbon storage in a diversified tropical forest of Panama. This is exactly the strategy of conventional agricultural systems – a singular focus on the most productive species which has led to the use of strategies focused on the sampling effect: identify the species with the greatest production potential, provide the conditions that maximize the productivity of this singular species, often at the expense of others, and focus on it. This is similar to nutrition professionals focusing on fortification of vitamin A for example, a singular focus on the most limited nutritional element, and a targeted solution through fortification or enrichment.

Increasingly however there is recognition of the environmental harm that this strategy has caused in agricultural landscapes (Foley et al., 2011), and renewed interest in the notion of multifunctional landscapes (Hector and Bagchi, 2007). Agricultural landscapes, which currently occupy 38 per cent of terrestrial landscapes, must do more than provide abundant food sources. Farmers and those who work with them urgently need to recognize that agricultural landscapes must become multifunctional, producing water, sequestering carbon, supporting pollinators, and providing corridors for wild biodiversity amongst others. As we increase the number of services expected or desired from ecosystems, we find that the value or contribution of biodiversity also increases (Isbell et al., 2011). That is, while we might find a singular species that is ideally suited for carbon sequestration, such as the eucalyptus, we would be hard pressed to find a single species ideally suited to providing multiple ecosystem services. The eucalyptus plantation mentioned above is ideally suited for carbon sequestration, but is particularly poor at providing important hydrological services, or habitat for species other than koalas.

Nutrient enrichment can also affect species richness and composition of ecological communities. Species are able to partition their niches when there are multiple limiting resources, or multiple niches to be occupied. Flooding a system with one of these limiting resources can alter community composition, favouring a limited number of species and driving biodiversity loss (Harpole and Tilman, 2007). Although the total productivity of such systems can be increased, their resilience to change and the provision of multiple services is often lost. The effects of such nutrient enrichment have been studied in field-scale experiments but the impacts can be seen at landscapes scales, often crossing from terrestrial to aquatic systems; one of the most famous examples is the effects of nutrient run-off from mid-western, and southern California agriculture into the gulfs of Mexico and California which drive massive algal blooms that devastate the marine ecosystems and fisheries located hundreds to thousands of miles away from agricultural lands where the nutrients originated.

Eco-agricultural interventions try to reduce these types of effects by reducing run-off from agricultural fields with multispecies buffer strips placed between fields and waterways as well as by reducing the amounts of fertilizer applied to fields. From a multifunctional perspective, maintaining buffer strips along waterways not only improves water quality, but can also provide numerous additional services such as maintaining biological connectivity in agricultural landscapes, and ensuring the availability of pollinator and pest control services to adjacent fields.

There are at least two ways, if not more, in which the ecological study of biodiversity and ecosystem function can be compared with human nutrition. Each is unique in its own regard, and intellectually very exciting. The first was briefly mentioned above and ties the nutritional diversity of farm fields and landscapes to human health. The second, and more novel still, considers the human gut as an ecosystem, and considers how the diversity of the bacterial community that inhabits the human gut impacts the acquisition and availability of nutrients.

Sampling and complementary effects apply to human nutrition when considering the diversity of foodstuffs that make up the human diet. This can be tied to field and forest diversity in the case of subsistence systems (DeClerck et al., 2011b; Penafiel et al., 2012) or to the availability of nutrient diversity in urban neighbourhoods (Gordon et al., 2011). Nutrition interventions cannot singularly focus on providing caloric requirements, or vitamin A enrichment. As important as these interventions are in crisis situations, they lack long-term sustainability. As with the management of eco-agricultural landscapes, interventions must be multifunctional (Remans et al., 2011b). Certain foods are important for providing specific nutritional requirements; for example grasses such as maize, rice and wheat are critical for providing calories, and legumes for providing plant-based proteins. However we also recognize that the human body cannot subsist on carbohydrates alone, that there is a need not only for high-energy foodstuffs, but also an essential need for those ingredients that provide vitamins and nutrients essential for human health. As a rule of thumb, the greater the diversity of species you eat, the more likely you are to cover all your nutritional bases including complementarity effects. This is evident in the indigenous Mayan three-sisters agriculture example described above; the complementarity between the three species plus lime ensures that all nutritional bases are covered.

The second example, very different from the first, considers the human gut as an ecosystem (Figure 1.1). Turnbaugh et al. (2006) studied the gut microflora of obese and lean mice and found that the relative abundance of two dominant bacterial divisions, the *Bacteroidetes* and the *Firmicutes*, are associated, with the obese dominated by *Firmicutes*. The change in gut microflora is due to change in diet where diets excessively high in sugars and carbohydrates favour the *Firmicutes* which are more effective at processing these food types and converting them to calories. Interestingly, Turnbaugh et al. (2006) use agricultural terminology suggesting that this community is more effective in 'harvesting' nutrients. The results of several studies from this research group demonstrate that the organismal assemblage in the human gut consists of a highly diversified (many species) core microbiome and deviations from this core such as a reduction of species richness are associated with obesity (Turnbaugh et al., 2006, 2009; Jumpertz et al., 2011). It is worth providing Turnbaugh et al.'s (2009) own words here:

> Across all methods, obesity was associated with a significant decrease in the level of diversity. This reduced diversity suggests an analogy: the obese gut microbiota is not like a rainforest or reef, which are adapted to high energy flux and are highly diverse; rather, it may be more like a fertilizer runoff where a reduced-diversity microbial community blooms with abnormal energy input.

Turnbaugh et al. imply that the impact of an 'obese' diet is not unlike flooding an ecological system with phosphorus and nitrogen fertilizer, with impacts similar to natural systems, which reduce the diversity of organisms in the systems and reduce their multifunctionality.

Conclusions

From the human gut to agricultural fields and landscapes (Figure 1.1), we find evidence that the species diversity or composition of an ecosystem operates in similar ways. Interactions between species provide us with multiple functions and are central to the stability of those functions. Ecology, with its focus on complex systems, can make contributions to several global issues of concern, primarily related to agriculture, environment and nutrition. Ecology is but one element of any cross-disciplinary solution. Effective solutions require a continued dialogue between a diversity of fields, and more is gained initially by focusing on process rather than context. Cross-disciplinary thinking is an effective means of discovering novel perspectives on humanity's pervasive problems, further leading to new and sustainable solutions to these problems.

Acknowledgements

The author wishes to thank an anonymous reviewer and particularly Dr Roseline Remans for their critical review of this chapter. Their comments have greatly improved the manuscript. Any remaining errors remain the author's. Work on this chapter was partially funded by the CGIAR Collaborative Research Program on Water Land and Ecosystems (CRP5).

References

An, R.P. and Sturm, R. (2012) 'School and Residential Neighborhood Food Environment and Diet among California Youth', *American Journal of Preventive Medicine*, vol 42, no 2, pp.129–135.

Borer, E.T., Antonovics, J., Kinkel, L.L., Hudson, P.J., Daszak, P., Ferrari, M.J., Garrett, K.A., Parrish, C.R., Read, A.F., and Rizzo, D.M. (2012) 'Bridging taxonomic and disciplinary divides in infectious disease', *Ecohealth,* vol 8, no 3, pp.261–267.

Bunker, D.E., DeClerck, F., Bradford, J.C., Colwell, R.K., Perfecto, I., Phillips, O.L., Sankaran, M., and Naeem S. (2005) 'Species loss and aboveground carbon storage in a tropical forest', *Science,* vol 310, no 5750, pp.1029–1031.

Butchart, S.H.M., Walpole, M., Collen, B., Van Strien, A., Scharlemann, J.P.W., Almond, R.E.A., Baillie, J.E.M., Bomhard, B., Brown, C., Bruno, J., Carpenter, K.E., Carr, G.M., Chanson, J., Chenery, A.M., Csirke, J., Davidson, N.C., Dentener, F., Foster, M., Galli, A., Galloway, J.N., Genovesi, P., Gregory, R.D., Hocking, M., Kapos, V., Lamarque, J.F., Leverington, F., Loh, J., McGeoch, M.A., McRae, L., Minasyan, A., Morcillo, M.H., Oldfield, T.E.E., Pauly, D., Quader, S., Revenga, C., Sauer, J.R., Skolnik, B., Spear, D., Stanwell-Smith, D., Stuart, S.N., Symes, A., Tierney, M., Tyrrell, T.D., Vie, J.C., and Watson, R. (2010) 'Global biodiversity: indicators of recent declines', *Science,* vol 328, no 5982, pp.1164–1168.

Daily, G.C. (1997) *Nature's Services: societal dependence on natural ecosystems*, Washington DC: Island Press.

Deckelbaum, R.J. (2011) 'Econutrition: Integrating food-based human nutrition with ecology and agrodiversity preface', *Food and Nutrition Bulletin,* vol 32, no 1, p.S3.

Deckelbaum, R.J., Palm, C., Mutuo, P., and DeClerck, F. (2006) 'Econutrition: Implementation models from the Millennium Villages Project in Africa', *Food and Nutrition Bulletin,* vol 27, no 4, pp.335–342.

DeClerck, F.A.J. and Negreros-Castillo, P. (2000) 'Plant species of traditional Mayan homegardens of Mexico as analogs for multistrata agroforests', *Agroforestry Systems,* vol 48, pp.303–317.

DeClerck, F.A.J., Ingram, J.C., and Rumbaitis del Rio, C. (2011a) 'Integrated Ecology and Poverty Alleviation', in: J.C. Ingram, F.A.J. DeClerck, and C. Rumbaitis del Rio (eds) *Integrating Ecology and Poverty Alleviation and International Development Efforts: a practical guide,* New York: Springer.

DeClerck, F.A.J., Fanzo, J., Palm, C., and Remans, R. (2011b) 'Ecological approaches to human nutrition', *Food and Nutrition Bulletin,* vol 32, no 1, pp.S41–S50.

DeHaan, R.L. (2011) 'Teaching creative science thinking', *Science,* vol 334, no 6062, pp.1499–1500.

Flegal, K.M., Carroll, M.D., Kit, B.K., and Ogden, C.L. (2012) 'Prevalence of obesity and trends in the distribution of Body Mass Index among US adults, 1999–2010', *JAMA: The Journal of the American Medical Association*, vol 307, no 5, pp. 491–497.

Foley, J.A., Ramankutty, N., Brauman, K.A., Cassidy, E.S., Gerber, J.S., Johnston, M., Mueller, N.D., O'Connell, C., Ray, D.K., West, P.C., Balzer, C., Bennett, E.M., Carpenter, S.R., Hill, J., Monfreda, C., Polasky, S., Rockstrom, J., Sheehan, J., Siebert, S., Tilman, D., and Zaks, D.P.M. (2011) 'Solutions for a cultivated planet', *Nature,* vol 478, no 7369, pp.337–342.

Franco, M., Diez-Roux, A.V., Nettleton, J.A., Lazo, M., Brancati, F., Caballero, B., Glass, T., and Moore, L.V. (2009) 'Availability of healthy foods and dietary patterns: the Multi-Ethnic Study of Atherosclerosis', *American Journal of Clinical Nutrition,* vol 89, no 3, pp.897–904.

Gordon, C., Purciel-Hill, M., Ghai, N.R., Kaufman, L., Graham, R., and Van Wye, G. (2011) 'Measuring food deserts in New York City's low-income neighbourhoods', *Health & Place,* vol 17, no 2, pp.696–700.

Harpole, W.S. and Tilman, D. (2007) 'Grassland species loss resulting from reduced niche dimension', *Nature,* vol 446, no 7137, pp.791–793.

Hector, A. and Bagchi, R. (2007) 'Biodiversity and ecosystem multifunctionality', *Nature,* vol 448, no 7150: p.188–U6.

Hector, A., Schmid, B., Beierkuhnlein, C., Caldeira, M.C., Diemer, M., Dimitrakopoulos, P.G., Finn, J.A., Freitas, H., Giller, P.S., Good, J., Harris, R., Hogberg, P., Huss-Danell, K., Joshi, J., Jumpponen, A., Korner, C., Leadley, P.W., Loreau, M., Minns, A., Mulder, C.P.H., O'Donovan, G., Otway, S.J., Pereira, J.S., Prinz, A., Read, D.J., Scherer-Lorenzen, M., Schulze, E.D., Siamantziouras, A.S.D., Spehn, E.M., Terry, A.C., Troumbis, A.Y., Woodward, F.I., Yachi, S., and Lawton, J.H. (1999) 'Plant diversity and productivity experiments in European grasslands', *Science,* vol 286, no 5442, pp.1123–1127.

Hooper, D.U., and Dukes, J.S. (2004) 'Overyielding among plant functional groups in a long-term experiment', *Ecology Letters,* vol 7, no 2, pp.95–105.

Isbell, F., Calcagno, V., Hector, A., Connolly, J., Harpole, W.S., Reich, P.B., Scherer-Lorenzen, M., Schmid, B., Tilman, D., van Ruijven, J., Weigelt, A., Wilsey, B.J., Zavaleta, E.S., and Loreau, M. (2011) 'High plant diversity is needed to maintain ecosystem services', *Nature,* vol 477, no 7363, pp.199–203.

Jumpertz, R., Le, D.S., Turnbaugh, P.J., Trinidad, C., Bogardus, C., Gordon, J.I., and Krakoff, J. (2011) 'Energy-balance studies reveal associations between gut microbes, caloric load, and nutrient absorption in humans', *American Journal of Clinical Nutrition,* vol 94, no 1, pp.58–65.

Levin, S. (1999) *Fragile Dominion,* Santa Fe: Perseus Books.

Loreau, M., Naeem, S., and Inchausti, P. (eds) (2002) *Biodiversity and Ecosystem Functioning, Synthesis and Perspectives, Oxford Biology,* Oxford: Oxford University Press.

McNeely, J.A., and Scherr, S.J. (2003) *Ecoagriculture: Strategies to feed the world and save wild biodiversity,* Washington: Island Press.

Millennium Ecosystem Assessment (MEA) (2005) *Ecosystems and Human Well-Being: Current State and Trends,* Island Press.

Naeem, S., Duffy, J.E., and Zavaleta, E. (2012) 'The functions of biological diversity in an age of extinction', *Science* 336, 1401–1406.

Naeem, S., Bunker, D.E., Hector, A., Loreau, M., and Perrings, C. (2009) *Biodiversity, ecosystem functioning, and human well-being: an ecological and economic perspective,* Oxford: Oxford Biology.

Nugent, R. (chair) (2011) *Bringing Agriculture to the Table: How agriculture and food can play a role in preventing chronic disease,* The Chicago Council on Global Affairs, www.thechicagocouncil.org, accessed August 2012.

Ogden, C.L., Carroll, M.D., Kit, B.K., and Flegal, K.M. (2012) 'Prevalence of obesity and trends in Body Mass Index among US children and adolescents, 1999–2010', *JAMA: The Journal of the American Medical Association*, vol 307, no 5, pp. 483–490.

Penafiel, D., Lachat, C., Espinel, R., Van Damme, P., and Kolsteren, P. (2012) 'A systematic review on the contributions of edible plant and animal biodiversity to human diets', *Ecohealth,* vol 8, no 3, pp.381–399.

Pollan, M. (2009) *Food Rule: An Eater's Manual,* New York: Penguin Books.

Remans, R., Flynn, D.F.B., DeClerck, F., Diru, W., Fanzo, J., Gaynor, K., Lambrecht, I., Mudiope, J., Mutuo, P.K., Nkhoma, P., Siriri, D., Sullivan, C., and Palm, C.A. (2011a) 'Assessing nutritional diversity of cropping systems in African villages', *Plos One,* vol 6, no 6, pp.1–11.

Remans, R., Fanzo, J., Palm, C., and DeClerck, F.A. (2011b) 'Ecological approaches to human nutrition', in J.C. Ingram, F.A.J. DeClerck and C. Rumbaitis del Rio (eds) *Integrating Ecology and Poverty Alleviation and International Development Efforts: a practical guide,* New York: Springer.

Rockstrom, J., Steffen, W., Noone, K., Persson, A., Chapin, F.S., Lambin, E.F., Lenton, T.M., Scheffer, M., Folke, C., Schellnhuber, H.J., Nykvist, B., de Wit, C.A., Hughes, T., van der Leeuw, S., Rodhe, H., Sorlin, S., Snyder, P.K., Costanza, R., Svedin, U., Falkenmark, M., Karlberg, L., Corell, R.W., Fabry, V.J., Hansen, J., Walker, B., Liverman, D., Richardson, K., Crutzen, P., and Foley, J.A. (2009) 'A safe operating space for humanity', *Nature,* vol 461, no 7263, pp.472–475.

Termote, C., Meyi, M.B., Djailo, B.D., Huybregts, L., Lachat, C., Kolsteren, P., and Van Damme, P. (2012) 'A biodiverse rich environment does not contribute to a better diet: a case study from DR Congo', *Plos One,* vol 7, no 1.

Tilman, D. (1999a) 'Global environmental impacts of agricultural expansion: The need for sustainable and efficient practices', *Proceedings of the National Academy of Sciences of the United States of America,* vol 96, no 11, pp.5995–6000.

Tilman, D. (1999b) 'The ecological consequences of changes in biodiversity: A search for general principles', *Ecology,* vol 80, no 5, pp.1455–1474.

Tilman, D., Balzer, C., Hill, J., and Befort, B.L. (2011) 'Global food demand and the sustainable intensification of agriculture', *Proceedings of the National Academy of Sciences of the United States of America,* vol 108, no 50, pp.20260–20264.

Turnbaugh, P.J., Ley, R.E., Mahowald, M.A., Magrini, V., Mardis, E.R., and Gordon, J.I. (2006) 'An obesity-associated gut microbiome with increased capacity for energy harvest', *Nature*, vol 444, no 7122, pp.1027–1031.

Turnbaugh, P.J., Hamady, M., Yatsunenko, T., Cantarel, B.L., Duncan, A., Ley, R.E., Sogin, M.L., Jones, W.J., Roe, B.A., Affourtit, J.P., Egholm, M., Henrissat, B., Heath, A.C., Knight, R., and Gordon, J.I. (2009) 'A core gut microbiome in obese and lean twins', *Nature*, vol 457, no 7228: p.480-U7.

Wilcox, B., Aguirre, A.A., Daszak, P., Horwitz, P., Martens, P., Parkes, M., Patz, J., and Waltner-Toews, D.(2004) EcoHealth: A transdisciplinary imperative for a sustainable future, *Ecohealth*, vol 1, no. 1: 3–5.

Wilson, E.O. (1994) *Naturalist*, New York: Warner Books.

2 Overview of agricultural biodiversity and its contribution to nutrition and health

Vernon H. Heywood

Introduction

> Agricultural biodiversity is the first link in the food chain, developed and safeguarded by indigenous people throughout the world, and it makes an essential contribution to feeding the world.
>
> (Nakhauka, 2009)

The world's agriculture and its ability to provide food for the ever-growing human population can be regarded as one of the great success stories of human civilization. It developed from our use of the natural capital of wild plant and animal biodiversity through a long period of natural and human selection and breeding of crops and the development of agronomic skills. The use of the diversity of wild species is at the very basis of human development. Across the world, our ancestors' hunter-gatherer nutritional regime depended on local wild species of plants and animals for food while others, mainly plants, provided materials for shelter, fibre and fuel and medicine. The transition from hunting-gathering to agriculture (Neolithic revolution) started some 12,500 years ago when the domestication of a small number of wild plant species in various parts of the world led to the first agricultural revolution that provided us with a relatively secure source of food.[1] This in turn allowed human communities to grow and adopt a more sedentary way of life that paved the way for the development of villages, towns and cities that increasingly dominate our way of life and all the social and cultural changes that this involves. The diversity we have today in these crops and domesticated animals is the result of the interaction between countless generations of farmers and the plants and animals they domesticated, either through farming or aquaculture, and their environment.

The connection between this diversity – agricultural biodiversity – and human nutrition and health is intrinsic, multifaceted and constantly changing. It is complex – reflecting the many dimensions of nutrition, health and agricultural biodiversity – and there is no necessary direct link between the amount or quality of agricultural biodiversity and provision of nutritional and health benefits. While it is incontestable that some elements of agricultural biodiversity such as crop diversity and wild-harvested plants and animals have made and continue to make appreciable contributions to human diets, detailed evidence of their importance in terms of energy intake, micronutrient intake and dietary diversification is scarce and correlating agricultural biodiversity with human nutrition is generally difficult for a number of reasons including human diversity (DeClerck et al., 2011).

Overall, the exploitation of agricultural biodiversity has provided enormous nutrition and health benefits despite the dramatic population growth of the human population during the past 150 years, more recently through agricultural intensification. Yet as we will see, this has incurred overexploitation of some resources and extensive habitat loss as a result of land cleared for agriculture with considerable but largely undocumented loss of species and massive soil erosion. Some of these changes have also had negative impacts on dietary diversity, nutrition and health of some groups of society (Nakhauka, 2009). We are now faced with attempting to assess these impacts, learn lessons and seek a sustainable way forward (IAASTD, 2009). New approaches will be explored in this overview, including what is termed 'econutrition' (see Chapter 1) which aims to integrate environmental and human health, focusing especially on the many interactions between agriculture, ecology and human nutrition (Blasbalg et al., 2011).

Despite the success of the agricultural revolution in providing enough food to feed the world, today we are faced with issues of over- and undernutrition – both forms of malnutrition: more than a billion people today are chronically underfed thus making them more disease-prone while much of the developed world is at the same time facing a crisis of obesity caused by overnutrition aggravated by an unhealthy lifestyle, leading to diet-related diseases, such as cardiovascular disease, hypertension, cancer, diabetes and non-alcoholic fatty-liver disease. This tendency is not confined to the developed world but is also spreading to countries undergoing rapid societal transition – so-called development-driven obesity.[2] Worldwide 30 per cent more people are now obese than those who are underfed. The causes of these nutritional challenges are many and complex as are possible solutions.

It will be argued in this chapter that healthy human nutrition is best achieved by an approach to agriculture that is biodiverse, providing a varied food supply, and ecologically sustainable but as Blasbalg et al. (2011) noted, while such an approach is sound in theory, clear evidence is scarce because of the multiple variables that contribute to such an econutrition model. Such a biodiverse food-based approach should be seen as an element in an overall strategy that also includes continuing improvement of agricultural production, breeding cultivars that are more resistant to disease and stress, nutritional enhancement of crops, industrial fortification, vitamin supplementation and other nutrition–agriculture linkages (Chung et al., 2010).

It is time to broaden our approach even further and explore the linkages between agriculture, food production, nutrition, ethnobiology and ethnopharmacology and the resource base of wild and agricultural biodiversity in the context of accelerating global change (Heywood, 2011). At an institutional level, both globally and nationally, these issues are very loosely (or not at all) coordinated. Such a strategy for agricultural biodiversity and nutrition is proposed by Frison et al. (2011): it requires several different kinds of undertaking, including:

- an evidence-based approach to nutrition and health and sustainable agriculture by small-scale farmers;
- the evaluation and use of local foods and their variety;
- traditional cuisines;
- culturally sensitive methods;
- nutrition education;
- research on novel and improved methods of food storage and processing;
- enhanced attention to marketing.

Agricultural biodiversity defined

Agricultural biodiversity is the variety and variability of living organisms (plants, animals, microorganisms) that are involved in food and agriculture. Such a definition is however too general to be of much practical value and needs to be expanded and analysed if agricultural biodiversity is to be quantified. It can be considered at three main levels – those of ecological diversity, organismal diversity and genetic diversity (Heywood, 1999a), each of which forms a hierarchy of elements (Table 2.1). It is not just a subset of biodiversity but represents an extension of it so as to embrace units (such as cultivars, pure lines, breeds and strains) and habitats (agroecosystems such as farmers' fields and fisheries) that are not normally considered or even accepted by some conservation biologists as properly part of biological diversity. It includes all those species (including crop wild relatives) and the crop varieties, animal breeds and races, and microorganism strains, that are used directly or indirectly for food and agriculture, both as human nutrition and as feed (including grazing) for domesticated and semi-domesticated animals, and the range of environments in which agriculture is practised. It includes not just food as such but diets, food intake and nutritional considerations. Also covered are ingredients such as flavourings, colourants, preservatives, etc. that are used in food preparation, cooking, processing and storage.

Agricultural biodiversity also includes habitats and species outside of farming systems that benefit agriculture and enhance ecosystem functions (Heywood, 2003). In addition to the elements of agricultural biodiversity that are directly managed to supply the goods and services used by humans, other elements are vital because of their contributions to ecosystem services such as pollination (Klein et al., 2007), control of greenhouse gas emissions and soil dynamics (Frison et al., 2011). Production of at least one third of the world's food, including 87 of the 113 leading food crops, depends on pollination carried out by insects, bats and birds (IUCN, 2012). As Westerkamp and Gottsberger (2001) note, 'Pollinator diversity is mandatory for crop diversity' and pollination services have been estimated to contribute €153 billion worldwide in 2005 (Gallai et al., 2009).

Table 2.1 The components of agricultural biodiversity (modified from Heywood 1999a)

Agroecological diversity	Organismal diversity	Genetic diversity
biomes	kingdoms	gene pools
agroecological zones	phyla	populations
agroecosystems	families	individuals
polycultures	genera	genotypes
monocultures	species	genes
rangelands	subspecies	nucleotides
mixed systems	varieties	breeds
pastures	cultivar groups	strains
fallows	cultivars	pure lines
agroforestry systems	landraces	
agrosylvicultural		
sylvopastoral		
agrosylvopastoral		
home gardens		
forest		
ecosystems		
managed forests		
plantation forests		
seed forests		
fisheries		
fresh water systems		
marine systems		
habitats		
fields		
plots		
crops		

Socio-cultural diversity: human interactions with the above at all levels, including dietary and culinary diversity, food preparation and storage.

Likewise, agricultural biodiversity includes elements that affect crops and food production negatively such as pests and diseases, weeds and alien invasive species.

Agricultural biodiversity is by definition the result of the deliberate interaction between humans and natural ecosystems and the species that they contain, often leading to major modifications or transformations: the resultant agroecosystems are the product, therefore, of not just the physical elements of the environment and biological resources but vary according to the cultural and management systems to which they are subjected. Agricultural biodiversity thus includes a series of social, cultural, ethical and spiritual variables that are determined by farmers at the local community level. These factors played a key role in the process of selection and evolution of new cultivars or of local crops and in the ways in which they are grown and managed. It is important to recognize that 'the relationship that people have with their environment is complex and locally specific. Consequently, environment and development problems may need to be dealt with at the local scale so that remedies can be designed in ways that are culturally, socio-politically and environmentally suited to each local context' (Thomas, 2011).

This chapter will focus on components of agricultural biodiversity that impact most directly on nutrition and health and are directly managed to provide us with goods and services such as:

- the diversity of wild and domesticated plant and animal species used in agriculture, including underutilized and wild-gathered species;
- the ecosystems in which they grow and are grown;
- plant and animal genetic resources, including crop wild relatives (CWR) and domesticated animal wild relatives and the landraces, cultivars and breeds developed from these wild species.

The simplification of agriculture

A remarkable feature of the agricultural revolution was the relatively small number of plant species that were successfully domesticated and of these, the even smaller number which were selected over time because of their relative ease of cultivation, reliability and their ability to be grown in a range of habitats, as well as their nutritional value (Padulosi et al., 2002). On the other hand, over the past 12,000 years, farmers have developed a bewildering diversity of local varieties or landraces of these staples and of minor crops resulting from 'interactions with wild species, adaptations to changing farming conditions, and responses to the economic and cultural factors that shape farmers priorities' (Tripp and van der Heide, 1996). Landraces or primitive cultivars are the products of breeding or selection carried out by farmers, either deliberately or not, over many generations and natural selection. As noted by Harlan (1975), they 'are recognizable morphologically; farmers have names for them, and different landraces are understood to differ in adaptation to soil type, time of seeding, date of maturity, height, nutritive value, use and other properties'.

The number of animal species that were fully domesticated was even smaller and today only some 40-plus livestock species contribute to agriculture and food production. Likewise, the number of breeds that were developed in these domesticates was very much smaller than in the case of plants – FAO's Global Databank for Animal Genetic Resources for Food and Agriculture contains information on a total of 7,616 livestock breeds from 180 countries. Furthermore, as *The State of the World's Animal Genetic Resources for Food and Agriculture* (FAO, 2007) notes, 'With the exception of the wild boar (*Sus scrofa*) the ancestors and wild relatives of major livestock species are either extinct or highly endangered as a result of hunting, changes to their habitats, and in the case of the wild red jungle fowl, intensive cross-breeding with the domestic counterpart. In these species, domestic livestock are the only depositories of the now largely vanished diversity'. It has been estimated that 30 per cent of the world's animal breeds are at risk of extinction.

Agriculture and sedentism gradually led to a significant reduction in our dietary diversity (Ogle and Grivetti, 1985; Diamond, 1987) through our increased reliance on domesticated species and new and improved crops varieties (cultivars) which increased yields and led to intensification of agriculture. Eventually only a tiny number of crop species – the staples – came to dominate our nutritional and calorific intake, and globally the number of wild species that we depended upon directly was dramatically diminished. As Diamond (1987) noted 'While farmers concentrate on high carbohydrate crops like rice and potatoes, the mix of wild plants and animals in the diets of surviving hunter-gatherers provides more protein and a better balance of other nutrients'. While many would cavil at his suggestions that the adoption of agriculture was 'the worst mistake in the history of the human race', there is some evidence that initially it had an adverse effect on human health. For example, in their *Paleopathology at the Origins of Agriculture*, Cohen and Armelagos (1984) reported empirical studies of societies shifting their subsistence from foraging to primary food production which showed that there was evidence for deteriorating health due to an increase in infectious diseases and a rise in nutritional deficiencies that could be attributed to reliance on single crops deficient in essential minerals, amongst other factors (see also review by Mummert et al., 2011). But on the whole, agricultural intensification has been one of the main factors that has allowed much of the human population to enjoy unprecedented levels of health and reduced mortality.

This process of simplification of agriculture led eventually to today's model of food production in which we rely on only around 100 crop species for about 90 per cent of national per capita supplies of food from plants. Of these only 20–30 make up the bulk of human nutrition – the so-called staples (Prescott-Allen and Prescott-Allen, 1990), such as wheat, barley, maize, rice, millet, sorghum, rye, cassava, yams, potato and sweet potato. Modern intensive agriculture not only reduces agricultural biodiversity but, as Frison et al. (2011) point out, is predicated on such a reduction.

The gradual substitution of locally adapted landraces or cultivars by more advanced high-yielding cultivars that were resistant to disease or other factors resulted in the erosion of this pool of diversity and represented a further simplification of agriculture. This genetic erosion of our crop species led to the development of the plant genetic resource movement by pioneers such as Vavilov, Bennett, Frankel, Harlan, Hawkes and others (Bennett 1964, 1965; Frankel and Bennett, 1970; Pistorius, 1997) as an attempt to conserve the remaining diversity in crops and their wild relatives. The scale of loss of landraces reported has been dramatic in some cases although it is not easy to verify due to lack of reliable baseline data and consistent standards of recording. In rice (*Oryza sativa*), for example, 40,000 to 50,000 landraces are estimated to exist but many reports have been published indicating extensive national or local loss of cultivar diversity in the crop. Genetic erosion was reported by about 60 countries in national reports for the *Second Report on the State of the World's Plant Genetic Resources for Food and Agriculture* (FAO, 2010b) although few concrete examples were given. On the other hand, a study by Ford-Lloyd et al. (2008) of germplasm and genetic data in the IRRI genebank collected throughout South and Southeast Asia from 1962 to 1995 was unable to detect a significant reduction of available genetic diversity in the study material, contrary to popular opinion. Likewise, despite the massive loss of landraces reported for several crops, a review by Jarvis et al. (2008) revealed that as measured by richness, evenness and divergence of cultivars, considerable crop genetic diversity continues to be maintained on farm, in the form of traditional crop varieties for a finite number of crops in a small number of countries. Major staples had higher richness in terms of the number of different kinds of individuals regardless of their frequencies and evenness (measuring how similar the frequencies of the different variants are) than non-staples. And in a study of genetic erosion in maize within smallholder agriculture in southern Mexico, van Heerwarden et al. (2009) found that despite the dominance of commercial seed, the informal seed system of local farmers persisted. True landraces were, however, rare and most of the informal seed was derived from modern 'creolized' varieties – developed as a result of exposing improved varieties to local conditions and management and continually selecting seed for replanting and promoting their hybridization with landraces (Bellon et al., 2003). They also showed that genetic erosion was moderated by the distinct features offered by modern varieties.

While acknowledging the undoubted success of modern agriculture, it should be remembered that the great majority of farmers in the developing world are traditional or peasant farmers who rely in varying degrees on small-scale cultivation of staples and various forms of traditional agriculture, including raised fields, terraces, swidden fallows, agroforestry polycultures (e.g. home gardens), semi-domesticated species and wild harvesting of fruits, fibres, medicinals and so on, and on the natural and semi-natural ecosystems that border or are adjacent to the cultivated fields (Altieri, 1999; Altieri and Koohafkan, 2008).

Globally, small-scale agriculture is the dominant form of food provision (IAASTD, 2009). It is estimated that about 60 per cent of the world's agriculture consists of traditional subsistence farming systems in which there is both a high diversity of crops and species grown and of ways in which they are grown, such as polycropping and intercropping, that leads to the maintenance of variation within the crops (FAO, 2010a; Vigouroux et al., 2011). Such traditional agricultural landscapes are estimated to provide as much as 20 per cent of the world's food supply. They are rich in agricultural biodiversity, especially in polycultures and agroforestry systems, thus contrasting with modern intensive industrial agriculture, and are often the product of complex farming systems that have developed in response to the unique physical conditions of a given location, such as altitude, slopes, soils, climates and latitude, as well as cultural and social influences (Phillips and Stolton, 2008). Many of the species grown in such systems are local 'underutilized species' as discussed below and provide nutritional balance to the diet, complementing the staple crops that are grown and providing micronutrients and vitamins. Another advantage of growing a diversity of crops and maintaining genetic diversity within local production systems is that it also favours the conservation of local knowledge (FAO, 2010b).

Home gardens (also known as homestead gardens, yard gardens, kitchen gardens, etc.) are a long-established tradition and offer great potential for improving household food security and alleviating micronutrient deficiencies. The home garden can be defined as a farming system which combines different physical, social and economic functions on the area of land around the family home (FAO, 1995, 1996). They occur in most parts of the world but especially in tropical and subtropical regions (Eyzaguirre and Watson, 2002; Wezel and Bender, 2003; Gebauer, 2005; Kabir and Webb, 2008) and it has been estimated that nearly 1 billion people in the tropics live from the produce of home gardens supported by subsistence agriculture. The essence of such systems is the diversity of species they contain – up to 100 or more species per garden – and their two- to four-layered structure that allows different ecological niches to be exploited by the species planted. Several organizations such as FAO and the Centre for Sustainable Development offer training courses or manuals on home gardens. Home gardens may also provide animal products such as chickens, eggs and livestock, as in the case of the homestead gardens promoted by Bioversity International and Helen Keller International (see Case Studies 2 and 7 in this volume) (Iannotti et al., 2009).

Although numerous reports on the role of home gardens in nutrition are found in the literature, there is little reliable evidence of their value. A systematic review of agricultural interventions, including many on home gardens, that aim to improve the nutritional status of children by improving the incomes and the diet of the rural poor, based on a systematic search of the published and unpublished literature (Masset et al., 2011), concluded that the interventions were as expected successful in promoting consumption of specific foods – in the case of home gardens fruit and vegetables – but very little evidence was available on their effects on nutritional status. On the other hand, the authors note that the absence of any reported statistically significant impact of agricultural interventions on nutritional status found in their review, as well as by other earlier reviews, 'should not be attributed to the inefficacy of these interventions. Rather it is the lack of power of the studies reviewed that could have prevented the identification of such impact, if any'.

The importance of plant diversity for nutrition

> Adequate human nutrition involves regular intake of a wide range of nutrients, some of which must be consumed on a frequent basis, even if in small quantities. As such, dietary diversity (DD), typically measured in the form of a count of food groups or food group frequency, has been suggested as a proxy indicator for nutrient adequacy.
>
> (Coates et al., 2007)

We have at our disposal some 400,000 species of plants but, as we have seen, only a small number of these are the staples on which global nutrition depends. This is, however, only part of the picture. The number of cultivated crop species (excluding ornamentals) has been estimated at about 7,000 (Khoshbakht and Hammer, 2008), most of them grown locally and on a small scale. In addition there are many locally used species that are scarcely or only partially domesticated and many thousands more are gathered from the wild (Heywood, 1999b).

The nutritional importance of dietary diversity (DD) is now widely recognized (WHO/FAO, 2003). Growing a range of local crops supplemented by wild-harvested species helps provide such diversity in the diet, especially of poor rural families, and complements the nutrition provided by staples such as maize, rice and cassava. Balanced nutrition in the human diet depends not just on growing a diversity of crops but on the diversity within the crops (Mouillé et al., 2010). The micronutrient superiority of some lesser-known cultivars and wild varieties over other, more extensively utilized cultivars, has been confirmed by recent research. For example, recent analyses have shown that beta-carotene content can differ by a factor of 60 between sweet potato cultivars and the pro-vitamin A carotenoid of banana cultivars can range between 1 μg and 8,500 μg/100 grams (Burlingame et al., 2009; Lutaladio et al., 2010), while the protein content of rice varieties can range from 5 to 13 per cent (Kennedy and Burlingame, 2003). As they observe, 'Intake of one variety rather than another can be the difference between micronutrient deficiency and micronutrient adequacy'. Unfortunately, we lack detailed information about such diversity within most crops at the cultivar level and the role it plays in nutrition because of the general neglect by professionals (Burlingame et al., 2009) and much of the evidence is anecdotal.

Underutilized or orphan crops

The term 'underutilized species' refers to those species whose potential to improve people's livelihoods, as well as food security and sovereignty, is not being fully realized because of their limited competitiveness with commodity crops in mainstream agriculture. While their potential may not be fully realized at national level, they are of significant importance locally, being highly adapted to marginal, complex and difficult environments and contributing significantly to diversification and resilience of agroecosystems. This means they are also of considerable interest for future adaptation of agriculture to climate change (Padulosi et al., 2011).

The importance of underutilized species is now receiving more recognition. The IAASTD (2009) report, for example, recognizes that investments in agricultural knowledge, science and technology 'can increase the sustainable productivity of major subsistence foods including orphan and underutilized crops, which are often grown or consumed by poor people'. Likewise, the Ministerial Declaration 'Action Plan on Food Price Volatility and Agriculture', issued by the G20 Agriculture Ministers from their meeting in Paris on 22–23 June 2011 recognized the importance of making the best use of all available plant genetic resources for food and agriculture, including research on underutilized crops. Underutilized species also received qualified endorsement in the Commission on Sustainable Agriculture and Climate Change's report *Achieving food security in the face of climate change* (Beddington et al., 2012).

Wild-gathered plant species

Despite the simplification of agriculture, wild species still represent a major resource today and form an important part of the diet of societies in both the developed and developing worlds, providing not only variety but also essential vitamins and micronutrients in the form of bushmeat, fruits, vegetables, herbs and spices, beverages and intoxicants, not to mention their use as fibres, fuel, ornament and medicines (Bharucha and Pretty, 2010; Heywood, 1999b, 2008, 2011; Turner et al., 2011). These range from locally consumed species such as leaf greens and wild fruits to economically important non-timber forest products obtained by extractivism, such as palm hearts, Brazil nuts and rubber and the trade – most of it uncontrolled and much of it illegal – in ornamentals including cycads, orchids, cacti and succulents and bulbs. The use of wild plants in most societies forms part of indigenous knowledge systems and practices that have been developed over many generations and which play an important part in decision-making in local agriculture, food production, human and animal health and management of natural resources (Slikkerveer, 1994). Growing vegetables in home gardens and other plots is often supplemented in traditional rural and farming communities by wild harvesting of local greens, fruits, nuts and fungi. The term 'wild food', therefore, is used to describe all plant resources that are harvested or collected for human consumption outside agricultural areas in forests, savannah and other bush-land areas.

The consumption of traditional leafy vegetables ('wild or leafy greens') as an important source of micronutrients is attracting a great deal of attention, notably in the tropics (Etkin, 1994; Chweya and Eyzaguirre, 1999; Price and Ogle, 2008; Afolayan and Jimoh, 2009; Grivetti and Ogle, 2000; Pretty, 2007b; Heywood, 1999b; Flyman and Afolayan, 2006; Uusiku et al., 2010). Often they provide rural poor with most of their daily requirements of essential vitamins and minerals, particularly folate, and vitamins A, B complex, E and C (Guarino, 1997; FAO, 2010a) and in many cases they also have medicinal properties and form part of local health care systems (Etkin, 2006). They are especially important in small children's diets to ensure normal growth and intellectual development (FAO, 2010a).

In the Mediterranean region, the habit of consuming wild food plants is still prevalent, especially for rural people, although it is 'ageing', with fewer traditional vegetables consumed than in previous decades. A circum-Mediterranean ethnobotanical field survey for wild food plants as part of the EU-supported RUBIA project (Hadjichambis et al., 2008) documented 294 wild food taxa. In particular, traditional leafy vegetables ('wild or leafy greens') are widely consumed in several Mediterranean countries such as France, Greece, Italy, Spain and Turkey (Pieroni et al., 2005; Heywood, 2009). They are especially important in Greece (where they are known as *xorta*), especially Crete (where over 92 wild greens have been catalogued (Stavridakis, 2006) and several studies published) and other islands such as Cyprus, Sicily and Sardinia. In recent years, work on economically valuable wild plant species in the Mediterranean region has increasingly focused on the nutritional and health aspects of wild foods (Heinrich et al., 2006a,b). A recent ethnobotanical study showed that as many as 2,300 different plant and fungal taxa are gathered and consumed in the Mediterranean region (Rivera et al., 2006) where they play an important role in human nutrition and can supply most of the necessary daily requirements for vitamins A, B complex and C and provide minerals and trace elements. They may sometimes even be better nutritionally than introduced cultivated vegetables. The so-called Mediterranean diet (Keys and Keys, 1959) or more properly diets that are rich in fruit, vegetables, legumes and olive oil, as well as fish and poultry, but low in meat and animal fats (Heinrich et al., 2006a) often include a range of local wild-gathered plants such as 'wild greens'.

Forests can play an important part in human nutrition, particularly in developing countries (Hladik et al., 1993) and according to the Collaborative Partnership on Forests (CPF), the potential of forests and trees to improve food and nutritional security needs more attention from policymakers and development agencies (FAO, 2011c). It is estimated that at least 410 million people derive much of their food and livelihoods from forests while some 1.6 billion people get some portion of their food and livelihood from forests around the world (ETC Group, 2009). Non-Wood Forest Products (NWFP) include many types of food such as fruits, nuts, leafy vegetables and oils that are widely recognized as contributing to the livelihood of millions of people in many parts of the world, especially in the tropics and subtropics, and contribute to dietary diversity. A six-year global study by CIFOR (2011) has documented for the first time on a broad scale the role that forests play in poverty alleviation and the significant contribution they make to the livelihoods of millions of people in developing countries. The Poverty and Environment Network (PEN) study consists of data from more than 8,000 households from 40+ sites in 25 developing countries. It makes a strong argument for the sustainable management of natural ecosystems to provide health and nutritional benefits.

Domestication programmes are being developed to bring many wild species, both trees and herbs, into cultivation and integrate them into agroforestry systems (Leakey, 1997, 2011; Leakey and Tchoundjeu, 2001). Examples of such species are *Adansonia digitata*, *Barringtonia procera*, *Canarium indicum*, *Gnetum africanum*, *Irvingia gabonensis*, *Sclerocarya birrea* and *Vitellaria paradoxa*. As well as providing 'marketable timber and non-timber forest products that will enhance rural livelihoods by generating cash for resource-poor rural and peri-urban households' and restoring productivity through soil fertility improvement, these species can provide health and nutritional benefits.

Crop wild relatives

While crop wild relatives (CWR) may not play a significant direct role in human nutrition – although there are notable exceptions such as wild yams in Madagascar – they are an essential source of genetic material for the development of new and better adapted crops (Maxted et al., 2011). For example, a recent study using microsatellite markers showed that a wild rice in Vietnam has much greater genetic variation than cultivated rice, with a single wild population showing greater genetic variation than that found in 222 local Vietnamese varieties (Ishii et al., 2011). Moreover, it is now widely recognized that the wild relatives of crops will play a key role in future food security in the face of global change (Guarino, 2010; Maxted et al., 2010; Hunter and Heywood, 2011).

The importance of animal diversity for nutrition

Although much of the focus in this chapter is on plants, animal diversity also plays an important role in human nutrition and dietary diversity, mainly in terms of dairy products, eggs, meat and offal, fish and seafood (see Chapter 3) (Ruel, 2003). Animal products are excellent sources of high quality protein and fat and are an important source of vitamins and minerals such as zinc, iron and selenium as well as calcium and phosphorus. According to a recent FAO report on livestock in food security (FAO, 2011d), 'Livestock contribute around 12.9% of global calories and 27.9% of protein directly through provision of meat, milk, eggs and offal…'.

Although for many people in developing countries, animal food products are not a significant part of their diet, and dietary restrictions prohibit the consumption of certain animal foods, globally they are becoming increasingly important and this trend is expected to continue (von Kaufmann, 2000). In China, which is undergoing rapid nutritional transition, consumption of meat (mainly pork) has increased dramatically over the past 35 years and the country now eats more than a quarter of all the meat produced worldwide. High meat intake has been one of several factors, such as increasing consumption of fast food with a high sodium content and sugar-sweetened beverages and lack of physical exercise, that have been associated with an increase in obesity in the Chinese population (Cheng, 2004; Ko et al., 2010).

According to FAO (2010c), as demand for animal source foods increases, global production of meat is projected to more than double between 1990 and 2050. The Rome-based food agency warns, however, that current industrial livestock production practices may not be sustainable and notes that livestock is currently the single largest user of land in the world, accounting for 70 per cent of all agricultural land and 30 per cent of total land surface.

Wild meat/bushmeat and other wildlife

Although 'bushmeat' is the African term for the meat of wild animals it is now applied to animals that are hunted for subsistence or commercial purposes especially in the tropics of the Americas, Asia and Africa. It is also known as wild meat (as recommended by IUCN) or game. It may be defined as 'any non-domesticated terrestrial mammals, birds, reptiles and amphibians harvested for food' (Nasi et al., 2008) or more widely to include any type of terrestrial wild animal, including reptiles (tortoises, lizards, snakes), birds, mammals,

---

Box 2.1 Nutritional importance of wild meat

'Bushmeat represents an important protein source in the tropics while gathered plant foods are important dietary supplements to the starchy staple diet. In at least 62 countries world-wide, wildlife and fish constitute a minimum of 20% of the animal protein in rural diets. Wildlife provides significant calories to rural communities, as well as essential protein and fats. … Even where there has been a change from a hunter-gatherer lifestyle to pastoralism or agriculture, hunting and gathering remain important to a high proportion of rural households in tropical forests. Hunting provides between 30 to 80% of the overall protein intake of rural households in Central Africa (Koppert et al.,1996) and nearly 100% of animal proteins. What is known of the nutritional composition of bushmeat species suggests that these provide an equivalent or even greater quality of food than domestic meats with less fat and more protein. The average protein value of wild meat is estimated at around 30 g of protein per 100 g of meat (Ntiamoa-Baidu, 1997). These proteins cannot be substituted by available protein of vegetal origin, such as cassava or gnetum leaves, as they are poorer in amino acids (Pagezy, 1996). They could be replaced by other vegetal sources, dairy products, and/or meat from domesticated animals'.

Source: Nasi et al., 2008

---

some amphibious or semi-aquatic freshwater animals, such as frogs, turtles and crocodilians and marine mammals such as seals, walruses, whales, dolphins, porpoises and manatees (Roth and Merz, 1996).

The nutritional importance of wild meat, like domesticated livestock, is that it provides protein and fat as well as vitamins in the diet (Box 2.1). Detailed reviews of the importance and role of wildlife in nutrition are given by Hladik et al. (1989, 1996) and Froment et al. (1996). However it must be noted that excessive hunting of some wild animal populations is leading to a bushmeat crisis that is threatening the livelihoods of some forest communities (Nasi et al., 2008).

Fish and crustaceans

Fish and fish products and shellfish provide a major source of nutrition for coastal, lacustrine and riverine communities, especially in developing countries, and play an important role in the diets, livelihoods, and income of many poor population groups who suffer from vitamin and mineral deficiencies (see Chapter 4 and Case Study 4) (Roos et al., 2007). According to FAO about 2,000 fish, crustacean, mollusc, echinoderm and aquatic plant species or species groups are caught annually. But since about 10 million tonnes of unnamed marine fish alone are landed annually, the total number of species harvested is likely to be more than 5,000 (Williams, 2011). Today almost half of all fish eaten come from farmed sources, not wild capture.

In 2007, fish accounted for 15.7 per cent of the global population's intake of animal protein and 6 per cent of all protein consumed (FAO, 2010d). Globally, fish consumption per capita increased by 43 per cent from 11 kg in 1970 to 16 kg in 2000. Fish played an important role in doubling animal protein consumption per capita in developing countries in the same period – from 6.3 kg in 1970 to 13.8 kg in 2000, driven, especially in Asia, by urbanization, income and population growth, while in the developed world fish consumption increased by less than one half between 1970 and 2000 (Ahmed, 2004).

In West Africa fish accounts for 30 per cent of animal protein intake (Neiland, 2006), limited only by its availability, and in Bangladesh the rural population depends on a diet of fish and rice supplemented by small amounts of vegetables to such an extent that as Roos et al. (2007) note, the old proverb 'mache bhate bangali' (fish and rice make a Bengali) is still true today. They also report that while carp polyculture production has been highly successful, small indigenous fish species that are caught, sold, and consumed by the rural population and which contain high levels of protein, vitamins, iron, calcium, zinc and other minerals tend to be ignored and are not captured in official statistics so that the benefits derived from such local fish are poorly documented and their importance can be underestimated.

An interesting example of where a plant-based agroecosystem also provides substantial amounts of animal biodiversity that is used in local nutrition is rice paddies. Perfecto et al. (2009) note that the biodiversity in rice fields may be divided into aquatic invertebrates, terrestrial invertebrates, vertebrates and plants with some rice-based systems containing more than 100 species that are used by local communities.

Changing the paradigm

> The present paradigm of intensive crop production cannot meet the challenges of the new millennium.
>
> (Diouf, 2011)

> What we desperately need is another revolution, one that deals with agricultural productivity for the smallholders ... We need to answer these questions: Are we growing the right foods? Are we growing them in the most efficient way with respect to inputs, water and land? Are we growing them in the most suitable way? And what foods are consumers actually eating in terms of quality and quantity, nutrition and food safety?
>
> (Andersen, 2011)

Agricultural intensification continues to pose a serious threat to biodiversity in many parts of the world. For example, a recent study of the impact of crop management and agricultural land use on the threat status of plants adapted to arable habitats in 29 European countries showed a positive relationship between national wheat yields and the numbers of rare, threatened or recently extinct arable plant species in each country (Storkey et al., 2012). This current paradigm of intensive high input, high output intensification of agriculture is now being questioned because of (1) growing concerns about its present impacts on biodiversity; (2) the predicted impacts of global change on agriculture and wild biodiversity; (3) serious issues over energy and water security; and (4) changes in dietary patterns.

Proposals for new paradigms are emerging (Lang, 2009; Thompson and Scoones, 2009; Brussaard et al., 2010; Pretty, 2002, 2007a; Pretty et al., 2010; Clay, 2011; Collette et al., 2011; Brown, 2011). As Frison et al. (2011) point out, 'Almost all of the approaches used to date in agricultural intensification strategies, for example the substitution and supplementation of ecosystem function by human labour and petrochemical products, contain the seeds of their own destruction in the form of increased release of greenhouse gases, depletion of water supplies and degraded soils. We need to build production systems that deliver intensification without simplification.' Sustainable intensification of agricultural production – 'producing more output from the same area of land while reducing the negative environmental impacts and at the same time increasing contributions to natural capital and the flow of environment' (Pretty, 2011; Pretty et al., 2011) – is now widely advocated (Royal Society, 2009; Godfray et al., 2010a, b).

Recent volatility in food prices together with extreme weather events and the projected impacts of climate change have intensified the search for alternative ways of addressing the problem of achieving food security through employing more sustainable and intelligent management of production and consumption as outlined in the UNEP rapid response assessment *The Environmental Food Crisis* (Nellemann et al., 2009). As Achim Steiner writes in the preface to the report, 'Simply cranking up the fertilizer and pesticide-led production methods of the 20th century is unlikely to address the challenge'.

Pretty et al. (2010) consider that 'The goal for the agricultural sector is no longer simply to maximize productivity, but to optimize across a far more complex landscape of production, rural development, environmental, social justice and food consumption outcomes'. For example, FAO has published a policymaker's guide to what is termed 'sustainable intensification of smallholder crop production' (Collette et al., 2011) in which more is produced from the same area of land while conserving resources, reducing negative impacts on the environment and enhancing natural capital and the flow of ecosystem services (see also Pretty et al., 2011). This approach involves:

- building crop production intensification on farming systems that offer a range of productivity, socio-economic and environmental benefits to producers and to society at large;
- using a genetically diverse portfolio of improved crop varieties that are suited to a range of agroecosystems and farming practices, and resilient to climate change;

- rediscovering the importance of healthy soil, drawing on natural sources of plant nutrition, and using mineral fertilizer wisely;
- smarter, precision technologies for irrigation and farming practices that use ecosystem approaches to conserve water;
- achieving plant protection by integrated pest management and avoiding overuse of pesticides;
- bringing about fundamental changes in agricultural development policies and institutions so as to encourage smallholders to adopt sustainable crop production intensification.

The need to maintain and manage ecosystems sustainably so that they continue to provide us with goods and services is critical: as Munang et al. (2011) observe, 'Healthy ecosystems provide a diverse range of food sources and support entire agricultural systems'. Although not new, there are increasing calls today for a more ecological approach to agriculture – sometimes called ecological agriculture (Kiley-Worthington, 1981), eco-agriculture (McNeely and Scherr, 2003; Buck et al., 2004; Scherr and McNeely, 2007; Buck and Scherr, 2011),[3] or regenerative agriculture (LaSalle, 2008) – and also to human nutrition (DeClerck et al., 2011). Such approaches look beyond a focus on production to sustainability, biodiversity protection and the complex dynamics of the agroecosystem in terms of plants, animals, insects, water and soil. A diversity of crops (and where appropriate livestock) is also a characteristic as is a focus on the role of indigenous communities.

So far, calls to promote a more food-based approach to nutrition and health (Levin et al., 2003) have met with resistance from policymakers and governments and as discussed below, the role of species diversity in nutrition and alleviation of poverty has been largely disregarded by mainstream agricultural policy although it is now a subject of considerable discussion.

Assessing the role of biodiversity in alleviating hunger and malnutrition

> …a wider deployment of agricultural biodiversity is an essential component in the sustainable delivery of a more secure food supply.
>
> (Frison et al., 2011)

Although the link between biodiversity and alleviating poverty, including food poverty and malnutrition, has been pointed out by many authors in recent years (e.g. Etkin, 1994; Batello et al., 2004; World Bank, 2007; Chivian and Bernstein, 2008; IAASTD, 2009; Kuhnlein et al., 2009; Lutaladio et al., 2010; Frison et al., 2011; DeClerck et al., 2011) and has been eloquently argued by distinguished figures such as M.S. Swaminathan, the Father of the Green Revolution in India and World Food Prize winner (Swaminathan, 2011), it is much more difficult to convince governments and policymakers and provide clear scientific evidence of a direct link between protecting the natural environment and promoting the interests of poor communities and more specifically between biodiversity and poverty (Roe et al., 2010).

An international symposium on 'Linking biodiversity conservation and poverty reduction: what, why and how?', organized by IIED, UNEP-WCMC and the African Wildlife Foundation, held at the Zoological Society of London, on 28–29 Apr 2010, debated these issues and several speakers questioned the robustness of the scientific evidence for the linkages between biodiversity and poverty (Roe et al., 2010). Some commentators take a more extreme position such as 'Biodiversity doesn't feed people, but GM crops do' which has evoked many responses to the effect that socially it is well documented that biodiversity and poverty are closely related.

It is clear from such exchanges that there is a need to recognize the importance of providing or actually generating good solid evidence on which policy can be based. As a recent editorial in *Science and Development Network* (Dickson and Lewis, 2010) notes, 'without solid evidence that biodiversity conservation can alleviate poverty, politicians simply won't buy into the idea of protecting biodiversity, or will take action that however well meaning, ends up unfocused and ineffective'.

One of the commonest criticisms of advocating a greater use of local agricultural biodiversity in the form of traditional crops, underutilized species and wild-harvested species to address under- or malnutrition is precisely that it is local and it is assumed therefore will have little impact on the global picture. Yet, at least 20 per cent of the world food supply comes from traditional multiple cropping systems, most of them small farm units often of 2 ha or less (Altieri, 2009).[4] There is ample evidence on the ground that local biodiversity and ecosystem services play an essential role in the lives of communities throughout the developing world, by providing a social safety net for food, medicine, fibre, fuel wood etc. that can act as route out of poverty and a source of income generation, prevent people falling further into poverty or in extreme cases as an emergency lifeline through the provision of 'famine food' (Roe et al., 2010). It can also play a major part in addressing some issues of malnutrition (see below).

The main reasons for the lack of attention given to underutilized or wild-gathered species include:

- a lack of information and reliable methods for measuring their contribution to farm households and the rural economy;
- low productivity compared with staples;
- the lack of guaranteed markets, except for a small number of products;
- the irregularity of supply of wild plant products;
- the lack of quality standards;
- lack of standardization of the product;
- the lack of storage and processing technology for many of the products;
- the availability of substitutes;
- the bias in favour of large-scale agriculture

(Heywood, 2006, 2008; Padulosi et al., 2008)

But perhaps the main problem is their low profile with the general public caused by lack of knowledge about what they are and what are their characteristics and value. Solid scientific evidence on the nutritional benefits of indigenous foods is often lacking and much further work is needed to provide a sounder basis for their possible development.

Knowledge gaps

In the case of both underutilized crops and wild-harvested species, much of the evidence on the nutritional or health benefits of particular species is partial or anecdotal and there is a need for critical scientific assessments. A systematic review of the literature on the contributions of edible plant and animal diversity to human diets concluded that local food biodiversity makes an important contribution to nutritious diets, although strong evidence is lacking, and the findings were limited to communities living in areas with high biodiversity (Penafiel et al., 2011). They comment that 'Only future multidisciplinary research, incorporating appropriate biodiversity and nutritional assessment methodologies, would lead to a better understanding of the dietary contributions of local food biodiversity and diets'. Also, as Flyman and Afolayan (2006) comment, 'the chemical, nutritional and toxicological properties of … local wild vegetables, the bioavailability of micronutrients present in these, and their modification by various processing techniques still need to be properly established and documented before their use as an alternative dietary source can be advocated'. This poses a major challenge not just for the proponents of these species but also for ethnopharmacologists and ethnobiologists (Heywood, 2011). A recent report (CIFOR, 2011) notes that 'Many existing tools for assessing poverty and income – such as poverty reduction strategy plans, poverty surveys, the World Bank's Living Standard Measurement Survey and national income accounting systems – fall short of capturing the importance of the income from natural resources, so that its true value in the livelihoods of the world's rural poor remains largely invisible'.

For most wild-collected species, whether for food, medicine or fuel, we have little knowledge of the amount of material that is harvested from the wild or of the effect that such gathering has on the health and survival of populations of these wild plants. Only a few countries have made detailed inventories of these species and the literature is scattered in numerous papers and reports and is often of only local importance. Few syntheses have been published such as *The Hidden Harvest* (Scoones et al., 1992), which is a literature review and annotated bibliography of wild foods and agricultural systems but now rather dated. A review of the roles and values of wild foods in agricultural systems by Bharucha and Pretty (2010) includes some information on the diversity of wild species used. In 22 countries in Asia and Africa, the mean use of wild foods by agricultural and forager communities is '90–100 species per location' while the figures for individual countries such as India, Ethiopia and Kenya can be as much as 300–800 species.

Agricultural biodiversity, nutrition and global change

> Agricultural biodiversity will also be absolutely essential to cope with the predicted impacts of climate change, not simply as a source of traits but as the underpinnings of more resilient farm ecosystems.
>
> (Frison et al., 2011)

The future impacts of the various components of global change – demographic, climatic, land use – on agricultural biodiversity and nutrition will be enormously complex and correspondingly difficult to decipher and predict. What is certain is that inexorable demographic growth during the remainder of this century will require a vast increase in agricultural production and productivity to feed the extra billions. Not only that but it will have to attempt to do so in ways that are sustainable and that address increasing environmental concerns at the multiple impacts of agriculture on our environment and on biodiversity (Foley et al., 2005, 2011) and do not exacerbate already rising world food prices, while also addressing the problems of hunger and malnutrition, satisfying rapidly escalating bioenergy use and tackling the problems of restoring degraded lands and soils. The question has been raised as to whether all these factors will converge, leading to what some authors have called 'a perfect storm' (Buchanan et al., 2010; Hertel, 2011) for global agriculture or whether practical solutions can be devised and implemented successfully (Foley et al., 2011).

The growing human population will inevitably lead to further overexploitation of resources and increase the pressure to convert further land for agriculture. What is much less clear is how the shifts in the climatic components of global change such as temperature, rainfall and greenhouse gases (carbon dioxide, methane, ozone and nitrous oxide) will interact with agricultural production. Global warming is predicted to pose significant threats to agricultural production and trade (UNCTAD, 2010) and to the ability of ecosystems and agroecosystems and their component species to adapt to these changes. The impacts of climate change will vary from region to region.

A report by the International Food Policy Research Institute on the impact of climate change on agriculture and the costs of adaptation (Nelson et al., 2009) draws stark conclusions: 'Crop yields will decline, production will be affected, crop and meat prices will increase, and consumption of cereals will fall, leading to reduced calorie intake and increased child malnutrition'. The report notes that:

- higher temperatures eventually reduce yields of desirable crops while encouraging weed and pest proliferation;
- changes in precipitation patterns increase the likelihood of short-run crop failures and long-run production declines;
- although there will be gains in some crops in some regions of the world, the overall impacts of climate change on agriculture are expected to be negative, threatening global food security.

As regards human nutrition, the report also suggests that:

- calorie availability in 2050 will not only be lower than in the no-climate-change scenario – it will actually decline relative to 2000 levels throughout the developing world;
- by 2050, the decline in calorie availability will increase child malnutrition by 20 per cent relative to a world with no climate change. Climate change will eliminate much of the improvement in child malnourishment levels that would occur with no climate change.

Modelling studies have shown that many wild species, including crop wild relatives, will be unable to track climate change and migrate successfully. The expected degradation of ecosystems is also likely to increase the vulnerability of populations to the consequences of natural disasters and climate change impacts (Munang et al., 2011).

Food and nutrition insecurity and climate change, the two major global challenges facing humanity, are inextricably linked. For this reason, the Committee on World Food Security (CFS) has requested its High Level Panel of Experts on Food Security and Nutrition (HLPE) to conduct a study on climate change to 'review existing assessments and initiatives on the effects of climate change on food security and nutrition, with a focus on the most affected and vulnerable regions and populations and the interface between climate change and agricultural productivity, including the challenges and opportunities of adaptation and mitigation policies and actions for food security and nutrition'.

Given that an estimated 70 per cent of the world population (nearly 4.7 billion people) is fed with food produced locally, mostly by small-scale farming, fishing or herding (ETC Group, 2009), it is important to look at the impacts of climate change on traditional farming communities. As Clements et al. (2011) note, 'Strengthening the livelihoods of rural populations is intrinsically linked to poverty reduction efforts and is a key area to focus climate change adaptation strategies in the agriculture sector.'

The role of agricultural biodiversity and its interaction with human nutrition in facing up to the challenges of global change will be vital. Some of the key factors are:

- Increased diversification of crops and livestock will not only enhance nutritional possibilities but will allow farmers to have a greater number of options to face the uncertain weather conditions associated with the increased climate variability (Lotze-Campen, 2011).
- Underdeveloped species are another source of potentially valuable food resources that can be developed for use in a wider range of farming systems and as a source of biofuels.
- The major crops contain many thousands of cultivars with wide variation in their capacity to adapt to a range of climatic conditions.

- Breeders and agronomists will have to make considerable efforts to identify and develop cultivars that will help provide the productivity increases needed for food production.
- In addition, the changing climates will require a massive effort in breeding cultivars that show better adaptation to the new eco-climatic conditions (including drought) that are predicted and crop wild relatives will be an important source of the genetic variation needed (see discussion in Hunter and Heywood, 2011, chapter 14).
- Extension workers will have to assist farmers to evaluate these new cultivars and facilitate their supply and cultivation.
- Major efforts will be needed to assess the adaptive capacity of local crops and wild species that play a significant role in human nutrition to changing climates.
- The support of international and regional aid and development agencies and national governments will be needed to support the efforts of local communities in developing adaptation strategies that help them strengthen their capacity to improve their agronomic and land-management skills, and to diversify their livelihoods through maintaining diversified cropping systems and increasing the productivity of local crops.
- A considerable investment in both *ex situ* and *in situ* conservation of crop wild relatives will be needed.

Conclusions

This chapter has shown the manifold ways in which agricultural biodiversity contributes to food, nutrition and health. While recognizing the enormous human benefits that agricultural intensification has provided, it highlights how traditional food systems that are characterized by rich agricultural biodiversity play an important role in the nutrition of hundreds of millions of people across the world and continue to provide options and resilience for building sustainable livelihoods (Johns and Sthapit, 2004). Local communities seldom depend on local crops and wild biodiversity alone except in extreme famine conditions but depend on a mix of one or more staples, local crops and semi-domesticates and a range of wild species of plants, and animals that add variety to the diet as well as providing micronutrients. Local biodiversity should be recognized as a significant contribution to a sustainable agriculture–food–nutrition strategy alongside improvements in agricultural productivity and agronomic practice, nutritional enhancement of crops, industrial fortification, vitamin supplementation and other nutrition–agriculture interventions.

There is abundant evidence that edible plant and animal diversity contributes substantially to human diets in terms of energy intake and also helps alleviate problems of malnutrition in developing countries through the supply of vitamins and micronutrients. There is also ample evidence that increased production of fruit, vegetables, eggs, poultry and other animal foods in traditional agricultural systems and in particular home/homestead gardens not only raises access to energy, protein and fat but also greatly improves the quality and micronutrient content of diets.

However, there is still a lack of knowledge about the species that are involved. Much of the evidence on their nutritional or health benefits of particular species is partial or anecdotal and there is a need for more critical and well-designed scientific reviews and analyses. Much more attention needs to be given to investigating the composition and nutrient contributions of local foods and the plant and animal resources that have in the past provided many of the nutrients and micronutrients in traditional diets and that are now increasingly deficient in today's diets. Likewise much more work is needed to assess the nutritional diversity of crop cultivars.

Assessments are also urgently needed of the impacts and effectiveness of biofortification, industrial fortification and vitamin supplementation on the lives of the local communities to which they have been applied and also of the contribution that local foods such a leafy green vegetables make so as to help situate such approaches within the larger context of sustainable food-based approaches. An integrated approach, involving the biological, social and environmental dimensions, is needed to address the issues of micronutrition deficiency and the underlying causes, and the role of agricultural biodiversity and community participatory approaches that identify local food resources with nutritional, agronomic and economic advantages to small-scale farmers (Johns and Eyzaguirre, 2007).

Agricultural biodiversity will be an important resource in assuring the availability of adequate nutrition in response to the challenges of global change, such as massive population growth and adapting to changing climatic conditions (temperature, nubosity, rainfall). The genetic diversity present in wild species, especially crop wild relatives, and in the cultivars of both staple and local or underutilized crops will be invaluable in developing new adapted cultivars for the future. As Guarino and Lobell (2011) put it succinctly 'Feeding a growing population in a hotter world will require exploiting a far broader range of crop diversity than now – and that means valuing wild genes'.

Notes

1 Both the transition to agriculture and the domestication process were in fact highly complex (Gepts, 2004; Price and Bar-Yosef, 2011).
2 Lustig et al. (2012) point out that obesity is not the cause of the metabolic syndrome but rather a marker for metabolic dysfunction.
3 See also the website of Ecoagriculture Partners: http://www.ecoagriculture.org/, accessed August 2012.
4 The ETC Group (2009) estimate that at least 70% of the world's population is fed by local people: 12.5% from hunting/gathering; 7.5% share urban food produced by city-dwellers; 50% share world's cultivated food produced by local farmers.

References

Afolayan, A.J. and Jimoh, F.O. (2009) 'Nutritional quality of some wild leafy vegetables in South Africa', *International Journal of Food Sciences and Nutrition,* vol 60, pp.424–431, doi:10.1080/09637480701777928.

Ahmed, M. (2004) 'Outlook for Fish to 2020: A Win-Win-Win for Oceans, Fisheries and the Poor?' in R. Kearney (ed.) *Fish, Aquaculture and Food Security, Conference Proceedings 2004*, pp. 66–74, Crawford Fund, Kingston, ACT, Australia.

Altieri, M.A. (1999) 'The agroecological dimensions of biodiversity in traditional farming systems', in D.A. Posey (eds) *Cultural and Spiritual Values of Biodiversity,* pp.291–297. For UNEP, Intermediate Technology Publications, London.

Altieri, M.A. (2009) 'Agroecology, Small farms, and food sovereignty', *Monthly Review*, vol 61, no 3.

Altieri, M.A. and Koohafkan, P. (2008) *Enduring farms: Climate change, smallholders and traditional farming communities*, Third World Network, Penang.

Andersen, I. (2011) *IFPRI (International Food Policy Research Institute). 2011. Leveraging Agriculture for Improving Nutrition and Health: Highlights from an International Conference*, p2, Washington, DC.

Barrett, C.R., Travis, A.I. and Dasgupta, P. (2011) 'On biodiversity conservation and poverty traps', *Proceedings National Academy of Sciences,* vol 108, pp.13907–13912.

Batello, C., Marzot, M. and Touré, A. H. (2004) *The future is an ancient lake: traditional knowledge, biodiversity and genetic resources for food and agriculture in Lake Chad Basin ecosystems*, FAO Interdepartmental Working Group on biological diversity for food and agriculture, Rome, 2004.

Beddington, J., Asaduzzaman, M., Clark, M., Fernández, A., Guillou, M., Jahn, M., Erda, L., Mamo, T., Van Bo, N., Nobre, C.A., Scholes, R., Sharma, R. and Wakhungu, J. (2012) *Achieving food security in the face of climate change: Final report from the Commission on Sustainable Agriculture and Climate Change*, CGIAR Research Program on Climate Change, Agriculture and Food Security (CCAFS), Copenhagen.

Bellon, M.R., Adato, M., Becerril, J. and Midex, D. (2003) *The impact of improved maize germplasm on poverty alleviation: the case of Tuxpeño-derived in Mexico*, IFPRI Discussion Paper Briefs, Discussion Paper 162, International Food Policy Research Institute, Washington DC.

Bennett, E. (1964) 'Historical perspectives in genecology', *Scottish Plant Breeding Station Record* 1964, pp. 29–115.

Bennett, E. (1965) 'Plant introduction and genetic conservation: genecologica; aspects of an urgent world problem', *Scottish Plant Breeding Station Record* 1964, pp. 27–113.

Bharucha, Z. and Pretty, J. (2010) 'The roles and values of wild foods in agricultural systems', *Philosophical Transactions of the Royal Society B: Biological Sciences* September 27, 365, pp.2913–2926, doi:10.1098/rstb.2010.0123.

Blasbalg, T.L., Wispelwey, B. and Deckelbaum, R.J. (2011) 'Econutrition and utilization of food-based approaches for nutritional health', *Food and Nutrition Bulletin* 32, pp. S4–S13.

Brown, A.G. (eds) (2011) *Biodiversity and world food security, nourishing the planet and its people: the Crawford Fund sixteenth annual development conference,* Parliament House, Canberra, 30 August – 1 September, pp.44–51.

Brussaard, L., Caron P., Campbell, B., Lipper L., Mainka, S., Rabbinge, R., Babin, D., and Pulleman, M. (2010) 'Reconciling biodiversity conservation and food security: scientific challenges for a new agriculture', *Current Opinion in Environmental Sustainability,* vol 2, pp.34–42.

Buchanan, G., Herdt, R. and Tweeten, L. (2010) *Agricultural Productivity Strategies for the Future -- Addressing U.S. and Global Challenges.* Issue Paper No. 45. Council for Agricultural Science and Technology.

Buck, L.E., and Scherr, S.J. (2011) 'Moving ecoagriculture into the mainstream', Chapter 2 in *2011 State of the World. Innovations that Nourish the Planet*, The Worldwatch Institute, Earthscan, London.

Buck, L.E., Gavin, T.A., Lee, D.R. and Uphoff, N.T. (2004) *Ecoagriculture, A Review and Assessment of its Scientific Foundations*, Cornell University, Ithaca, New York.

Burlingame, B., Charrondière, R. and Mouille, B. (2009) 'Food composition is fundamental to the cross-cutting initiative on biodiversity for food and nutrition', *Journal of Food Composition and Analysis*, vol 22, pp.361–365.

CBD (2010) Conference of the Parties to the Convention on Biological Diversity, Tenth meeting, Nagoya, Japan, 18–29 October 2010. Agenda item 4.4, Decision adopted by the Conference of the Parties to the Convention on Biological Diversity at its tenth meeting, X/2, The Strategic Plan for Biodiversity 2011–2020 and the Aichi Biodiversity Targets, http://www.cbd.int/doc/decisions/cop-10/cop-10-dec-02-en.pdf, accessed August 2012.

Cheng, T.O. (2004) 'Obesity in Chinese children', *Health Place*, 10, pp.395-396.

Chivian, E. and Bernstein, A. (2008) *Sustaining Life, How Human Health Depends on Biodiversity*, Oxford University Press, Oxford and New York.

Chung, M., Balk, E.M., Ip, S. et al. (2010) 'Systematic review to support the development of nutrient reference intake values: challenges and solutions', *The American journal of Clinical Nutrition*, 92(2), pp. 273–276.

Chweya, J.A. and Eyzaguirre, P.B. (eds) (1999) *The biodiversity of traditional leafy vegetables*, IPGRI [Bioversity International], Rome.

CIFOR (2011) *New global study shows high reliance on forests among rural poor*, http://www.cifor.cgiar.org/fileadmin/fileupload/media-release/PEN-New-global-study-shows-high-reliance-on-forests-among-rural-poor.pdf, accessed August 2012.

Clay, J. (2011) 'Freeze the footprint of food', *Nature* 475, pp. 287–289. doi:10.1038/475287a.

Clements, R., Haggar, J., Quezada, A. and Torres, J. (2011) *Technologies for Climate Change Adaptation – Agriculture Sector*, X. Zhu (ed.), UNEP Risø, Centre, Roskilde.

Coates, J., Rogers, B.L., Webb, P., Maxwell, D., Houser, R. and McDonald, C. (2007) *Diet Diversity Study*, World Food Programme, Emergency Needs Assessment Service (ODAN), Rome.

Cohen, M.N. and Armelagos, G.J. (eds) (1984) *Paleopathology at the Origins of Agriculture*, Academic Press, Orlando, FL.

Collette, L., Hodgkin, T., Kassam, A. et al. (2011) *Save and grow. A policymaker's guide to the sustainable intensification of smallholder crop production*, FAO, Rome.

Cunningham, I.S. (1989) 'Erna Bennett: her career and convictions', *Diversity*, vol 5, no 2&3, pp.60–63.

Diamond, J. (1987) 'The worst mistake in the history of the human race', *Discover Magazine* May, pp.64–66.

DeClerck, F.A.J., Fanzo, J., Palm, C. and Remans, R. (2011). 'Ecological approaches to human nutrition', *Food and Nutrition Bulletin*, 32(Suppl.1), pp.41S–50S.

Dickson, D. and Lewis, S. (2010) 'More research needed into biodiversity–poverty links', *Science and Development Network* 21 May.

Diouf, J. (2011) Foreword in *Save and Grow. A policymaker's guide to the sustainable intensification of smallholder crop production* ppiii–iv, FAO, Rome.

ETC Group (2009) 'Who will feed us? Questions for the Food and Climate Crises', *Communiqué* Issue #102, November.

Etkin, N.L. (eds) (1994) *Eating on the Wild Side, The Pharmacologic, Ecologic and Social Implications of Using Noncultigens*, University of Arizona Press, Tucson.

Etkin, N.L. (2006) *Edible medicines: An Ethnopharmacology of Food*, University of Arizona Press, Tucson.

Eyzaguirre, P. and Watson, J. (2002) 'Home Gardens and Agrobiodiversity: an Overview Across Regions'. In Home Gardens and in situ Conservation of Plant Genetic Resources in Farming Systems, in *Proceedings of the Second International Home Gardens Workshop, 17-19 July, Witzenhausen, Federal Republic of Germany*. Eds. J.W. Watson and P.B. Eyzaguirre. Rome: International Plant Genetic Resources Institute, pp.10–13.

FAO (Food and Agriculture Organization of the United Nations) (1995, 1996) *Improving nutrition through home gardening – A training package for preparing field workers in Southeast Asia*, FAO, Rome.

FAO (Food and Agriculture Organization of the United Nations) (2007) *The State of the World's Animal Genetic Resources for Food and Agriculture*, Commission on Genetic Resources for Food and Agriculture, FAO, Rome.

FAO (Food and Agriculture Organization of the United Nations) (2010a) *The State of Food Insecurity in the World. Addressing food insecurity in protracted crises*, FAO, Rome.

FAO (Food and Agriculture Organization of the United Nations) (2010b) *Second Report on the State of the World's Plant Genetic Resources for Food and Agriculture*, FAO, Rome.

FAO (Food and Agriculture Organization of the United Nations) (2010c) *The state of food and agriculture 2009: livestock in the balance*, FAO, Rome.

FAO (Food and Agriculture Organization of the United Nations) (2010d) *The State of World Fisheries and Aquaculture 2010*, FAO, Rome.

FAO (Food and Agriculture Organization of the United Nations) (2011a) *Biodiversity for Food and Agriculture Contributing to food security and sustainability in a changing world, Outcomes of an Expert Workshop held by FAO and the Platform on Agricultural biodiversity Research from 14–16 April 2010 in Rome, Italy*, FAO, Rome.

FAO (Food and Agriculture Organization of the United Nations) (2011b) *Report International Scientific Symposium Biodiversity and Sustainable Diets United Against Hunger, Rome, 3–5 November 2010*, FAO, Rome.

FAO (Food and Agriculture Organization of the United Nations) (2011c) *Forests, potential solution in the fight against hunger*, FAO Media Centre, http://www.fao.org/news/story/en/item/93236/icode/, accessed August 2012.

FAO (Food and Agriculture Organization of the United Nations) (2011d) *World Livestock 2011 – Livestock in food security,* FAO: Rome.

Flyman, M.V. and Afolayan, A.J. (2006) 'The suitability of wild vegetables for alleviating human dietary deficiencies', *South African Journal of Botany,* vol 72, pp.492–497.

Foley, J.A., Defries, R., Asner, G.P., Barford, C., Bonan, G., Carpenter, S.R., Chapin, F.S., Coe, M.T., Daily, G.C., Gibbs, H.K., Helkowski, J.H., Holloway, T., Howard, E.A., Kucharik, C.J., Monfreda, C., Patz, J.A., Prentice, I.C., Ramankutty, N. and Snyder, P.K. (2005) 'Global Consequences of Land Use', *Science*, vol 309, pp.570–574.

Foley, J.A., Ramankutty, N., Brauman, K.A., Cassidy, E.S., Gerber, J.S., Johnston, M., Mueller, N.D., O'Connell, C., Ray, D.K., West, P.C., Balzer, C., Bennett, E.M., Carpenter, S.R., Hill, J., Monfreda, C., Polasky, S., Rockström, J., Sheehan, J., Siebert, S., Tilman, D. and Zaks, D.P.M. (2011) 'Solutions for a cultivated planet', *Nature,* vol 478, pp.337–342 (20 October), doi:10.1038/nature10452.

Ford-Lloyd, B., Brar, D., Khush, G., Jackson, M. and Virk, P. (2008) 'Genetic erosion over time of rice landrace agricultural biodiversity', *Plant Genetic Resources,* vol 7, pp.163–168.

Frankel, O. H. and Bennett, E. (1970) *Genetic Resources in Plants: Their Exploration and Conservation*, Blackwell, Oxford.

Frison, E.A., Cherfas, J. and Hodgkin, T. (2011) 'Agricultural biodiversity is essential for a sustainable improvement in food and nutrition security', *Sustainability 2011*, vol 3, pp.238–253, doi: 10.3390/su3010238.

Froment, A., de Garine, I., Binam Bikoi, Ch. and Loung, J.F. (eds) (1996) *Bien Manger et Bien Vivre: Anthropologie alimentaire et développement en Afrique intertropicale: du biologique au social*, L'Harmattan-ORSTOM, Paris.

Gallai, N., Salles, J.M., Settele, J. and Vaissière, B.E. (2009) 'Economic valuation of the vulnerability of world agriculture confronted with pollinator decline', *Ecological Economics,* vol 68, pp.810–821.

Galluzzi, G., van Duijvendijk, C., Collette, L., Azzu, N. and Hodgkin, T. (2011) 'Biodiversity for Food and Agriculture. Contributing to food security and sustainability in a changing world', PAR platform, FAO, Rome.

Gebauer, J. (2005) 'Plant species diversity of home gardens in El Obeid, Central Sudan', *Journal of Agriculture and Rural Development in the Tropics and Subtropics* 106, pp. 97–103.

Gepts, P. (2004) 'Crop domestication as a long-term selection experiment', *Plant Breeding Reviews*, vol 24, no 2, pp.1–44.

Godfray, H.C. J., Crute, I.R., Haddad, L., Lawrence, D., Muir, J.F., Nisbett, N., Pretty, J., Robinson, S., Toulmin, C. and Whiteley, R. (2010a) 'The future of the global food system', *Philosophical Transactions of the Royal Society B: Biological Sciences,* vol 365, pp.2769–2777, doi: 10.1098/rstb.2010.0180.

Godfray, H.C.J., Beddington, J.R., Crute, I.R., Haddad, L., Lawrence, D., Muir, J.F., Pretty, J., Robinson, S., Thomas, S.M. and Toulmin, C. (2010b) 'Food Security: The Challenge of Feeding 9 Billion People', *Science*, vol 327, pp.812–818.

Green, R.E., Cornell, S.J., Scharlemann, J.P.W. and Balmford, A. (2005) 'Farming and the fate of wild nature', *Science,* vol 307, pp.550–555.

Grivetti, L.E. and Ogle, B.M. (2000) 'Value of traditional foods in meeting macro- and micronutrient needs: the wild plant connection', *Nutrition Research Reviews,* vol 13, pp.31–46, doi:10.1079/095442200108728990.

Guarino, L. (ed.) (1997) *Traditional African Vegetables. Promoting the Conservation and Use of Underutilized and Neglected Crops, 16,* Proceedings of the IPGRI International Workshop on Genetic Resources of Traditional Vegetables in Africa: Conservation and Use, 29–31 August 1995, ICRAF-HQ, Nairobi, Kenya, Institute of Plant Genetics and Crop Plant Research, Gatersleben/International Plant Genetic Resources Institute, Rome, Italy.

Guarino, L. (2010) 'Adapting agriculture to climate change: The role of crop wild relatives', Summary Statement from a Bellagio Meeting 6–10 September 2010, http://iis-db.stanford.edu/pubs/23098/Bellagio_2_statement_draft_final_with_all_comments.pdf, accessed August 2012.

Guarino, L. and Lobell, D.B. (2011) 'A walk on the wild side', *Nature Climate Change,* vol 1, pp.374–375, doi:10.1038/nclimate1272.

Hadjichambis, A.C.H., Paraskeva-Hadjichambi, D., Della, A., Giusti, M., Pasquale, D.E., Lenzarini, C., Censorii, E., Gonzales-Tejero, M.R., Sanchez-Roja, C.P., Ramiro-Gutierrez, J., Skoula, M., Johnson, C.H., Sarpakia, A., Hmomouchi, M., Jorhi, S., El-Demerdash, M., El-Zayat, M. and Pioroni, A. (2008) 'Wild and semi-domesticated food plant consumption in seven circum-Mediterranean areas', *International Journal of Food Sciences and Nutrition,* vol 59, pp.383–414.

Harlan, J.R. (1975) 'Our vanishing genetic resources', *Science* 188, pp. 618–621.

van Heerwaarden, J., Hellin, J., Visser, R.F. and Van Eeuwijk, F.A. (2009) 'Estimating maize genetic erosion in modernized smallholder agriculture', *Theoretical and Applied Genetics* 119, pp.875–888.

Heinrich, M., Müller, W.E. and Galli, C. (eds) (2006a) *Local Mediterranean Food Plants and Nutraceuticals, Forum of Nutrition.* Vol. 59, Karger, Basel.

Heinrich, M., Nebel, S., Leonti, M., Rivera, D. and Obón, C. (2006b) 'Local foodnutraceuticals: bridging the gap between local knowledge and global needs', in M. Heinrich, W.E. Müller and C. Galli (eds) *Local Mediterranean Food Plants and Nutraceuticals. Forum Nutr.*, 59. pp1–17, Karger, Basel.

Hertel, T.W. (2011) 'The Global Supply and Demand for Agricultural Land in 2050: A Perfect Storm in the Making?', *American Journal of Agricultural Economics,* vol 93, no 2, pp.259–275.

Heywood , V.H. (1999a) 'Trends in agricultural biodiversity', in J. Janick (ed.) *Perspectives on New Crops and New Uses,* pp.2–14, ASHS Press, Alexandria, VA.

Heywood, V. H (1999b) *Use and Potential of Wild Plants in Farm Households*, FAO Farm System Management Series, No. 15, Food and Agriculture Organization of the United Nations, Rome, Italy.

Heywood, V.H. (2003) 'Conservation strategies, plant breeding, wild species and land races', in K. Ammann, Y. Jacot and R. Braun, (eds) *Methods for Risk Assessment of Transgenic Plants IV. Biodiversity and Biotechnology*, pp.143–159, Birkhäuser Verlag, Basel/Switzerland.

Heywood, V.H. (2006) 'Human use of plant resources – the knowledge base and conservation needs', in Z.F. Ertuğ (ed.) *Proceedings of the IVth International Congress of Ethnobotany (ICEB, 2005),* pp.365–372, Ege Yaynilari, Istanbul.

Heywood, V.H. (2008) 'The use and economic potential of wild species – an overview', in N. Maxted, B.V. Ford-Lloyd, S.P. Kell, J.M. Iriondo, M.E. Dulloo and J. Turok (eds) *Crop Wild Relative Conservation and Use,* pp.585–604, CABI, Wallingford.

Heywood, V. (2009) 'Introduction: perspectives for economically important wild species and neglected crops in the Mediterranean', *Bocconea,* vol 23, pp.107–114.

Heywood, V.H. (2011) 'Ethnopharmacology, food production, nutrition and biodiversity conservation: Towards a sustainable future for indigenous peoples', *Journal of Ethnopharmacology,* vol 137, pp.1–15, doi:10.1016/j.jep.2011.05.027.

Heywood, V.H. and Dulloo, M.E. (2005) *In Situ Conservation of Wild Plant Species – A Critical Global Review of Good Practices*, IPGRI Technical Bulletin, no 11, FAO and IPGRI, IPGRI, Rome, Italy.

Hladik, C.M., Bahuchet, S. and de Garine, I. (eds) (1989) *Se nourrir en forêt équatoriale,* UNESCO-CNRS, Paris.

Hladik, C.M., Hladik, A., Linares, O.F., Oagezy, H., Semple, A. and Hadley, M. (eds) (1993) *Tropical Forests, People and Food, Biocultural interactions and applications to development*, Man and the Biosphere Series 13, UNESCO, Paris and The Parthenon Publishing Group, Carnforth, UK.

Hladik, C.M., Hladik., A., Pagezy, H., Linares, O.F., Koppert, G.J.A. and Froment, A. (eds) (1996) *L'alimentation en forêt tropicale, interactions bioculturelles et perspectives de développement.* Volume I: *Les ressources alimentaires : production et consommation*; Volume II: *Bases culturelles des choix alimentaires et stratégies de développement*, UNESCO, Paris.

Hunter, D. and Heywood, V. (eds) (2011) *Crop Wild Relatives, A manual of* in situ *conservation*, Earthscan, London.

IAASTD (International Assessment of Agricultural Knowledge, Science and Technology for Development) (2009) *Agriculture at a Crossroads, International Assessment of Agricultural Knowledge, Science and Technology for Development: Global Report*, Island Press, Washington DC.

Iannotti, L., Cunningham, K. and Ruel, M. (2009), 'Diversifying into healthy diets. Homestead food production in Bangladesh', Chapter 21 in D.J. Spielman and Rajul

Pandya-Lorch (eds), *Millions fed: proven successes in agricultural development,* International Food Policy Research Institute, Washington DC.

IFFRI (International Food Policy Research Institute) (2011) 'Leveraging Agriculture for Improving Nutrition and Health', Highlights from an International Conference, IFFRI, Washington DC, http://content.yudu.com/Library/A1ry9d/Leveragingagricultur/resources/index.htm?referrerUrl=http%3A%2F%2Fwww.ifpri.org%2Fpublication%2Fleveraging-agriculture-improving-nutrition-and-health, accessed August 2012.

Ishii, T., Hiraoka, T., Kanzaki, T., Akimoto, M., Shishido. R. and Ishikawa, R. (2011) 'Evaluation of Genetic Variation Among Wild Populations and Local Varieties of Rice', *Rice,* vol 4, no 3–4, pp.170–177, doi: 10.1007/s12284-011-906.

IUCN (2012) 'Securing the web of life', 19 June 2012. News story, http://www.iucn.org/?uNewsID=10173 (accessed 19 October 2012).

Jarvis, D.I., Brown, A.H., Cuong, P.H., Collado-Panduro, L., Latournerie- Moreno, L., Gyawali, S., Tanto, T., Sawadogo, M., Mar, I., Sadiki, M., Hue, N.T., Arias-Reyes, L., Balma, D., Bajracharya, J., Castillo, F., Rijal, D., Belqadi, L., Rana, R., Saidi, S., Ouedraogo, J., Zangre, R., Rhrib, K., Chavez, J.L., Schoen, D., Sthapit, B., De Santis, P., Fadda, C. and Hodgkin, T. (2008) 'A global perspective of the richness and evenness of traditional crop-variety diversity maintained by farming communities', *Proc. Natl. Acad. Sci. U.S.A.,* vol 105, pp.2101–2103.

Johns, T. and Eyzaguirre, P.B. (2006) 'Linking biodiversity, diet and health in policy and practice', *Proceedings of the Nutrition Society,* vol 65, pp.82–189.

Johns, T. and Eyzaguirre, P.B. (2007) 'Biofortification, biodiversity and diet: a search for complementary applications against poverty and malnutrition', *Food Policy,* vol 32, pp.1–24.

Johns, T. and Sthapit, B.R. (2004) 'Biocultural diversity in the sustainability of developing-country food systems', *Food and Nutrition Bulletin,* vol 25, pp.143–155.

Kabir, M.E. and Webb, E.L. (2008) 'Can homegardens conserve biodiversity in Bangladesh?', *Biotropica* 40, pp. 95–103, doi:10.1111/j.1744-7429.2007.00346.x.

von Kaufmann, R. (2000) Preface, in E.F. Thomson, R. von Kaufmann, H. Li Pun, T. Treacher and H. van Houten (eds) *Global Agenda for Livestock Research. Proceedings of a Consultation on Setting Livestock Research Priorities in West Asia and North Africa (WANA) Region, ICARDA, Aleppo, Syria, 12–16 November 1997,* ILRI (International Livestock Research Institute), Nairobi, Kenya and ICARDA (International Center for Agricultural Research in the Dry Areas), Aleppo, Syria.

Kenmore, P. and Collette, L. (2011) 'Foreword. Biodiversity for food and agriculture. Contributing to food security and sustainability in a changing world', in *Outcomes of an Expert Workshop held by FAO and the Platform on Agricultural Biodiversity Research from 14–16 April 2010 in Rome, Italy,* FAO and the Platform for Agricultural Biodiversity Research, Rome.

Kennedy, G. and Burlingame, B. (2003) 'Analysis of food composition data on rice from a plant genetic resources perspective', *Food Chemistry,* vol 80, pp.589–596.

Keys, A. and Keys, M. (1959) *How to eat well and stay well: the Mediterranean way,* Doubleday, New York.

Khoshbakht, K. and Hammer, K. (2008) 'How many plant species are cultivated?' *Genetic Resources and Crop Evolution,* vol 55, pp.925–928.

Kiley-Worthington, M. (1981) 'Ecological agriculture: what it is and how it works', *Agriculture and Environment,* vol 6, pp.349–381.

Klein, A.M., Vaissière, B.E., Cane, J.H., Steffan-Dewenter, I., Cunningham, S.A., Kremen, C. and Tscharntke, T. (2007) 'Importance of pollinators in changing landscapes for world crops', *Proc. Roy. Soc. B.*, vol 274, pp. 303–313.

Ko, G.T., So, W.Y., Chow, C., Wong, P.T., Tong, S.D., Hui, S.S. et al. (2010) 'Risk associations of obesity with sugar-sweetened beverages and lifestyle factors in Chinese: the "Better Health for Better Hong Kong" health promotion campaign', *European Journal of Clinical Nutrition*, 64, pp1386–1392.

Koppert, G., Dounias, E., Froment, A. and Pasquet, P. (1996) 'Consommation alimentaire dans trois populations forestières de la région côtière du Cameroun: Yassa, Mvae et Bakola', in C.M. Hladik, A. Hladik, H. Pagezy, O. F. Linares, G.J.A. Koppert and A. Froment (eds) *L'alimentation en forêt tropicale, interactions bioculturelles et perspectives de développement* pp. 477–496. Volume I, Les ressources alimentaires: production et consommation, UNESCO: Paris.

Kuhnlein, H.V., Erasmus, B. and Spigelski, D. (2009) *Indigenous Peoples' Food Systems: the Many Dimensions of Culture, Diversity and Environment for Nutrition and Health*, United Nations Food and Agriculture Organization, Rome.

Lang, T. (2009) 'Reshaping the Food System for Ecological Public Health', *Journal of Hunger & Environmental Nutrition,* vol 4, no 3, pp.315–335.

LaSalle, T.J. (2008) *Regenerative Organic Farming: A Solution to Global Warming*, Rodale Institute, Kutztown, PA. http://www.rodaleinstitute.org/files/Rodale_Research_Paper-07_30_08.pdf.

Leakey, R.R.B. (1997) 'Domestication and Commercialization of Non-timber Forest Products', in *Agroforestry Systems: International Conference Proceedings (Non-wood Forest Products), FAO*, Rome.

Leakey, R. (2011) 'NWFPS: Cultivation – the key to better agriculture and improved livelihoods', *Non-Wood News,* vol 22, pp.3–4.

Leakey, R.R.B. and Tchoundjeu, Z. (2001) 'Diversification of tree crops: domestication of companion crops for poverty reduction and environmental services', *Experimental Agriculture,* vol 37, pp.279–296.

Lenné, J.M. and Wood, D. (2011) *Agricultural biodiversity Management for Food Security: A critical review*, CAB International, Wallingford.

Levenstein, H. (2003) *Paradox of Plenty: A Social History of Eating in Modern America*, University of California Press, Berkeley and Los Angeles.

Levin, C.E., Long, J., Simler, K.R. and Johnson-Welch, C. (2003) 'Cultivating Nutrition: A Survey of Viewpoints on Integrating Agriculture and Nutrition', Discussion Paper, Food Consumption and Nutrition Division, International Food Policy Research Institute: Washington DC.

Lotze-Campen, H. (2011) 'Climate Change, Population Growth, and Crop Production: An Overview', in D.S. Yadav, R.J. Redden, J.L. Hatfield, H. Lotze-Campen and A.E. Hall (eds) *Crop Adaptation to Climate Change,* pp.1–11, John Wiley and Sons, London.

Lustig, R.H., Schmidt, L.A. and Brindis, C.D. (2012) 'The toxic truth about sugar', *Nature,* vol 482, pp.27–29.

Lutaladio, N., Burlingame, B. and Crews, J. (2010) 'Horticulture, biodiversity and nutrition', *Journal of Food Composition and Analysis*, vol 23, no 6, pp.481–485.

Masset, E., Haddad, L., Cornelius, A. and Isaza-Castro, J. (2011*) A systematic review of agricultural interventions that aim to improve nutritional status of children*, EPPI-Centre, Social Science Research Unit, Institute of Education, London, University of London.

Maxted, N., Kell, S. and Magos Brehm, J. (2011) *Options to promote food security: on farm management and in situ conservation of plant genetic resources for food and agriculture.* Food and Agriculture Organization of the United Nations, Rome, Italy.

Maxted, N., Kell, S., Toledo, A., Dulloo, E., Heywood, V., Hodgkin, T., Hunter, D., Guarino, L., Jarvis, A. and Ford-Lloyd, B. (2010) 'A global approach to crop wild relative conservation: securing the gene pool for food and agriculture', *Kew Bulletin* 65, *Plant Conservation for the Next Decade: A Celebration of Kew's 250th Anniversary*, no 4, pp.561–576, doi: 10.1007/s12225-011-9253-4.

McNeely, J.A. and Scherr, S.J. (2003) *Ecoagriculture: Strategies to Feed the World and Save Wild Biodiversity*, Island Press, Washington DC.

Misra, S., Maikhuri, R.K., Kala, C.P., Rao, K.S. and Saxena, K.G. (2008) 'Wild leafy vegetables: a study of their subsistence dietetic support to the inhabitants of Nanda Devi Biosphere Reserve', *Indian Journal of Ethnobiology and Ethnomedicine* 4, 15, p.9.

Mouillé, B., Charrondière, U.R. and Burlingame, B. (2010) *The Contribution of Plant Genetic Resources to Health and Dietary Diversity. Thematic Background Study*, FAO, Rome, available at: http://typo3.fao.org/fileadmin/templates/agphome/documents/PGR/SoW2/Dietary_Diversity_Thematic_Study.pdf, accessed August 2012.

Mummert, A., Esche, E., Robinson, J. and Armelagos, G.J. (2011) 'Stature and robusticity during the agricultural transition: Evidence from the bioarchaeological record', *Economics and Human Biology,* vol 9, pp.284–301.

Munang, R.T., Thiaw, I. and Rivington, M. (2011) 'Ecosystem Management: Tomorrow's Approach to Enhancing Food Security under a Changing Climate', *Sustainability,* vol 3, pp.937–954, doi: 10.3390/su3070937.

Muñoz, E. (2009) *New Hope for Malnourished Mothers and Children*, Briefing paper no. 7 October, Bread for the World Institute, Washington DC.

Nakhauka, E.B. (2009) 'Agricultural biodiversity for food and nutrient security: The Kenyan perspective', *International Journal of Biodiversity and Conservation,* vol 1, pp.208–214.

Nasi, R., Brown, D., Wilkie, D., Bennett, E., Tutin, C., van Tol, G. and Christophersen, T. (2008) *Conservation and use of wildlife-based resources: the bushmeat crisis*, Secretariat of the Convention on Biological Diversity, Montreal and Center for International Forestry Research (CIFOR), Bogor, Technical Series no 33.

Neiland, A.E. (2006) *Contribution of Fish Trade to Development, Livelihoods and Food Security in West and Central Africa: Making Trade Work for Poverty Reduction and Responsible Fisheries*, Report to the DFID/FAO Sustainable Fisheries Livelihoods Programme, FAO, Rome.

Nellemann, C., MacDevette, M., Manders, T., Eickhout, B., Svihus, B., Prins, A. G. and Kaltenborn, B. P. (eds) (2009) *The environmental food crisis – The environment's role in averting future food crises.* A UNEP rapid response assessment. United Nations Environment Programme, GRID-Arendal, www.grida.no.

Nelson, G.C., Rosegrant, M.W., Koo, J., Robertson, R., Sulser, T., Zhu, T., Ringler, C., Msangi, S., Palazzo, A., Batka, M., Magalhaes, M., Valmonte-Santos, R., Ewing, M. and Lee, D. (2009) *Climate Change, Impact on Agriculture and Costs of Adaptation*, International Food Policy Research Institute, Washington DC, updated October 2009.

Ntiamoa-Baidu, Y. (1997) *Wildlife and Food Security in Africa.* FAO Conservation Guide, No. 33, FAO, Rome.

Ogle, B.M. and Grivetti, M.E. (1985) 'Legacy of the chameleon. Edible wild plants in the kingdom of Swaziland, Southern Africa, A cultural, ecological, nutritional study. Part 2, Demographics, species availability and dietary use, analysis by ecological zone', *Ecology of Food and Nutrition,* vol 17, pp.1–30.

Padulosi, S., Hodgkin, T., Williams, J.T. and Haq, N. (2002) 'Underutilized crops: trends, challenges and opportunities in the 21st century', in J.M.M. Engels et al. (eds) *Managing Plant Genetic Resources*, pp.323–338, CAB International, Wallingford, UK and IPGRI, Rome, Italy.

Padulosi, S., Hoeschle-Zeledon, I. and Bordoni, P. (2008) 'Minor crops and underutilized species: lessons and prospects', in N. Maxted, B.V. Ford-Lloyd, S.P. Kell, J.M. Iriondo, M.E. Dulloo and J. Turok (eds) *Crop Wild Relatives Conservation and Use*, pp.605–624, CAB International, Wallingford, UK.

Padulosi, S., Heywood, V., Hunter, D. and Jarvis, A. (2011) 'Underutilized Species and Climate Change: Current Status and Outlook', Chapter 26 in S.S. Yadav, B. Redden, J.S. Hatfield, H. Lotze-Campen and A. Hall (eds) *Crop Adaptation to Climate Change*, John Wiley and Sons.

Pagezy, H. (1996) 'Importance des ressources naturelles dans l'alimentation du jeune enfant en forêt tropicale inondée', in C.M. Hladik, A. Hladik, H. Pagezy, O. F. Linares, G.J.A. Koppert and A. Froment (eds) *L'alimentation en forêt tropicale, interactions bio culturelles et perspectives de développement*. Volume I, Les ressources alimentaires: production et consummation, pp. 569-588 UNESCO, Paris.

Penafiel, D., Lachat, C., Espinel, R., Van Damme, P. and Kolsteren, P. (2011) 'A systematic review on the contributions of edible plant and animal biodiversity to human diets', *EcoHealth,* vol 8, no 3, pp.381–399.

Perfecto, I., Vandermeer, J. and Wight, A. (2009) *Nature's Matrix, Linking agriculture, conservation and food sovereignty*, Earthscan, London.

Phalan, B., Balmford, A., Green, R.E. and Scharlemann, J.P.W. (2011a) 'Minimisimg the harm to biodiversity of producing more food globally', *Food Policy,* vol 36, pp.562–571.

Phalan, B., Onial, M., Balmford, A. and Green, R.E. (2011b) 'Reconciling food production and bodiversity conservation: land sharing and land sparing compared', *Science,* vol 333, pp.1289–1291, doi: 10.1126/science.1208742.

Phillips, A. and Stolton, S. (2008) 'Protected landscapes and biodiversity values: an overview', in Amend T., Brown J., Kothari A., Phillips A. and Stolton S. (eds) *Protected Landscapes and Agrobiodiversity Values* pp. 8–22, Volume 1 in the series, *Protected Landscapes and Seascapes*, IUCN & GTZ, Kasparek Verlag, Heidelberg.

Pieroni, A., Nebel, S., Santoro, R.F. and Heinrich, M. (2005) 'Food for two seasons: culinary uses of non-cultivated local vegetables and mushrooms in a south Italian village', *International Journal of Food Science and Nutrition*, vol 56, pp.245–272.

Pistorius, R. (1997) *Scientists, Plants and Politics, A history of the plant genetic resources movement*, IPGRI, Rome.

Prescott-Allen, R. and Prescott-Allen, C. (1990) 'How many plants feed the world?' *Conservation Biology,* vol 4, pp.365–374.

Pretty, J. (2002) *Agri-Culture: Reconnecting People, Land and Nature*, Earthscan, London.

Pretty, J. (ed.) (2007a) *Sustainable Agriculture and Food. Volume I: History of Agriculture and Food; Volume II: Agriculture and the Environment; Volume III: Agriculture and Food Systems; Volume IV: Polices, Processes and Institutions*, Earthscan, London.

Pretty, J. (2007b) *The Earth Only Endures*, Earthscan, London.

Pretty, J. (2011) 'Editorial: Sustainable intensification in Africa', *International Journal of Agricultural Sustainability,* vol 9, no 1, pp.3–4.

Pretty, J., Sutherland, W.J., Ashby, J., Auburn, J., Baulcombe, D., Bell, M., et al. (2010) 'The top 100 questions of importance to global agriculture', *International Journal of Agricultural Sustainability,* vol 8, pp.219–236, doi:10.3763/ijas.2010.0534.

Pretty, J., Toulmin, C. and Williams, S. (eds) (2011) 'Sustainable Intensification, Increasing Productivity in African Food and Agricultural Systems', *International Journal of Agricultural Sustainability,* vol 9, no 1.

Price, T.D. and Bar-Yosef, O. (2011) 'The Origins of Agriculture: New Data, New Ideas. An Introduction to Supplement 4', *Current Archaeology,* vol 52, no S4, pp.163–174.

Price, L.P. and Ogle, B. (2008) 'Chapter 11. Gathered Indigenous Vegetables in Mainland Southeast Asia: A Gender Asset', in B.P. Resurreccion and R. Elmhirst (eds) *Gender and Natural Resource Management. Livelihoods, Mobility and Interventions*, Earthscan/IDRC, London.

Rivera, D., Obón, C., Heinrich, M., Inocencio, C., Verde, A. and Fajardo, J. (2006) 'Gathered Mediterranean Food Plants – Ethnobotanical Investigations and Historical Development', in M. Heinrich, W.E. Müller and C. Galli (eds) *Local Mediterranean Food Plants and Nutraceuticals. Forum of Nutrition Basel, Karger*, vol 59, pp.18–74.

Roe, D., Walpole, M. and Elliot, J. (2010) 'Symposium. Linking biodiversity conservation and poverty reduction: What, Where and How?', *Biodiversity*, vol 11, pp.107–124.

Roos, N., Wahab Md, A., Hossain, M.A.R. and Thilsted, S.H.(2007) 'Linking human nutrition and fisheries: Incorporating micronutrient-dense, small indigenous fish species in carp polyculture production in Bangladesh', *Food and Nutrition Bulletin*, vol 28, no 2 (supplement), pp.S280–S293.

Roth, H.H. and Merz, G. (1996) *Wildlife Resources: a global account of economic use*, Springer Verlag, Berlin.

Royal Society (2009) *Reaping the benefits: science and the sustainable intensification of global agriculture, RS Policy document 11/09* Issued: October 2009 RS1608, The Royal Society, London.

Ruel, M.T. (2003) 'Animal source foods to improve micronutrient nutrition and human function in developing countries. Operationalizing Dietary Diversity: A Review of Measurement Issues and Research Priorities', *Journal of Nutrition*, vol 133, pp.3911S–3926S.

Scherr, S.J. and McNeely, J.A. (2007) *Farming with Nature: The Science and Practice of Ecoagriculture*, Island Press, Washington, DC.

Scoones, I., Melnyk, M. and Pretty, J.N. (1992) *The Hidden Harvest. Wild foods and agricultural systems: A literature review and annotated bibliography*, IIED, SIDA and WWF International, London.

Slikkerveer, L. (1994) 'Indigenous agricultural knowledge systems in developing countries: a bibliography', *Indigenous Knowledge Systems Research and Development Studies*, no. 1. Special Issue: INDAKS Project Report 1 in collaboration with the European Commission DG XII. Leiden Ethnosystems and Development Programme (LEAD), Leiden.

Stavridakis, K.G. (2006) *Wild Edible Plants of Crete*, Rethymno.

Storkey, J., Meyer, S., Still, K.S. and Leuschner, C. (2012) 'The impact of agricultural intensification and land-use change on the European arable flora', *Proc R Soc Biol Sci.* 279, pp. 1421–1429.

Swaminathan, M.S. (2011) 'In Search of Biohappiness: Biodiversity and Food, Health and Livelihood Security', World Scientific Publishing and Cambridge University Press, India.

Thomas, D. (2011) *Poverty, Biodiversity and Local Organisations: Lessons from BirdLife International*, Gatekeeper Series no 152, International Institute for Environment and Development, London.

Thompson, J. and Scoones, I. (2009) 'Addressing the Dynamics of Agri-Food Systems: An Emerging Agenda for Social Science Research', *Environmental Science and Policy* 12, pp. 386–397.

Thomson, E.F., von Kaufmann, R., Li Pun, H., Treacher, T. and van Houten, H. (eds) (2000) *Global Agenda for Livestock Research*. Proceedings of a Consultation on Setting Livestock Research Priorities in West Asia and North Africa (WANA) Region, ICARDA, Aleppo, Syria, 12–16 November 1997, ILRI (International Livestock

Research Institute), Nairobi, Kenya, and ICARDA (International Center for Agricultural Research in the Dry Areas), Aleppo, Syria.

Tripp, R. and van der Heide, W. (1996) 'The erosion of crop genetic diversity: challenges, strategies and uncertainties', *Natural Resource Perspectives*, no 7, March, Overseas Development Institute, London.

Turner, N.J., Łuczaj, Ł.J., Migliorini, P., Pieroni, A., Dreon, A.L., Sacchetti, L.E. and Paoletti, M.G. (2011) 'Edible and Tended Wild Plants, Traditional Ecological Knowledge and Agroecology', *Critical Reviews in Plant Sciences*, vol 30, pp.198–225.

UNCTAD (2010) 'Agriculture at the crossroads: guaranteeing food security in a changing global climate', *UNCTAD Policy Briefs*, no 18, December.

UNISDR (2011) *Global Assessment Report on Disaster Risk Reduction*, United Nations International Strategy for Disaster Reduction, Geneva, Switzerland.

United Nations General Assembly (2010) *Report submitted by the Special Rapporteur on the right to food, Olivier De Schutter*, A/HRC/16/49, United Nations, New York.

UNSCN (2010) *Progress in Nutrition*, 6th Report on the World Nutrition Situation, UNSCN, Geneva.

Uusiku, N.O., Oelofs, A., Duodu, K.G., Bester, M.J. and Faber, M. (2010) 'Nutritional value of leafy vegetables of sub-Saharan Africa and their potential contribution to human health: A review', *Journal of Food Composition and Analysis*, vol 23, pp.499–509.

Veenemans, J., Milligan, P., Prentice, A.M., Schouten, L.R.A., Inja, N., van der Heijden, A.C., de Boer, L.C.C., Jansen, E.J.S., Koopmans, A.E., Enthoven, W.T.M., Kraaijenhagen, R.J., Demir, A.Y., Uges, D.R.A., Mbugi, E.V., Savelkoul, H.F.J. and Verhoef, H. (2011) 'Effect of Supplementation with zinc and other micronutrients on malaria in Tanzanian Children: A Randomised Trial', *PLoS Med*, vol 8, no 11: e1001125, doi:10.1371/journalpmed.1001125.

Vigouroux, Y., Barnauda, A., Scarcellia, N. and Thuilleta, A.-C. (2011) 'Biodiversity, evolution and adaptation of cultivated crops', *Comptes Rendus Biologies*, vol 334, pp.450–457.

Westerkamp, C. and Gottsberger, G. (2001) 'Pollinator diversity is mandatory for crop diversity', in P. Benedek and K.W. Richards (eds) *Proceedings 8th Pollination Symposium*, *Acta Horticulturae*, vol 561, pp.309–316.

Wezel, A. and Bender, S. (2003) 'Plant species diversity of homegardens of Cuba and its significance for household food supply', *Agroforestry Systems* 57, pp. 39–49.

WHO/FAO (World Health Organization/ Food and Agriculture Organization) (2003) *Diet, nutrition and the prevention of chronic diseases*, Report of a joint WHO/FAO expert consultation, Geneva, 28 January–1 February 2002, WHO Technical Report Series No. 916, Geneva, Switzerland.

Williams, M.J. (2011) 'Food from the Water: How the Fish Production Revolution Affects Aquatic Biodiversity and Food Security', in A.G. Brown (ed.) *Biodiversity and world food security, nourishing the planet and its people: the Crawford Fund sixteenth annual development conference*, Parliament House, Canberra, 30 August – 1 September, 2010, pp.44–51.

Wolfe, M.S. (2000) 'Crop strength through diversity,' *Nature*, vol 406, pp.681–682.

World Bank (2007) *From Agriculture to Nutrition: Pathways, Synergies and Outcomes*, The World Bank Agriculture and Rural Development, Department Report, no 40196-Glb, Washington DC.

Youyong Zhu, Y., Chen, H., Fan, J., Wang, Y., Li, Y., Jianbing, Chen, Fan, J., Yang, S., Hu, L., Leung, H., Mew, T.W., Teng, P.S., Wang, Z. and Mundt, C.C. (2000) 'Genetic diversity and disease control in rice', *Nature*, vol 406, pp.718–722 (17 August), doi:10.1038/350210468.

3 The role of livestock and livestock diversity in sustainable diets

Irene Hoffmann and Roswitha Baumung

Introduction

Sustainability is a complex and sometimes contested concept. While the overall concept is widely accepted and used, a clear definition is still problematic as different stakeholders – and stakeholders at different levels – have different interpretations. The Johannesburg Declaration on Sustainable Development states that there are three fundamental 'pillars' to sustainable development: environmental protection, economic growth and social equity, both in an inter- and intra-generational equity perspective. However, the 'three-pillars' model is imperfect because it is based on the assumption that trade-offs can be made between the environmental, social and economic dimensions of sustainability.

Growing demands for ecosystem services, particularly for food, water, timber, fibre and fuel, were the direct or indirect drivers of ecosystem changes. The Millennium Ecosystem Assessment (MEA, 2005a,b) estimated that human activities have resulted in approximately 60 per cent of the ecosystem services examined being degraded or used unsustainably. UNEP (2010) states that 'Agriculture and food consumption are identified as one of the most important drivers of environmental pressures, especially habitat change, climate change, water use and toxic emissions'. They further confirm FAO's (2006a) assessment of the livestock sector's environmental impact, due to the high trophic level of livestock in the food web and the related high land use.

Although the increased utilization of the provisioning services contributed substantially to net gains in human well-being and economic development, the global community seems now to have reached a point where the loss of some of the supporting, regulating and cultural ecosystem services appears to exceed 'planetary boundaries' and increase the vulnerability of resource supply systems (Rockström et al., 2009; McKinsey Global Institute, 2011). Food systems, from production over-processing to consumption, are an obvious area of vulnerability.

Several recent studies identified food production and consumption patterns as key factor for achieving sustainability (UNEP, 2010; Foresight, 2011; Grethe et al., 2011; McKinsey Global Institute, 2011; UNEP, 2011; Westhoek et al., 2011). Heller and Keoleian (2003) stated that 'A sustainable food system must be founded on a sustainable diet'. In 2010, FAO experts agreed on a general concept for sustainable diets being 'those diets with low environmental impacts which contribute to food and nutrition security and to healthy life for present and future generations. Sustainable diets are protective and respectful of biodiversity and ecosystems, culturally acceptable, accessible, economically fair and affordable; nutritionally adequate, safe and healthy; while optimizing natural and human resources.' With this definition, biodiversity is linked with human diets and with the diversity of livestock and livestock systems. However, trade-offs between the different pillars of sustainability, and temporal and spatial dimensions, are not addressed (Hoffmann, 2011b).

FAO (2011a) has started to develop a method for sustainability assessments of food and agriculture systems. Main criteria are environmental integrity (energy, climate, air, water, soil, material cycles, waste and biodiversity), economic resilience (strategic management, operating profit, vulnerability, local economy and decent livelihood), social well-being (human rights, equity, occupational health and safety, capacity building, food and nutrition security, product quality) and good governance (participation, accountability, rule of law, fairness and evaluation). This chapter addresses mainly environmental aspects of sustainable diets but touches also briefly on social and economic aspects. It describes the links between human diets, expected changes in lifestyle, livestock sector trends and their combined impact on animal genetic resources. Specifically, the focus is on the genetic resources of domesticated avian and mammalian species that contribute to food production and agriculture.

Products and services provided by livestock

Livestock are used by humans to provide a wide range of products and services. Foods derived from animals are an important source of nutrients (Givens, 2010) that provide a critical supplement and diversity to staple plant-based diets (Murphey and Allen, 2003; Randolph et al., 2007). However, there are other reasons for keeping livestock, which include providing manure, fibre for clothes and resources for temporary and permanent shelter, producing power, and serving as financial instruments and enhancing social status. This range of products and services supporting livelihoods – especially of the poor – is a key feature of livestock. Until recently, a large proportion of livestock in developing countries was not kept solely for food. Due to an ongoing trend away from backyard and smallholder livestock production to more intensive and larger-scale systems (FAO, 2010b), many purposes for which livestock are kept, are vanishing and being replaced by an almost exclusive focus on generating food.

Animal source foods (ASF), mainly meat, milk and eggs, provide concentrated, high quality sources of essential nutrients for optimal protein, energy and micronutrient nutrition (esp. iron, zinc and vitamin B12). Access to ASF is believed to have contributed to the evolution of the human species' unusually large and complex brain and its social behaviour (Milton, 2003; Larsen, 2003). Today, ASF contribute a significant proportion to the food intake of Western

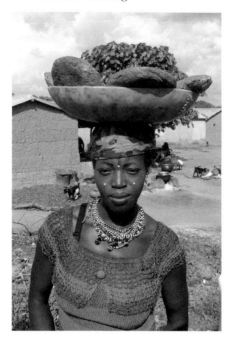

Figure 3.1 Fulani woman with traditional cheese in Northern Benin. By Frédéric Lhoste

societies (MacRae et al., 2005), but also play an increasingly role in developing countries.

Since the early 1960s, ASF consumption has increased in all regions except sub-Saharan Africa. The greatest increases occurred in East and Southeast Asia, and in Latin America and the Caribbean (FAO, 2010b). Structural changes in food consumption patterns occurred in South Asia, with consumer preference shifts towards milk and in East and Southeast Asia towards meat, while no significant changes could be detected in the other developing regions (Pica-Ciamarra and Otte, 2009). The growing demand for livestock products, a development termed the 'livestock revolution' (Delgado et al., 1999; Pica-Ciamarra and Otte, 2009), has been driven mostly by population growth in developing countries, while economic growth, rising per-capita incomes and urbanization were major determinants for increasing demand in a limited number of highly populated and rapidly growing economies. This has translated into considerable growth in global per capita kcal intake derived from livestock products, but with significant regional differences.

World population is projected to surpass 9 billion people by 2050. Most of the additional people will be based in developing countries while the population of developed regions is expected to remain stable (UNDP, 2009). About 3 billion new middle class consumers may emerge in the next 20 years (McKinsey, 2011). The concomitant 'nutrition transition' results in diet changes from staples to higher value foods such as fruit, vegetables and livestock products. Longer and more complex food chains have increased food diversity available for consumers, but also resulted in more common diets (Nugent, 2011).

FAO projects that by 2050, global average per-capita food consumption could rise to 3130 kcal per day. Agricultural production in the next 30 years will therefore present unprecedented challenges; it would need to increase by 60 per cent by 2050, with increases in crop and livestock production. Compared with 2005/07, this requires an additional production of 1 billion tonnes of cereals and 200 million tonnes of meat annually. Approximately half of the total increase in grain demand is predicted to be for animal feed. Globally, meat consumption per capita per year will increase from 41 kg in 2005 to 52 kg in 2050, reaching an average of 44 kg in developing countries and 95 kg in developed countries (OECD-FAO, 2009; Bruinsma, 2011; FAO, 2010b). Despite the absolute increase, growth rates in overall agricultural production are expected to decelerate as a consequence of the slowdown in population growth and because a growing share of population will reach medium to high levels of food consumption (Bruinsma, 2011).

Although global average production has increased, under- and malnutrition remains a large problem for those without access to animal source food and with food insecurity (Neumann et al., 2010), especially for poor children and their mothers. High rates of undernutrition and micronutrient deficiency among the rural poor suggest that, although often keeping livestock, they consume very little ASF. As iron, zinc and other important nutrients are more readily available in ASF than in plant-based foods, increased access to affordable ASF could significantly improve nutritional status, growth, cognitive development and physical activity and health for many poor people (Neumann et al., 2003). On the other hand, excessive consumption of livestock products is associated with increased risk of obesity, heart disease and other non-communicable diseases (WHO/FAO, 2003; Popkin and Du, 2003; Nugent, 2011). However, the nutritional aspects of animal products as part of human diets are not the main focus of this chapter.

Livestock production and the environment

The livestock sector has seen impressive production increases. Between 1980 and 2007, global beef output per animal grew at 0.4 per cent/year, milk at 0.3 per cent, pork at 0.8 per cent and poultry at 1.1 per cent (FAO Statistical Database [http://faostat.fao.org/default.aspx], accessed July 2012). These general trends mask high variation in productivity between species and livestock production systems, both within and between regions. The differences are larger in ruminants than in monogastrics for which industrial systems prevail in both developed and developing regions (FAO, 2010b). The most revolutionary change in the meat sector is in poultry; its share in world meat production increased from 13 per cent in the mid-1960s to 31 per cent in 2007 (FAO, 2010b).

The most important supply drivers over recent decades were cheap grain and cheap energy, technological change, especially in biotechnology, feeding and transport, together with a policy environment, including incentives, favourable to intensive production (FAO, 2010b). The growing demand for animal food products is being met increasingly through industrial systems, where meat production is no longer tied to a local land base for feed inputs or to supply animal power or manure for crop production (Naylor et al., 2005). There was a general shift from pasture-based ruminant species to feed-dependent monogastric species (Pingali and McCullough, 2010). In parallel, the non-food uses of livestock are in decline and are being replaced by modern substitutes (FAO, 2010b). Not only is animal draft power replaced by machinery and organic farm manure by synthetic fertilizers, but also insurance companies and banks replace more and more the risk management and asset functions of livestock.

The sector is also changing in regard to its contribution to poverty alleviation and income growth. While traditional livestock systems contribute to the livelihoods of 70 per cent of the world's rural poor, the dichotomy between large numbers of small-scale livestock keepers and pastoralists, and intensive large-scale commercial livestock production is growing. Generally, this goes hand-in-hand with shifts from multifunctional to commodity-specific production, local to globally integrated markets and from dispersed to clustered production. While livestock provide multiple roles and functions for the livelihoods of the poor, the same poor are especially vulnerable to environmental hazards and zoonotic diseases (FAO, 2010b).

Satisfying the growing demand for animal products while at the same time sustaining productive assets of natural resources is one of the major challenges for agriculture (Pingali and McCullough, 2010). Resource competition is likely to increase, for example through the decreasing availability of and competition for land and water (including from other land uses such as production of biofuels, urbanization and industrial development). Poor soil fertility and reduced access to fertilizer, overgrazing and deforestation, and loss of wild and agricultural biodiversity are further challenges. Thornton (2010) gives a comprehensive overview on possible modifiers of future livestock production and consumption trends, listing competition for resources, climate change, socio-cultural modifiers, ethical concerns and technological development. Many countries, especially in Africa, and small countries in Asia and Latin America are already struggling to adapt to current environmental degradation and climate variability. Climate change will exacerbate the existing challenges faced by the livestock sector. Hoffmann (2010a,b) gives a comprehensive overview on the consequences of climate change for animal genetic diversity, discussing the differences between developing and developed countries. Thornton (2010) and Hoffmann (2010b) illustrate the complex interaction of livestock and environment. At the same time as the livestock sector is a major contributor to greenhouse gas emissions, climate change itself may have substantial impact on livestock production systems.

The environmental footprint of agriculture, and particularly livestock production, has raised concerns in global assessments (e.g. MEA, 2005a,b; FAO, 2006a, 2010b; UNEP, 2007, 2010, 2011; Rockström et al., 2009; Foresight, 2011;

Grethe et al., 2011; McKinsey Global Institute, 2011; Westhoek et al., 2011) and in many studies (e.g. Gerbens-Leenes and Nonhebel, 2002; Pelletier and Tyedmers, 2010; Wirsenius et al., 2010). Livestock are the biggest land-user; they currently use about 30 per cent of the earth's entire land surface. This is mostly permanent pasture; but 33 per cent of global arable land is used to produce livestock feed. The sector also accounts for about 8 per cent of global water use, mainly for irrigation of feed crops. However, in arid areas, water consumed directly by animals or for product processing can represent a considerable share of total water use. Furthermore, the sector is a large producer of greenhouse gases (GHG), accounting for 18 per cent of GHG emissions, as measured in CO_2 equivalent – via enteric fermentation, land use and land-use change (directly for grazing or indirectly through production of feed crops) and manure management (FAO, 2010a).

The environmental impacts of livestock production occur at local, regional and global levels (FAO, 2006a). The rapid growth of the sector implies that much of the projected additional cereal and soybean production will be used for feeding enlarging livestock populations, resulting in increasing competition for land, water and other productive resources. This in turn puts upward pressure on prices for staple grains, potentially reducing food security (FAO, 2010b). A further concern in relation to products of animal origin is livestock's contribution to climate change and pollution. The projected need for additional cropland and grassland areas implies further risks of deforestation and other land-use changes, e.g. conversions of semi-natural grasslands. This will most likely not only lead to loss of biodiversity, but also to greenhouse gas and nitrogen emissions (FAO, 2010b; Westhoek et al., 2011). More research is needed related to livestock–water interactions. Such concerns are highly relevant when talking about sustainable diets.

Trends in breed diversity

The diversity of breeds is closely related to the diversity of production systems and cultures. Local breeds are usually based in grassland-based pastoral and small-scale mixed crop–livestock systems with low to medium use of external inputs. Over the past decades, agriculture has achieved substantial increases in food production, but accompanied by loss of biodiversity, including in animal genetic resources, and degradation of ecosystems, particularly with respect to their regulating and supporting services (MEA, 2005b). *The State of the World's Animal Genetic Resources for Food and Agriculture* (FAO, 2007) describes the link between livestock biodiversity and food security. Genetically diverse livestock populations provide society with a greater range of options to meet future challenges. Therefore animal genetic resources are the capital for future developments and for adaptation to changing environments. If they are lost, the options for future generations will be severely curtailed.

Diversity in livestock populations is measured in different forms: livestock breeds belong to different avian and mammalian species; thus species diversity can simply be measured as the number of species. Only about 40 of the about 50,000 known avian and mammalian species have been domesticated. On a global scale, just five species show a widespread distribution and particularly large numbers. Those species are cattle, sheep, chickens, goats and pigs, the 'big five' (FAO, 2007). Therefore, the majority of products of animal origin are based on quite narrow species variability.

The diversity presently observed within farm animal species is the result of a long history of human practice. At the sub-species level, diversity within and between breeds and the interrelationships between populations of a breed can be distinguished. Over millennia, a variety of breeds have been developed in a wide range of production environments. For livestock keepers, animal genetic diversity is a resource to be drawn upon to select stocks and develop (new) breeds. The term 'breed' does not have a universally accepted biological or legal definition. It originated in Europe and was linked to the existence of breeders' organizations. The term is now applied widely in developing countries, but it tends to refer to a socio-cultural concept rather than a distinct physical entity. FAO uses a broad definition of breeds which accounts for social, cultural and economic differences between animal populations and which can therefore be applied globally in the measurement of livestock diversity. According to FAO (2007) breeds can be categorized as local (reported by only one country) or transboundary (reported by several countries). The latest assessment identifies 7,001 local breeds and 1,051 transboundary breeds (FAO, 2010a).

Simply measuring breed diversity on the basis of number of breeds leads to biases due to the socio-cultural nature of the breed concept. However, between-breed diversity is classically considered as a major criterion to be taken into account when setting priorities for conservation. It has also been argued that additional criteria are needed for establishing those priorities, including within-breed variation (Barker, 2001; Caballero and Toro, 2002). The within-breed diversity may be lost due to random genetic drift and inbreeding in small populations, usually local breeds. However, within-breed diversity is also threatened within international transboundary breeds as a side effect of efficient breeding programmes, usually focusing on rather narrow breeding goals.

Various drivers influence the between- and within-breed diversity. Those drivers overlap with drivers of change in global agriculture and livestock systems including population and income growth, urbanization, rising female employment, technological change and the liberalization of trade for capital and goods. Those drivers had and have direct impact on human diets where a shift away from cereal-based diets is at the same time the cause and consequence of change in agriculture.

Together with increasing urbanization and globalization, market requirements are expected to change in the next decades. As many markets require standardized products and allow for little differentiation, some traditional and rare breeds might face increasing marketing difficulties. For example, the loss of small-scale abattoirs, often due to food safety regulation, can reduce the ability for breeds to enter niche markets or product differentiation. Developing countries' national strategies for livestock production aim at increasing food production rather than reflect the need for a genetic pool of breeding stock, although this is slowly changing due to the implementation of the Global Plan of Action for Animal Genetic Resources. Although breeding has to focus on what the market wants (mass or niche market), other factors also have to be taken into account. The choice of breeds/breeding used in the livestock sector needs to ensure the profitability of the farm, safeguard animal health and welfare, focus on conserving genetic diversity and promote human health.

Globally, about one-third of cattle, pig and chicken breeds are already extinct or currently at risk (FAO, 2010a). According to the last status and trends report on animal genetic resources (FAO, 2010a) a total of 1,710 (or 21 per cent) of all reported breeds are classified as being 'at risk'. Taking into account countries' different levels of breed population reporting, Woolliams et al. (2007) assume even higher shares of breeds at risk. Intensification of livestock production systems, coupled with specialization in breeding and the harmonizing effects of globalization and zoosanitary standards, has led to a substantial reduction in the genetic diversity within domesticated animal species (MEA, 2005b; FAO, 2007). Economic and market drivers were most frequently mentioned as threats for breed survival (FAO, 2009). The rate of breed extinction in the past was highest in regions that have the most highly-specialized livestock industries with fast structural change and in the species kept in such systems; however, several economically advanced countries have recently taken conservation action and broadened breeding goals (Hoffmann, 2011b).

Breeds adapted optimally to their habitat, in most cases not tailored to maximum meat or milk output, are increasingly being displaced by high-performance breeds – usually transboundary breeds for use in high external input, often large-scale, systems under more or less globally standardized conditions. In contrast to many local breeds, transboundary breeds provide single products for the market at high levels of output. Holstein-Friesian cattle – one of the most successful international dairy breeds – are reported to be present in at least 163 countries (http://dad.fao.org/, accessed July 2012). Large White pigs are present in 139 countries (http://dad.fao.org/, accessed July 2012); while in chicken commercial strains dominate the worldwide distribution. Extrapolating the figures of FAO (2006a) and assuming that the production increase between the early 2000s and 2009 is 100 per cent attributable to industrial systems, it can be estimated now that industrial systems provide 79 per cent of global poultry meat, 73 per cent of egg and 63 per cent of global pork production. This shows the increasing importance of transboundary breeds. Although the majority of milk is produced in small farms with an average herd size of three cows (IFCN, 2011), the share of transboundary dairy breeds or their crosses with local breeds is increasing. Unless selection within the local breed is incorporated in a structured crossbreeding programme, this may lead to the genetic 'dilution' of the local breed.

In parallel, consolidation in the breeding industry, especially in poultry and pigs, is ongoing (Gura, 2007). Breed utilization, genetic improvement and industry consolidation have major impacts on the genetic composition of transboundary breeds. A study in commercial chickens (Muir et al., 2008) indicated that more than 50 per cent of the original genetic diversity found in non-commercial breeds is absent in commercial pure lines. The genetic basis of a major commodity is reduced and may limit the capacity to respond to future needs. Due to global use of a few prominent bulls and a related fast increase in inbreeding, the effective population size of international dairy breeds, especially Holstein-Friesian, has declined (Fikse and Philipsson, 2007; Mrode et al., 2009; Philipsson et al., 2009).

In the case of crop diversity, FAO (2010d) noted that reliance on a smaller number of species and varieties not only results in erosion of genetic resources but can also lead to an increased risk of diseases when a variety is susceptible to new pests and diseases. This means increased food insecurity. The same arguments regarding increased risks hold for animal genetic resources. It should be considered that a rapid spread of pathogens, or even small spatial or seasonal changes in disease distribution, possibly driven by climate change, may expose livestock populations with a narrow genetic basis to new disease challenges.

A reduction of species and breed variety may also affect nutrition diversity. Meat quality is influenced by breed differences (e.g. Marshall, 1994; Suzuki et al., 2003; Bozzi et al., 2007; Lo Fiego et al., 2007; Sirtori et al., 2007), and species and breed differences are being exploited in many crossbreeding and selection schemes (e.g. Anderson, 1990; Beef CRC; Sheep CRC). For cattle milk, various interactions exist between breed, diet and location (including altitude) that contribute to the characteristic fatty acid profile of the milk (Bartl et al., 2008). Genetic differences also influence milk protein (e.g. casein) and processing quality. A review of milk composition for minor dairy species has shown large differences for macro- and micronutrients in different species and among breeds within the same species (Medhammar et al., 2011).

Meat quality is also heavily influenced by feeding and other environmental effects. Usually, grass-fed ruminants have higher levels of a-tocopherol, b-carotene, ascorbic acid, glutathione and nutritionally important long chain poly-unsaturated fatty-acids than feedlot-fed animals (Descalzo and Sancho, 2008; Wood et al., 2008). Meat from pasture feeding contains higher levels of antioxidants which in turn maintain the overall quality of meat and secondary products. Diet also affects meat flavour in both sheep and cattle but the components involved seem to be different. Meat from cattle raised on pasture is reported to be darker than meat from animals raised on concentrates (Priolo et al., 2001).

Reducing the environmental footprint – possible implications for breed diversity

Land and water availability are considered important future resource constraints for food security (FAO, 2011b). McKinsey (2011) estimated that more than 70 per cent of the opportunities to boost resource use efficiency lies in developing countries. Modelling results indicate that main points of intervention to reduce the environmental impacts of livestock production are: changes in nutrient management, crop yields and land management, grassland soil carbon restoration, husbandry systems and animal breeds, and feed conversion and feed composition on the supply side. On the demand side, shifts in consumption and reduction in food losses have been mentioned.

Due to the many synergies between enhancing production and reducing costs, it is already common practice to improve production efficiency. Comparisons for the USA indicate that improvements in genetics, feeding, health and management have reduced the carbon footprint for milk by 37 per cent if comparing a unit of milk produced in 2007 with that in 1944 (Capper et al., 2009) and for beef by 16.3 per cent if comparing a unit of beef produced in 2007 with that in 1977 (Capper, 2011). However, despite impressive relative efficiency improvements, life-cycle assessments show that the rebound effect of increased production and the absolute scale of the intensive landless livestock production still leads to considerable associated environmental impacts – beyond GHG emissions – and at different spatial and temporal scales (Pelletier, 2008; FAO, 2010b; Pelletier et al., 2010).

The future expected changes will most likely favour intensive livestock systems in which good feed conversion efficiency leads to reduced greenhouse gas emissions per unit of produce, which can be judged positively with regard to contributing products to sustainable diets. It is expected that breeding strategies using genomic information and transgenic approaches will in some sectors become more important to make farm animals more feed efficient and reduce the environmental footprint, thereby contributing to sustainability (Golovan et al., 2001; Niemann et al., 2011). However, the first 'beneficiaries' of such new technologies will most likely be the highly specialized transboundary breeds, such as the already dominating Holstein-Friesian cattle. Many recent scientific publications in the field of genomic selection focus on this breed (e.g. Hayes et al., 2009; Qanbari et al., 2010; Chen et al., 2011). Increasing concentrate feed efficiency will most likely lead not only to a shift towards highly productive and specialized breeds but also to a shift with regard to the species: away from ruminants towards monogastric species like poultry and pigs (FAO, 2010a,b). Except in marginal areas and extensive grazing systems, it can be expected that at the breed level, local breeds will more and more be replaced by transboundary breeds, leading to a further loss of local breeds and their manifold functions (Hoffmann, 2011b). Besides the loss of between-breed diversity an additional loss of within-breed diversity can be expected due to the further pressure on increasing yields of transboundary breeds by applying effective breeding programmes focusing on rather narrow breeding goals. Such losses due to effective breeding programmes might even be faster than in the past due to application of new biotechnologies.

From a biological conversion point of view, animal production systems consume more energy in feed than they generate in animal products. This is less of an issue in grazing systems where animals do not compete with humans over edible protein. Limited land availability for food production and the inefficiencies inherent in biological feed conversion have raised the importance of consumption and diets (Goodland, 1997; Gerbens-Leenes and Nonhebel, 2002). Studies following the recent attention to climate change propose to curtail the consumption of ASF in order to reduce anthropogenic greenhouse gas emissions (Stehfest et al., 2009; Wirsenius et al., 2010; Garnett, 2011; Grethe et al., 2011; Westhoek et al., 2011). Most studies propose to lower meat demand in industrialized countries only. Although such reductions would have only a small positive effect on food security in developing countries, they would have positive effects for human health, result in a less unequal per capita use of global resources, lower greenhouse gas emissions and could ease the introduction of higher animal welfare standards. The need for a broader view on sustainability, beyond a single focus on reducing GHG emissions, has been stressed by several authors (e.g. MacMillan and Durrant, 2009; Deckers, 2010).

A further option to fulfil the globally growing demand for animal source products could be the use of 'artificial' meat or *in-vitro* produced meat. In this trajectory, changes in food composition could improve health characteristics, and closed industrial production technology may result in more hygienic and environmentally friendly characteristics than 'traditional' meat (Thornton, 2010). While this may contribute for example to the health aspect of a sustainable diet, it may possibly not fulfil the criterion of 'cultural acceptance' across all societies. Also, a large-scale development and uptake of *in-vitro* meat might have severe effects on the livestock sector including employment and most likely a negative effect on the diversity of animal genetic resources. *In-vitro* meat and food fortification also contradict the concept of sustainable diet which stresses the importance of food-based approaches (Allen, 2008).

Finally, the reduction of food losses and wastes will be critical, as they imply that large amounts of the resources used in, and emissions and pollution caused by food production are used in vain. ASF, being highly perishable and connected to food safety risks, incur high losses along the chain. Losses of meat and meat products in all developing regions are distributed quite equally throughout the chain, while in industrialized regions, about 50 per cent of losses occur at the end of the chain. Approximately 40–65 per cent of total milk food losses in industrialized regions occur at the consumption level, while in developing regions, milk losses during post-harvest handling and storage, as well as at the distribution level, is relatively high (FAO, 2011c). Food waste disposal finally releases more GHG and water pollution.

In summary, past efforts to increase intensive production system yields and productivity have been undertaken mainly within a framework that has aimed to control conditions and make production systems uniform (FAO and PAR, 2011), which tends to favour the use of uniform breeds and therefore tends to undermine animal genetic diversity. This has led to a narrow set of breeds and management practices. The actual trends in combination with the growing demand for products of animal origin for human diets continue to drive a further shift in agricultural systems towards more intensive systems. This will most likely favour international transboundary breeds instead of local breeds. At species level, the shift towards poultry and pigs will continue.

Whether products especially from intensive systems can contribute to a sustainable diet depends on the systems' compatibility with regard to the rather complex requirements of the sustainable diets concept, namely being protective and respectful of biodiversity and ecosystems, culturally acceptable, accessible, economically fair and affordable; nutritionally adequate, safe and healthy; while optimizing natural and human resources. However, even if many aspects do contribute to a sustainable diet, a loss of animal genetic diversity appears to be quite likely at a global level. Given the important role of biodiversity in the sustainable diet definition, breed loss constitutes a negative impact on sustainable diets.

Solutions with focus on sustainable diets favouring animal genetic diversity

Inevitably, cultural and social roles of livestock will continue to change, and the nutrition transition will continue, including its undesirable health effects (Thornton, 2010; Nugent, 2011). The scenarios described above do not give rise to a bright future for animal genetic diversity even if sustainable diets are propagated. However, there is hope because a wide range of agricultural practices are already available to improve production in sustainable ways (e.g. FAO and IAEA, 2010).

Arguments in favour of local, mostly low-input breeds are based on the multiple products and services they provide, mostly at regional and local level. Firstly, their ability to make use of low-quality forage results in a net positive human edible protein ratio (FAO, 2011d). Secondly, under appropriate management, livestock kept in low external input mixed and grazing systems provide several ecosystem services. Thirdly, as a result, and linked to local breeds' recognition as cultural heritage, linkages to nature conservation need to be further explored and strengthened (Hoffmann, 2011a). All this is in harmony with the qualities of a sustainable diet.

Aiming for the improvement of the livestock sector's environmental performance will lead to different, locally tailored solutions, favouring certain environmental goods over others. Such systems are a prerequisite for production of food for sustainable diets and may add value to breed diversity. Besides traditional systems, a range of different innovative approaches to agricultural production exist, seeking to combine productivity and increased farmer incomes with long-term sustainability (FAO and PAR, 2011). In European countries, there is an increased emphasis on, and economic support for, the production of ecosystems goods and services, with a possibly positive effect on the role of local breeds, rural employment and survival chances for small-scale abattoirs. However, the efficiency of the EU agri-environmental programmes to breed conservation has been questioned (Signorello and Pappalardo, 2003) as payments are often below opportunity costs and little prioritization is undertaken.

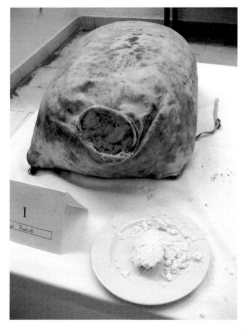

Figure 3.2 Cheese tasting in Mostar, Bosnia-Herzegovina. By Irene Hoffmann

In this context the ability of livestock, especially ruminants, to transform products not suitable for human consumption such as grass and by-products, into high-value products such as dairy and meat, plays a role. Grasslands have been identified as critical for C-sequestration, soil and vegetation restoration, and livelihoods for poor people, mostly pastoralists. Grasslands occupy about 25 per cent of the terrestrial ice-free land surface. In the early 2000s they harboured between 27 and 33 per cent of cattle and small ruminant stocks, respectively, and produced 23 per cent of global beef, 32 per cent of global mutton and 12 per cent of milk (FAO, 2006a). In Europe, so-called high nature value farmlands make up approximately 30 per cent of grasslands (EU-15 countries); they are considered to be part of Europe's cultural heritage and are mostly Natura 2000 sites. However, only an estimated 2–4 per cent of dairy production and around 20 per cent of beef production comes from high nature value grasslands (Westhoek et al., 2011).

One of the six priority targets of the 2011 EU Biodiversity Strategy is 'To increase EU contribution to global efforts to avoid biodiversity loss'. The accompanying impact assessment suggests that approximately 60 per cent of agricultural land would need to be managed in a way that supports biodiversity to meet this target, including both extensively and intensively managed areas under grass, arable and permanent crops. A mosaic of habitats with generation of positive co-benefits for production, biodiversity and local people would lead to what Scherr and McNeely (2008) called diverse types of 'eco-agriculture' landscapes. Also Benton et al. (2003) conclude that the re-creation of ecological heterogeneity at multiple spatial and temporal scales is key to restoring and sustaining biodiversity.

There is sufficient intensification potential in extensive systems without having to change the breed base. A recent life-cycle analysis for the dairy sector also showed a huge potential for moderate efficiency gains in developing countries (FAO, 2010c). On the contrary, well-adapted, hardy breeds are advantageous in utilizing the vast areas under rangelands (FAO, 2006b).

However, focusing on local and regional rather than global (i.e. GHG) aspects of sustainability also has its drawbacks. Measures such as improved animal welfare may lead to less efficient production, and thereby may just shift the negative environmental impact elsewhere; other measures may lead to higher costs for farmers. However, if done properly, measures taken locally at the supply and demand side would lead to lower societal costs by reducing local environmental impacts, animal welfare problems and public health risks (Grethe et al., 2011; Westhoek et al., 2011).

The main criticisms of ecological approaches were summarized during an expert workshop on biodiversity for food and agriculture as follows: (i) adoption of ecological approaches to farming reflects a romantic and backward-looking perspective, (ii) they will require even larger subsidies, and (iii) they are labour and knowledge intensive. To overcome this scepticism, innovation and development for new approaches will be essential, while a critical assessment of existing research results might be advisable, because most cost-benefit analyses comparing high-input systems with sustainable agricultural systems tend not to account for the manifold benefits agricultural systems can provide (FAO and PAR, 2011). In view of the existing agricultural subsidies in many countries it cannot be argued that commercial breeds are associated with some ideal free market equilibrium price. On the other hand, society cannot expect farmers to maintain breed diversity for the public good (ecosystem services or future option values) unless society is willing to compensate them up to the opportunity costs they incur for not using a more commercial breed (Drucker et al., 2005; Hoffmann, 2011b).

The recognition of the value of nutritional and dietary diversity is becoming an important entry point for exploring more ecologically sustainable food systems. Consumers may play a key role by improving their access to information and their control over what they choose to consume. Undoubtedly, use of diversity requires significant knowledge and skills. There are questions about the robustness of consumers' preferences regarding organic and local food, particularly in times of considerable economic uncertainty (Thornton, 2010). Limited economic resources may shift dietary choices towards cheap, energy-dense, convenient and highly palatable diets providing maximum energy (Drewnowski and Spencer, 2004). Consumption shifts, particularly a reduction in the consumption of livestock products, will not only have environmental benefits (Stehfest et al., 2009), but may also reduce the cardiovascular disease burden (Popkin and Du, 2003). However, changing consumption patterns is considered a longer-term process involving societal and cultural shifts.

Conclusions

In view of the uncertainty for future developments, a wide diversity of genetic resources is the best insurance to cope with unpredictable effects. There is no question that demands for animal products will continue to increase in the next decades and a further push to enhance livestock productivity across all production systems is needed to lower the environmental footprint of livestock production. At local level, there are many overlaps between environmental sustainability goals, sustainable production and providing sustainable diets. However, many of the required new technologies to increase resource efficiencies at global level will accelerate the structural change of the sector towards more intensive systems and thereby the losses of animal genetic diversity even if sustainable diets are aimed at. Taking into account the complexity of issues associated with the elements of a sustainable diet, more emphasis will need to be placed on avoiding the erosion of genetic diversity.

Providing sustainable diets can only be achieved with a combination of sustainable improvement of livestock production and a combination of policy approaches integrating the full concept of sustainable diets, accompanied by awareness raising for the value of biodiversity and investing in research as basis for sound decisions. Numerous research questions still require investigation, spanning different fields of science. With regard to livestock diversity and in view of uncertainty of future developments and climate change this implies the need to develop simple methods to characterize, evaluate and document adaptive and production traits in specific production environments. It also requires better identification of nutritional differences between ASF from different breeds and productions systems. The lack of such data is currently one of the constraints to effective prioritizing and planning for the best use of animal genetic resources measures in a sustainable development of the livestock sector and food systems. Intensifying research to develop life-cycle assessments and to include delivery of ecosystem services in the analysis recognizing and rewarding the sustainable use of biodiversity in well-managed rangelands with local breeds will also be one major task. Addressing the various spatial and temporal connections and trade-offs, and reaching out to different stakeholders in the value chain are considerable challenges. The concept of sustainable diet and the essential role of animal genetic diversity need to be addressed through awareness and educational programmes. Eating means not just ingesting food, but it is also a form of enjoyment and cultural expression.

Note

The views expressed in this publication are those of the author(s) and do not necessarily reflect the views of the Food and Agriculture Organization of the United Nations

References

Allen, L.H. (2008) 'To what extent can food-based approaches improve micronutrient status?' *Asia Pacific Journal of Clinical Nutrition*, vol 17, no S1, pp.103–105.

Anderson, P.T. (1990) 'Crossbreeding Systems for Beef Cattle' *University of Minnesota, Extension Service, FS-03926*, http://www.ansci.umn.edu/beef/beefupdates/bcmu03. pdf, accessed August 2012.

Barker, J.S.F. (2001) 'Conservation and management of genetic diversity: a domestic animal perspective' *Can. J. For. Res.*, vol 31, pp.588–595.

Bartl, K., Gomez, C.A., García, M., Aufdermauer, T., Kreuzer, M., Hess, H.D., Wettstein, H.R. (2008) 'Milk fatty acid profile of Peruvian Criollo and Brown Swiss cows in response to different diet qualities fed at low and high altitude', *Archives of Animal Nutrition*, vol 62, no 6, pp.468–484.

Benton, T.G., Vickery, J.A., Wilson, J.D. (2003) 'Farmland biodiversity: Is habitat heterogeneity the key?' *Trends in Ecology and Evolution*, 18:4, pp.182–188.

Bozzi, R., Crovetti, A., Nardi, L., Pugliese, C., Sirtori, F., Franci, O. (2007) 'Study on genes related to meat quality in Cinta Senese pig breed', *Proceedings of the 6th International Symposium on the Mediterranean Pig*, October 11–13, Messina-Capo d'Orlando, Italy, pp.41–45.

Bruinsma, J. (2011) 'The resources outlook: by how much do land, water and crop yields need to increase by 2050?', in FAO, (2011) *Looking ahead in world food and agriculture: Perspectives to 2050* (eds) P. Conforti, FAO, Rome, pp.233–278.

Caballero, A., Toro, M.A. (2002) 'Analysis of genetic diversity for the management of conserved subdivided populations', *Conserv. Genet.*, vol 3, pp.289–299.

Capper, J.L. (2011) 'The environmental impact of U.S. beef production: 1977 compared with 2007', *J Anim Sci*, vol 89, no 12, pp.4249–4261.

Capper, J.L., Cady, R.A., Bauman, D.E. (2009) 'The environmental impact of dairy production: 1944 compared with 2007', *J Anim Sci,* vol 87, pp.2160–2167.

Chen, J., Wang, Y., Zhang, Yi, Sun, D., Zhang, S., Zhang, Yu. (2011) 'Evaluation of breeding programs combining genomic information in Chinese Holstein', *Journal Agricultural Sciences in China*, vol 10, no 12, pp.1949–1957.

Co-operative Research Centre for Beef Genetic Technologies (Beef CRC) http://www.beefcrc.com.au/, accessed August 2012.

Cooperative Research Centre for Sheep Industry Innovation (Sheep CRC) http://www.sheepcrc.org.au/, accessed August 2012.

Deckers, J. (2010) 'Should the consumption of farm animal products be restricted, and if so, by how much?' *Food Policy* , vol 35, no 6, pp.497–503.

Delgado, C., Rosegrant, M., Steinfeld, H., Ehui, S., Courbois, C. (1999) 'Livestock to 2020. The next food revolution', in *Food, Agriculture and the Environment Discussion Paper,* 28, Washington, USA: IFPRI.

Descalzo, A.M., Sancho, A.M. (2008) 'A review of natural antioxidants and their effects on oxidative status, odor and quality of fresh beef produced in Argentina', *Meat Science,* vol 79, pp.423–436.

Drewnowski, A., Spencer, S.E. (2004) 'Poverty and obesity: The role of energy density and energy cost', *American Journal of Clinical Nutrition,* vol 79, no 1, pp.6–16.

Drucker, A.G., Smale, M., Zambrano, P. (2005) *Valuation and Sustainable Management of Crop and Livestock Biodiversity: A Review of Applied Economics Literature*, Published for the CGIAR System-wide Genetic Resources Programme (SGRP) by the International Food Policy Research Institute (IFPRI), the International Plant Genetic Resources (IPGRI), and the International Livestock Research Institute (ILRI).

FAO (2006a) *Livestock's long shadow – environmental issues and options*, H. Steinfeld, P. Gerber, T. Wassenaar, V. Castel, M. Rosales, and C. de Haan (eds), Rome, Italy: Food and Agriculture Organization of the United Nations.

FAO (2006b) *Breed diversity in dryland ecosystems*, Information Document 9, Fourth Session of the Intergovernmental Technical Working Group on Animal Genetic Resources for Food and Agriculture, Rome.

FAO (2007) *The state of the world's animal genetic resources for food and agriculture,* B. Rischkowsky, and D. Pilling (eds), Rome, Italy: Food and Agriculture Organization of the United Nations.

FAO (2009) *Threats to animal genetic resources – their relevance, importance and opportunities to decrease their impact,* CGRFA Background Study Paper, no 50, Rome.

FAO (2010a) *Status and trends report on animal genetic resources – 2010,* CGRFA/WG-AnGR-6/10/Inf. 3. Rome, Italy: Food and Agriculture Organization of the United Nations.

FAO (2010b) *The State of Food and Agriculture 2009, Livestock in the Balance,* Rome, Italy: Food and Agriculture Organization of the United Nations.

FAO (2010c) *Greenhouse Gas Emissions from the Dairy Sector, A Life Cycle Assessment,* Rome, Italy: Food and Agriculture Organization of the United Nations.

FAO (2010d) *Second Report on the State of the World's Plant Genetic Resources,* Rome, Italy: Food and Agriculture Organization of the United Nations.

FAO (2011a) *Sustainability Assessment of Food and Agriculture systems (SAFA),* Background Document for the E-Forum held in February–March 2011.

FAO (2011b) *The state of the world's land and water resources for food and agriculture (SOLAW) – Managing systems at risk,* Food and Agriculture Organization of the United Nations, Rome and Earthscan, London.

FAO (2011c) *Global food losses and food waste, Extent, causes and prevention,* J. Gustavsson, C. Cederberg, U. Sonesson, R. van Otterdijk, A. Meybeck, Rome, 2011, http://www.fao.org/fileadmin/user_upload/ags/publications/GFL_web.pdf, accessed August 2012.

FAO (2011d) *World Livestock 2011, Livestock in food security,* FAO, Rome.

FAO and IAEA (2010) 'Sustainable improvement of animal production and health', in *Proceedings of the International Symposium* organized by the joint FAO/IAEA Division of Nuclear Techniques in Food and Agriculture in cooperation with the Animal Production and Health Division of FAO, Rome.

FAO and PAR (2011) *Biodiversity for Food and Agriculture. Contributing to food security and sustainability in a changing world,* Rome, Italy: Food and Agriculture Organization and Platform for Agrobiodiversity Research.

Fikse, W.F., Philipsson, J. (2007) 'Development of international genetic evaluations of dairy cattle for sustainable breeding programs', *Animal Genetic Resources Information,* vol 41, pp.29–44.

Foresight (2011) *The Future of Food and Farming (2011) Final Project Report,* Government Office for Science, London.

Garnett, T. (2011) 'Where are the best opportunities for reducing greenhouse gas emissions in the food system (including the food chain)?' *Food Policy,* vol 36, pp.23–32.

Gerbens-Leenes, P.W., Nonhebel, S. (2002) 'Consumption patterns and their effects on land required for food', *Ecological Economics,* vol 42, pp.185–199.

Givens, D.I. (2010) 'Milk and meat in our diet good or bad for health?', *Animal,* vol 4, no 12, pp.1941–1952.

Golovan, S.P., Meidinger, R.G., Ajakaiye, A., Cottrill, M., Wiederkehr, M.Z., Barney, D.J., Plante, C., Pollard, J.W., Fan, M.Z., Hayes, M.A., Laursen, J., Hjorth, J.P., Hacker, R.R., Phillips, J.P., Forsberg, C.W. (2001) 'Pigs expressing salivary phytase produce low-phosphorus manure', *Nature Biotechnology,* vol 19, no 8, pp.741–745, doi:10.1038/90788.

Goodland, R. (1997) 'Environmental sustainability in agriculture: diet matters', *Ecological Economics,* vol 23, pp.189–200.

Grethe, H., Dembélé, A., Duman, N. (2011) *How to feed the world's growing billions? Understanding FAO world food projections and their implications,* Heinrich Böll Foundation and WWF: Berlin, Germany.

Gura, S. (2007) *Livestock Genetics Companies. Concentration and proprietary strategies of an emerging power in the global food economy*, League for Pastoral Peoples and Endogenous Livestock Development.

Hayes, B.J., Bowman, P.J., Chamberlain, A.J., Goddard, M.E. (2009) 'Genomic selection in dairy cattle: progress and challenges', *J Dairy Sci*, vol 92, no 2, pp.433–443.

Heller, M.C., Keoleian, G.A. (2003) 'Assessing the sustainability of the US food system: a life cycle perspective', *Agricultural Systems*, vol 76, pp.1007–1041.

Hoffmann, I. (2010a) 'Climate change and the characterization, breeding and conservation of animal genetic resources', *Animal Genetics*, vol 41 (Suppl. 1), pp.32–46.

Hoffmann, I. (2010b) 'Climate Change in Context: Implications for Livestock Production and diversity', in N.E. Odongo, M. Garcia, G.J. Vilojen (eds) *Sustainable improvement of Animal Production and Health* (pp.33–44), Rome, Italy: Food and Agriculture Organization of the United Nations.

Hoffmann, I. (2011a) 'Contribution of low-input farming to biodiversity conservation', in *First Low Input Breeds Workshop, 15–16 March 2011*, Wageningen, The Netherlands.

Hoffmann, I. (2011b) 'Livestock biodiversity and sustainability', *Livestock Science*, vol 139, Special Issue 'Assessment for sustainable development of animal production systems', pp.69–79.

International Farm Comparison Network (IFCN) (2011) *Dairy Report 2011. For a better understanding of milk production world-wide*, Kiel, Germany.

Larsen, C.S. (2003) 'Animal source foods and human health during evolution', *Journal of Nutrition*, vol 133, no 11, pp.3893S–3897S.

Lo Fiego, D.P., Ielo, M.C., Cornellini, M., Volpelli, L.A. (2007) 'Carcass and meat quality traits of pigs with different fraction of Mora Romagnola breed, reared outdoors', *Proceedings of the 6th International Symposium on the Mediterranean Pig*, October 11–13, 2007, Messina-Capo d'Orlando, Italy, pp.302–306.

MacMillan, T., Durrant, R. (2009) *Livestock consumption and climate change, A framework for dialogue*, WWF and Food Ethics Council, UK.

MacRae, J., O'Reilly, L., Morgan, P. (2005) 'Desirable characteristics of animal products from a human health perspective', *Livestock Production Science*, vol 94, no 1, pp.95–103.

Madalena, F. E. (2012) 'Animal breeding and development – South American Perspective', *J. Anim. Breed. Genet.* 171–172.

Marshall, D.M. (1994) 'Breed differences and genetic parameters for body composition traits in beef cattle', *J. Anim. Sci.*, vol 72, pp.2745–2755.

McKinsey Global Institute (2011) *Resource revolution: Meeting the world's energy, materials, food and water needs*, R. Dobbs, J. Oppenheim, F. Thompson, M. Brinkmann, M. Zornes, McKinsey Global Institute, p.210.

Medhammar, E., Wijesinha-Bettoni, R., Stadlmayr, B., Nilsson, E., Charrondiere, U.R., Burlingame, B. (2011) 'Composition of milk from minor dairy animals and buffalo breeds: a biodiversity perspective', *Journal of the Science of Food and Agriculture* 92:3, pp.445–474.

Millennium Ecosystem Assessment (MEA) (2005a) *Ecosystems and Human Well-being: Synthesis*, Island Press, Washington DC.

Millennium Ecosystem Assessment (MEA) (2005b) *Ecosystems and Human Well-being: Biodiversity Synthesis*, World Resources Institute, Washington DC.

Milton, K. (2003) 'The critical role played by animal source foods in human (homo) evolution', *Journal of Nutrition*, vol 133, no 11, pp.3886S–3892S.

Mrode, R., Kearney, J.F., Biffani, S., Coffey, M., Canavesi, F. (2009) 'Short communication: Genetic relationships between the Holstein cow populations of three European dairy countries', *Journal of Dairy Science*, vol 92, no 11, pp.5760–5764.

Muir, W.M., Wong, G.K.S., Zhang, Y., Wang, J., Groenen, M.A.M., Crooijmans, R.P.M.A., Megens, H.J., Zhang, H., Okimoto, R., Vereijken, A., Jungerius, A., Albers,

G.A.A., Lawley, C.T., Delany M.E., MacEachern, S., Cheng, H.H. (2008) 'Genome-wide assessment of worldwide chicken SNP genetic diversity indicates significant absence of rare alleles in commercial breeds', *PNAS* vol 105, no 45, pp.17312–17317, doi_10.1073_pnas.0806569105.

Murphey, S.P., Allen, L.H. (2003) 'Nutritional importance of animal source foods', *Journal of Nutrition*, vol 133, no 11, pp.3932S–3935S.

Naylor, R., Steinfeld, H., Falcon, W., Galloway, J., Smil, V., Bradford, E., Alder, J., Mooney, H. (2005) 'Agriculture: Losing the links between livestock and land', *Science,* vol 310, no 5754, pp.1621–1622.

Neumann, C.G., Bwibo, N.O., Murphy, S.P., Sigman, M., Whaley, S., Allen, L.H., Guthrie, D., Weiss, R.E., Demment, M.W. (2003) 'Animal source foods improve dietary quality, micronutrient status, growth and cognitive function in Kenyan school children: Background, study design and baseline findings', *Journal of Clinical Nutrition,* vol 133, no 11, pp.3941S–3949S.

Neumann, C.G., Demment, M.W., Maretzki, A., Drorbaugh, N., Galvin, K.A. (2010) 'Benefits, Risks, and Challenges in Urban and Rural Settings of Developing Countries', in H. Steinfeld, H.A. Mooney, F. Schneider, L.E. Neville (eds) *Livestock in a Changing Landscape, Vol. 1: Drivers, Consequences, and Responses*, pp.221–248, Washington, Covelo, London: Island Press.

Niemann, H., Kuhla, B., Flachowsky, G. (2011) 'Perspectives for feed-efficient animal production', *J Anim Sci,* vol 89, pp 4344–4363.

Nugent, R. (2011) *Bringing agriculture to the table, How agriculture and food can play a role in preventing chronic disease*, Chicago Council on Global Affairs, p.85.

OECD-FAO (2009) *Agricultural Outlook 2009–2018*, Rome, Italy: Food and Agriculture Organization of the United Nations.

Pelletier, N. (2008) 'Environmental performance in the US broiler poultry sector: Life cycle energy use and greenhouse gas, ozone depleting, acidifying and eutrophying emissions', *Agricultural Systems,* vol 98, pp.67–73.

Pelletier N., Tyedmers, P. (2010) 'Forecasting potential global environmental costs of livestock production 2000–2050', *PNAS* vol 107:43, pp.18371–18374.

Pelletier, N., Lammers, P., Stender, D., Pirog, R. (2010) 'Life cycle assessment of high- and low-profitability commodity and deep-bedded niche swine production systems in the Upper Midwestern United States', *Agricultural Systems,* vol 103, pp.599–608.

Philipsson, J., Forabosco, F., Jakobsen, J.H. (2009) 'Monitoring sustainability of international dairy breeds', *Interbull Bulletin* 40, 287–291.

Pica-Ciamarra, U., Otte, J. (2009) 'The "Livestock Revolution": Rhetoric and Reality' in *Pro-Poor Livestock Policy Initiative,* pp.05–09, Rome, Italy: Food and Agriculture Organization of the United Nations.

Pingali, P., McCullough, E. (2010) 'Drivers of Change in Global Agriculture and Livestock Systems', in H. Steinfeld, H.A. Mooney, F. Schneider, L.E. Neville (eds) *Livestock in a Changing Landscape, Vol 1: Drivers, Consequences, and Responses*, pp.5–10, Washington, Covelo, London: Island Press.

Popkin, B.M., Du, S. (2003) 'Dynamics of the nutrition transition toward the animal foods sector in China and its implications: A worried perspective', *Journal of Clinical Nutrition*, vol 133, no 11, pp.3898S–3906S.

Priolo, A., Micol, D., Agabriel, J., (2001) 'Effects of grass feeding systems on ruminant meat colour and flavour, A review', *Anim. Res.* 50, pp.185–200.

Qanbari, S., Pimentel, E.C., Tetens, J., Thaller, G., Lichtner, P., Sharifi, A.R., Simianer, H. (2010) 'A genome-wide scan for signatures of recent selection in Holstein cattle', *Anim. Genet.*, vol 41, no 4, pp.377–389, Epub 2010 Jan 21. PubMed PMID: 20096028.

Randolph, T.F., Schelling, E., Grace, D., Nivholson, C.F., Leroy, J.L., Cole, D.C., Demment, M.W., Omore, A., Zinsstag, J., Ruel, M. (2007) 'The role of livestock in human nutrition and health for poverty reduction in developing countries', *Journal of Animal Science*, vol 85, pp.2788–2800.

Rockström J. et al. (2009) 'A safe operating space for humanity', *Nature*, vol 461, no 24, pp.472–475.

Scherr, S.J., McNeely, J.A. (2008) 'Biodiversity conservation and agricultural sustainability: towards a new paradigm of "ecoagriculture" landscapes', *Philosophical Transactions of the Royal Society, B* 363, pp.477–494, doi:10.1098/rstb.2007.2165.

Signorello, G., Pappalardo, G. (2003) 'Domestic animal biodiversity conservation: a case study of rural development plans in the European Union', *Ecological Economics,* vol 45, no 3, pp.487–499.

Sirtori, F., Parenti, S., Campodoni, G., D'Adorante, S., Crovetti, A., Acciaioli, A. (2007) 'Effect of sire breed in Cinta Senese crossbreds: chemical, physical and sensorial traits of fresh and seasoned loin', *Proceedings of the 6th International Symposiom on the Mediterranean Pig*, October 11–13, Messina-Capo d'Orlando, Italy, pp.338–341.

Stehfest, E., Bouwman, L., van Vuuren, D.P., den Elzen, M.G.J., Eickhout, B., Kabat, P. (2009) 'Climate benefits of changing diet', *Climatic Change*, vol 95, pp.83–102.

Suzuki, K., Shibata, T., Kadowaki, H., Abe, H., Toyoshima, T. (2003) 'Meat quality comparison of Berkshire, Duroc and crossbred pigs sired by Berkshire and Duroc', *Meat Science*, vol 84, pp.35–42.

Thornton, P.K. (2010) 'Livestock production: recent trends, future prospects'. *Philosophical Transactions of the Royal Society, B*, vol 365, pp.2853–2867.

UNDP (2009) *World Population Prospects, The 2010 Revision*, http://esa.un.org/wpp/index.htm, accessed August 2012.

UNEP (2007) *Global Environment Outlook GEO 4 Environment for development*, Nairobi, p.540.

UNEP (2010) *Assessing the Environmental Impacts of Consumption and Production: Priority Products and Materials*, A Report of the Working Group on the Environmental Impacts of Products and Materials to the International Panel for Sustainable Resource Management, E. Hertwich, E. van der Voet, S. Suh, A. Tukker, M. Huijbregts, P. Kazmierczyk, M. Lenzen, J. McNeely, Y. Moriguchi.

UNEP (2011) *Vision for change, Recommendations for effective policies on sustainable lifestyles*, Paris.

Westhoek, H., Rood, T., van den Berg, M., Janse, J., Nijdam, D., Reudink, M., Stehfest, E. (2011) *The Protein Puzzle. The consumption and production of meat, dairy and fish in the European Union*, The Hague, The Netherlands: PBL Netherlands Environmental Assessment Agency.

WHO/FAO (2003) *Diet, nutrition and the prevention of chronic diseases, Report of a joint WHO/FAO Expert Consultation*, WHO Technical Report series 916. Geneva, Switzerland: WHO.

Wirsenius, S., Azar, C., Berndes, G. (2010) 'How much land is needed for global food production under scenarios of dietary changes and livestock productivity increases in 2030?' *Agricultural Systems,* vol 103, pp.621–638.

Wood, J.D., Enser, M., Fisher, A.V., Nute, G.R., Sheard, P.R., Richardson, R.I., Hughes, S., Whittington, F.M. (2008) 'Fat deposition, fatty acid composition and meat quality: A review', *Meat Science,* vol 78, pp.343–358.

Woolliams, J.A., Matika, O., Pattison, J. (2007) *Conservation of animal genetic resources: approaches and technologies for in situ and ex situ conservation*. Scientific Forum on Animal Genetic Resources, ITC-AnGR/07/Inf.2.

4   Valuing aquatic biodiversity in agricultural landscapes

Matthias Halwart

Introduction

This chapter deals with the role of aquatic organisms in agricultural landscapes and in particular their importance for food and nutrition security of rural livelihoods. In this context, aquatic organisms are usually derived from inland capture fisheries from wetlands, streams, rivers, or irrigation canals, and from aquaculture which means the farming of aquatic organisms including fish, molluscs, crustaceans and aquatic plants mostly in ponds, cages, tanks or rice fields.

Undernutrition is caused by an insufficient intake of food or of certain nutrients or by an inability of the body to absorb and use nutrients. Documented nutrient deficiencies in rural communities include vitamin A, several B vitamins, calcium, iron, zinc, iodine, sulphur-containing amino acids and lysine, and fatty acids of the n-3 series (Halwart et al., 2006). Undernutrition remains a huge and persistent problem, especially in many developing countries, with the bulk of undernourished people living in rural areas. The number of undernourished people in developing countries declined significantly in the 1970s, 1980s and early 1990s, in spite of rapid population growth (FAO, 2011a). However, the incidence of hunger and undernourishment in the world has been dramatically affected by two successive crises – the food crisis first, with basic food prices beyond the reach of millions of poor, and then the economic recession. These crises have had very severe consequences for millions of people, pushing them into hunger and undernourishment. FAO's current estimate of the number of undernourished people in the world in 2009 is 1.02 billion people, which represents more hungry people than at any time since 1970 (FAO, 2011a).

The food and agricultural system as a whole has a key role to play in reducing malnutrition in the world, and the availability of and access to fish is critically important for nutrition and diverse diets especially for the rural poor. Producers can be encouraged to grow a wider variety of crops, including fish, often reviving traditional species and varieties or breeds with high nutritive values. Fish is usually cited as an important source of nutrients and for wild and farmed fish alike often valued for its long-chained omega-3 fatty acids (e.g. Jensen et al., 2012) and fish should be, and in many parts of the world already is, part of a healthy diet. In some places, plants and animals including fish from the forest and the wild contribute variety and taste to otherwise poor rural diets (Ainsworth et al., 2008; Halwart and Bartley, 2005; Jarvis et al., 2007; MAF/ FAO, 2007). For those who consume out of their own production or from home or school gardens, diversity in the kinds of foods they grow, gather, fish, or raise is important (Tutwiler, 2012).

It will be argued in this chapter that a focus on the often cited nutritional value of proteins derived from fish (e.g. EC, 2000; ICTSD, 2006) for human nutrition *in agricultural landscapes* certainly is justified to some extent; however, even more important is the role of fish for avoiding micronutrient-related nutritional disorders in developing countries. Examples include anaemia caused by insufficient intake of iron (De Benoist et al., 2008), and impaired sight which is a severe problem because of inadequate intake of vitamin A (WHO, 2009). Such nutrition disorders can be particularly serious in children, since they interfere with growth and development, and may predispose to many health problems, such as infection and chronic disease. Safe and nutritious aquatic foods, selected by nutrition-conscious consumers and caregivers, are therefore critically important in the battle against undernutrition.

Fish availability in inland waters

Fish and other aquatic organisms make an important contribution to food security for many people in agricultural landscapes where they are collected or farmed providing valuable sources of highly nutritious food to all household members. Generally, inland capture fisheries from a wide range of aquatic environments such as swamps, rivers, flood plains and lakes, but also modified habitats such as rice fields or reservoirs produce a large variety of aquatic organisms usually directly consumed and, to a much lesser extent, bartered or sold (Figure 4.1). A recent review on trends of catches is provided by Welcomme (2011a). Aquatic products coming from aquaculture, often farmed in ponds or cages, can also contribute significantly to household nutrition (Swaminathan, 2012). In farming systems where fish are principally intended to be sold they can also provide important benefits indirectly by increasing the purchasing power of farming households for food or for investment in education, access to health services or improvements in household hygiene, all having positive indirect effects on nutrition. There are significant differences in the nutritional value of aquatic food items depending on available species and sizes or developmental form of the organisms. The integration of fisheries, aquaculture and agriculture, innovatively practised by many farmers around the globe, provides numerous options for the sustainable exploitation of a rich diversity of food items that can cover to a large extent the nutritional needs of the different members of the household and the society at large.

The aquatic biodiversity of inland waters useful to humans includes plants, fish, amphibians, reptiles, molluscs, crustaceans and insects. FAO Fisheries and

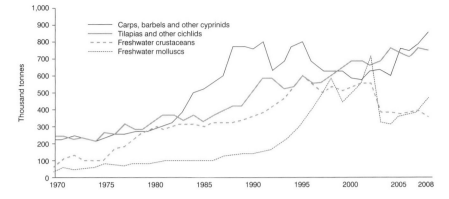

Figure 4.1 Catch trends by major inland waters species group

Aquaculture Department information contributed by member countries in 2010 officially indicates that 10.2 million tonnes were harvested from inland capture fisheries and 36.9 million tonnes from inland aquaculture (FAO, 2012a). However, accurate information on small-scale inland capture fisheries and rural aquaculture is extremely difficult to obtain because of the informal and diffuse nature of these subsectors. Additionally, much of what is caught or produced by small-scale fishers/farmers is consumed by them or bartered locally, and therefore does not enter the formal economy and accounting of national governments. In-depth work has revealed that real production from inland waters is several times higher than that officially reported. It is clear that inland aquatic biodiversity is an important resource for rural communities and often provides a 'safety net' to rely on in the face of other crop and food shortages.

Inland fisheries

In most rural areas of many developing countries, especially landlocked ones, inland fisheries from lakes, floodplains, streams, rivers, and other wetlands including rice fields are very important for food security and income generation. In 1950, inland fisheries produced about 2 million tonnes in terms of fish landings. The figure was about 5 million tonnes in 1980, and, after steady growth of 2–3 per cent per year, 10 million tonnes in 2008. This growth occurred mainly in Asia and Africa, with Latin America making a small contribution. Asia and Africa regularly account for about 90 per cent of reported landings. The remaining 10 per cent is split between North and South America and Europe. The bulk (about 90 per cent) of inland fish is caught in developing countries and 65 per cent is caught in low-income food-deficit countries (LIFDCs). However, much uncertainty surrounds both the trend in and the level of production.

The amount of food produced in inland waters in general (FAO/MRC, 2003) and rice fields (other than rice itself) in particular (Halwart, 2003) is generally

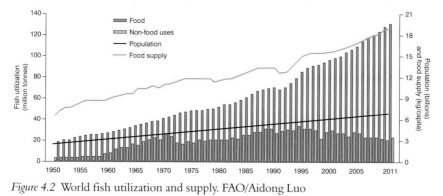

Figure 4.2 World fish utilization and supply. FAO/Aidong Luo

underestimated and undervalued, because it is small quantities (although collected by many individuals and in large areas) which are all locally consumed or marketed, and therefore not recorded in official statistics.

Using a model calculation, Welcomme (2011b) estimated that more than 93 million tonnes could be produced just from the world's lakes. Rice fields have been found to be another important source of origin for fish production. Indeed, the cultivation of rice in irrigated, rain-fed and deepwater systems often offers a suitable environment for fish and other aquatic organisms. Over 90 per cent of the world's rice, equivalent to approximately 134 million hectares, is grown under flooded conditions. It is quite clear that the actual global aquatic food production from inland waters could be much higher than what is currently reported.

Utilization

In developing countries, most of the catch from inland fisheries is processed in small-scale or medium-scale units and goes for domestic consumption (FAO, 2011b) (Figure 4.2). Many rural farmer and fisher families cannot obtain a sufficient variety of nutritious food in their local markets or are simply too poor to purchase it. Cultivated species may be complemented by harvested wild species that can be of particular significance for indigenous communities and for poor and vulnerable communities especially in times of shortage of main staples. Wild and gathered foods, including from the aquatic habitat, therefore provide important diversity, nutrition and food security (Halwart and Bartley, 2007). Trade in inland fish and products are constrained by lack of infrastructure and facilities needed to establish and operate cold chains. This often results in high post-harvest losses, especially quality losses that can amount to up to 40 per cent of the landings. Owing to the remoteness and isolated nature of many inland fishing communities and the high abundance of fish on a seasonal basis, large amounts of fish from inland capture are cured. In Africa, fish processing methods vary according to region and even subregion. Drying and smoking, and to a very small extent fermenting, are the main methods. Some processed freshwater products are considered a delicacy in some countries and are higher priced than similar products prepared using marine fish, e.g. in Ghana, where fresh and salted dried tilapia as well as smoked catfish or perch (*Lates*) are highly preferred. In Asia, a significant proportion of inland fish goes into fish sauce and fish paste. In Cambodia for example, the bulk of the fish caught from the Mekong River in the dai fishery is used for making fish paste (prahoc) and fish sauce (FAO, 2010).

Aquaculture

The farming of inland aquatic species has a much shorter history than farming of crops or livestock and issues, trends and prospects including its role for human nutrition have been comprehensively addressed in a recent Global Conference (FAO/NACA, 2012). Except for the common carp that was domesticated approximately 2,000 years ago, breeding of aquatic species for food is relatively recent. However, the sector is increasing rapidly and represents the fastest growing food producing sector: in 1985 only 73 freshwater species were farmed, in 2000 there were over 150. Today, aquaculture involves the farming of over 540 species of finfish, molluscs, crustaceans and other invertebrates (FAO, 2012a). Traditional animal breeding, chromosome-set manipulation and hybridization have used the genetic diversity of aquatic species such as tilapia, catfish, rainbow trout and common carp to create characteristic breeds of fish to suit environmental and consumer demands (Greer and Harvey, 2004; FAO, 2012b).

World production of food fish

Aquaculture is a growing, vibrant and important production sector. The reported global production of food fish from aquaculture, including finfish, crustaceans, molluscs and other aquatic animals for human consumption, reached 59.9 million tonnes in 2010 out of which 36.9 million tonnes came from inland waters (Table 4.1). In the period 1970–2010, the production of food fish from aquaculture increased at an average annual growth rate of 8.2 per cent, while the world population grew at an average of 1.6 per cent per year. The combined result of development in aquaculture worldwide and the expansion in global population is that the average annual per capita supply of food fish from aquaculture for human consumption has increased by 10 times, from 0.7 kg in 1970 to 7.8 kg in 2008, at an average rate of 6.6 per cent per year (FAO, 2012a).

Globally, aquaculture accounted for 46 per cent of the world's fish food production for human consumption in 2009, up from 42.7 per cent in 2006. Despite the long tradition of aquaculture practices in a few countries over many centuries, aquaculture in the global context is a young food production sector that has grown rapidly in the last five decades. World aquaculture output has increased substantially from less than 1 million tonnes of annual production

Table 4.1 Volume of world aquaculture production of food fish★ by major groups of aquatic animals (units: million tonnes). Source: FAO 2012a

Major species group	1980	1985	1990	1995	2000	2001	2002	2003	2004	2005	2006	2007	2008	2009	2010
Freshwater fishes	2.09	4.34	7.14	12.93	17.59	18.59	19.79	20.32	22.20	23.67	25.29	26.62	29.03	30.65	33.74
Molluscs	1.84	2.49	3.61	8.23	9.76	10.29	10.87	11.35	11.84	12.11	12.67	13.03	13.01	13.51	14.16
Crustaceans	0.09	0.26	0.75	1.08	1.69	1.98	2.22	3.00	3.39	3.78	4.26	4.80	5.02	5.34	5.73
Diadromous fishes	0.49	0.67	1.21	1.52	2.25	2.52	2.57	2.68	2.83	2.87	3.00	3.24	3.32	3.53	3.60
Marine fishes	0.19	0.23	0.32	0.55	0.98	1.05	1.16	1.23	1.28	1.44	1.64	1.74	1.95	1.95	1.83
Miscellaneous aquatic animals	0.01	0.03	0.05	0.08	0.16	0.18	0.19	0.33	0.38	0.43	0.42	0.51	0.62	0.73	0.81
World total	4.71	8.02	13.07	24.38	32.42	34.61	36.79	38.92	41.91	44.30	47.29	49.94	52.95	55.71	59.87

★ Farmed food fish = farmed finfish, crustaceans, molluscs, amphibians, reptiles (excluding crocodiles) and other aquatic animals (such as sea cucumber, sea urchin, etc.) for human consumption.

in 1950 to 59.9 million tonnes in 2010 (FAO, 2012a), demonstrating three times the growth rate of world meat production (2.7 per cent, from poultry and livestock together) in the same period.

The value of the harvest of world aquaculture, excluding aquatic plants, was estimated at US$119.4 billion in 2010. However, the actual total output value from the entire aquaculture sector should be significantly higher than this figure because the values of aquaculture hatchery and nursery production and the breeding of ornamental fishes have yet to be estimated and included. If aquatic plants are included, world aquaculture production in 2010 was 78.9 million tonnes, with an estimated value of US$125.1 billion (FAO, 2012a).

The above figures demonstrate impressively the increasing importance of aquaculture worldwide and the important role that the farming of fish will increasingly assume both for food security and poverty alleviation.

World production of aquatic plants

Aquaculture produced 19 million tonnes (live weight equivalent) of aquatic plants, mostly seaweeds, in 2010, with a total estimated value of US$5.7 billion. Of the world total production of aquatic plants in the same year, 95.5 per cent came from aquaculture. The culture of aquatic plants has consistently expanded its production since 1970, with an average annual growth rate of 7.7 per cent. The production is overwhelmingly dominated by seaweeds (over 99 per cent by quantity or value in 2010) (FAO, 2012a).

Not included in the above production figures, yet critically important in terms of production in agricultural landscapes and nutrition for national food security particularly in many Asian countries, are freshwater macrophytes such as water spinach, water Neptune, lotus, water caltrops, wild rice (*Zizania aquatica*), water chestnut, prickly water lily and arrow head (*Sagittaria sagittifolia*).

Fish in the diet

Fish diversity

Out of 32,200 fish species described in *FishBase* (Froese and Pauly, 2012), food, industrial (fishmeal and fish oil), ornamental, sport and bait fisheries target about one-sixth, equivalent to 5,000 species. Aquaculture farms over 540 species of finfish, molluscs, crustaceans and other invertebrates, about 50 species of microalgae and invertebrates as food organisms in hatcheries, about 35 species of seaweeds, and over 10 species of amphibians and aquatic reptiles.

Halwart and Bartley (2005) documented the rich variety of aquatic species found and utilized from rice-based systems in Southeast Asia (Box 4.1). A total of 64 aquatic animal species from farmer-managed systems were recorded as being consumed in northeast Thailand, compared with 34 and 19 species in southeast Cambodia and Red River Delta in Viet Nam, respectively (Morales et al., 2006).

Box 4.1 Aquatic species in Southeast Asia

For many rural populations in lowland Southeast Asia, rice and fish are the mainstay of their diet. Aquatic animals represent a significant, often the most important, source of animal protein and are also essential during times of rice shortages (Meusch et al., 2003). Wild and gathered foods from the aquatic habitat provide important diversity, nutrition and food security as food resources from ricefield environments supply essential nutrients that are not adequately found in the diet (Halwart, 2008).

Studies on the availability and use of aquatic biodiversity from rice-based ecosystems in Cambodia, China, Laos and Vietnam documented 145 species of fish, 11 species of crustaceans, 15 species of molluscs, 13 species of reptiles, 11 species of amphibians, 11 species of insects and 37 species of plants directly caught or collected from the rice fields and utilized by rural people during one season (Halwart and Bartley, 2005). Fish usually constitute the major part. Fish plays a major role in supplying food and some income among the groups encountered. Most of it is consumed fresh, but there are a number of ways to preserve it for periods when the supply of fresh fish is interrupted. Among these, drying and fermenting are the most common methods, but fish is also preserved in salt, or smoked; and some aquatic organisms are preserved in alcohol to be used as medicine (Halwart and Bartley, 2005).

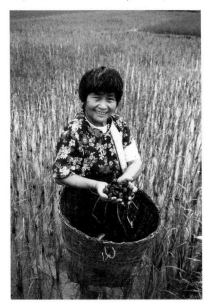

Figure 4.3 Snails are being collected regularly from flooded rice fields in P.R. China (Photo: FAO/Aidong Luo)

Fish consumption and composition

In 2009, fish accounted for 16.6 per cent of the global population's intake of animal protein and 6.4 per cent of all protein consumed. Globally, fish provides about 2.9 billion people with almost 20 per cent of their average per capita intake of animal protein, and 4.2 billion people with 15 per cent of such proteins. Annual per capita fish consumption grew from an average of 9.9 kg in the 1960s to 12.6 kg in the 1980s, and reached 17.8 kg in 2007. Of the 17.8 kg of fish per capita available for consumption about 75 per cent came from finfish. Shellfish supplied 25 per cent (or about 4.1 kg per capita), subdivided into 1.6 kg of crustaceans, 0.6 kg of cephalopods and 1.9 kg of other molluscs. Freshwater and diadromous species accounted for about 36.4 million tonnes of the total supply, whereas marine finfish species provided about 48.1 million tonnes (FAO, 2010).

In agricultural landscapes, fish consumption may vary between poorer and richer households. Studies conducted in several Asian countries found that low-income households depend largely on fish as their major animal protein source but generally consume less fish than high-income households (Dey et al., 2005). Another study found that fish in poorer households are often consumed in the 'low-income vegetable-scarce months', when other sources of micronutrients such as vegetables are not available or affordable (Islam, 2007). Significantly higher consumption of fish was found in Nigeria in households engaged in capture fisheries (Gomna and Rana, 2007). Seasonality is another important factor influencing fish harvests, processing and consumption, with cured products being critically important in the diets of rural households during times of low wild fish availability.

Inland aquaculture and integrated agriculture and aquaculture systems usually lead to an increase in household consumption of fish (Prein and Ahmed, 2000). However, as pointed out by Kawarazuka and Béné (2010), this relationship is not straightforward since farmed aquatic products are often viewed as a cash crop rather than a food crop, and the income generated from aquaculture is rarely used to buy smaller lower value fish from the market. Alim et al. (2004) stated that farmers should be given an option so that they could continue to sell their precious cash crop and feed their family with other fish of low market value. A technology of simultaneous culture of popular large carps (as a cash crop) and cheap but nutritious small fish (to feed the family) may satisfy both these needs (Thilsted, 2012). For capture fisheries, case studies from Laos and Papua New Guinea reveal big differences as to whether the majority of the fish caught are being kept for home consumption or not.

Reliable information from published sources on nutritional composition of consumed aquatic organisms is scarce. The importance of fish as a source of animal protein and essential fatty acids is well documented and often cited. A recent expert consultation on the risks and benefits of fish consumption highlighted the importance of fish consumption in order to secure an optimal development of the brain and neural system of children (FAO/WHO, 2011). Several more recent studies stress the role of fish as a source of micronutrients.

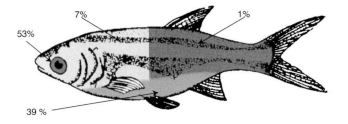

Figure 4.4 Distribution of vitamin A in *Amblypharyngodon mola* (with kind permission after Thorseng 2006, original data from Roos et al., 2002)

Small sized fish are of particular importance since they are consumed whole including bones, heads and organs where concentration of micronutrients is highest (Figure 4.4). Table 4.2 summarizes the data (modified after James, 2006).

DFID (2001) provided indications on the importance of proteins from aquatic organisms in the diet in Southeast Asia. In Northeast Thailand, 72–82 per cent of animal protein consumed in the wet season in Yasothon province comprises wild aquatic resources, derived from rice fields. In Cambodia, fish and fish products account for 70–75 per cent of the dietary protein intake of the population. In Lao PDR, fish had traditionally contributed 85 per cent of animal protein intake. A survey in Luang Prabang province found fish to represent 50–55 per cent of animal protein intake. Fish still represents the largest component of animal protein in the diet. In Viet Nam, fish in An Giang Province contributes nearly 76 per cent of the average person's supply of animal protein, although the role of aquatic resources in the diet of Northern Provinces is considerably less.

Aquatic organisms supply essential and limiting micronutrients that are not found in rice (or found in limited quantities), particularly calcium, iron, zinc and vitamin A. The nutrient content in different fish species may vary by several orders of magnitude (Tetens et al., 1998). As mentioned before, the small fish are of particular importance since they are usually eaten whole. Kawarazuka and Béné (2011) collected evidence from case studies which confirmed the high levels of vitamin A, iron and zinc in some of the small fish species in developing countries. These small fish are reported to be more affordable and accessible than the larger fish and other usual animal-source foods and vegetables. Evidence suggests that these locally available small fish have considerable potential as cost-effective food-based strategies to enhance micronutrient intakes or as a complementary food for undernourished children (Table 4.3).

Hansen et al. (1998) showed that small (4–10 cm) fish eaten with the bones as part of the everyday diet in many Asian countries contribute considerable amounts of calcium. The recommended daily calcium intake for adults can be met by eating 34–43 g of these fresh small fish daily, collecting them from rice fields, ponds and ditches. In Bangladesh, Roos et al. (2007) found that the consumption of small fish contributed 31 per cent of total calcium intake. Similar considerations apply for vitamin A, as this is found particularly in eyes

Table 4.2 Summary of compositional data, per 100 g fresh weight basis

	Protein (g)		Fat (g)		Ca (mg)		Fe (mg)		Vitamin A (μg)	
	Min	Max	Min	Max	Min	Max	Min	Max	Min	Max
Fish	9.7	22.7	0.8	8.0	17	1751	0.6	9.2	5	1800
Crustaceans	10.7	21.2	0.9	3.3	75	5000	0.6	7.5	0	133
Molluscs	7.0	20.2	0.3	1.4	16	2500	7.0	26.6	0	243
Frogs	15.1	20.2	0.2	2.0	19	1293	0.7	3.8	Low	
Insects	3.5	26.2	1.4	8.3	6	120	1.8	30.0	N/D	
Recommended intake, adults, per day*	0.79 g/kg body wt or 10–15% of energy		Min 15% of energy		600–1000 mg		5–24 mg		450–600 μg	

*Modified after James, 2006

Table 4.3 Content of vitamin A and calcium in small and big Bangladeshi fish species (per 100 g raw edible part).

Fish species	Vitamin A μg	Calcium mg
Small indigenous fish		
Mola (*Amblypharyngodon mola*)	1960	1071
Dhela (*Rohtee cotio*)	937	1260
Chanda (*Chanda* sp.)	341	1162
Puti (*Puntius* spp.)	37	1059
Big fish		
Hilsa (*Hilsa ilisha*)	69	126
Rui (*Labeo rohita*)	27	317
Silver carp (*Hypophthalmichthys molitrix*)	17	268

Source: Tetens et al., 1998

and viscera of small fish (Roos et al., 2002). In Bangladesh, it is commonly believed that the small fish mola (*Amblypharyngodon mola*) is 'good for your eyes', a perception that may have originated from indigenous knowledge that night blindness can be cured by eating mola. Roos et al. (2003) found that the consumption of small fish contributed up to 40 per cent of total vitamin A intake.

Iron deficiency is a widespread nutritional disorder in developing countries. In Cambodia, 16 fish species were screened for iron contents. One local small fish species, *Esomus longimanus,* which is found in ponds, canals and ditches has a higher iron content (451 mg Fe/kg dry matter, $SD = 155$, $n = 4$) than other species. In a field study, 30 rural women were interviewed about traditional use of this species and their cleaning and cooking practices were observed. The amounts of fish consumed were recorded and meal samples were collected for iron analysis. Calculations based on the iron content and a high bioavailability of Hm-Fe showed that a traditional fish meal (sour soup) covered 45 per cent of the daily iron requirement for women (Roos et al., 2007).

Another group of particular nutritional importance is the essential fatty acids which are critical for maternal, fetal and neonatal nutrition. The health attributes of fish are particularly due to long-chain n-3 polyunsaturated fatty acids. However, it has been noted that fish contain many other important nutrients that also contribute to the health benefits of fish, and the health effects of fish consumption may be greater than the sum of the individual constituents (FAO/WHO, 2011). Eating fish is also part of the cultural traditions of many peoples. In some countries, where viable options for substitute foods are extremely limited, fish is the major source of protein and other essential nutrients. A review of the potential benefits of fish for maternal, fetal and neonatal nutrition is provided by Elvevoll and James (2000).

Many rural farmer and fisher families in developing countries cannot obtain a sufficient variety of nutritious food in their local markets or are simply too poor to purchase it. Cultivated species may be complemented by harvested wild species that can be of particular significance for indigenous communities and for poor and vulnerable communities, especially in times of shortage of main staples. Wild and gathered foods, including from the aquatic habitat, therefore provide important diversity, nutrition and food security (Halwart and Bartley, 2007). Available information on nutrient composition of aquatic species and their consumption is limited, and sometimes inadequate (Halwart, 2006).

Case study: Laos

The role of aquatic ricefield species in rural Laotian diets has been underestimated, as almost 200 species are consumed, supplying a range of nutrients needed by the villagers. A recent consumption study in Laos shows that rice fields are the source of about two-thirds of all aquatic organisms consumed by rural households, whilst for fish alone it is about 50 per cent. About one-third of all consumed organisms are frogs and most of these come from rice fields (Box 4.2).

Nevertheless, national and regional food composition databases contain limited information on the nutritional composition of these species. The aquatic animals consumed on a daily basis contained high amounts of protein (11.6–19.7 per cent for fish, crustaceans, molluscs, amphibians and insects and 3.3–7.8 per cent for fermented fish), and a generally acceptable essential amino acid profile. They were also excellent sources of calcium, iron and zinc. However, they had low contents of fat (0.1–4.6 per cent), fatty acids and vitamin A. Essential amino acids, iron and zinc are nutrients that are scarce in rural Laotian diets. As the food supply of rural households in rice farming areas of Laos is critically dependent on the environment, the sustainable existence of the ricefield aquatic animals is a crucial factor for the nutritional status of the Laotians (Nurhasan et al., 2010).

Box 4.2 Aquatic biodiversity and nutrition: the contribution of rice-based ecosystems in the Lao PDR

A monthly household survey has been conducted in 240 households in three provinces of the Lao PDR which were selected to represent the different topographical and agro-ecological zones of the country. The survey yielded information on acquisition, amount and uses of fish and other aquatic animals (OAAs) based on 24-hour recall of the respondents over a one-year period ending October 2007. Data were obtained on catch and habitats, species and biodiversity, household consumption of fish and OAAs, and relationship between catches and village resources/village pesticide use.

The results of this survey show that rice fields contribute far more to people's livelihood and food security than just the rice alone: Two-thirds of all the aquatic animals and 50% of all fish consumed by the surveyed households come from the ricefield habitat:

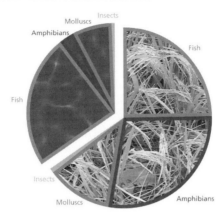

Generally, habitats outside the ricefield zone play a more important role as food source for rural people in the dry season, while the importance of habitats within the rice-based ecosystem increases significantly in the wet season. Exceptional in this respect are frogs which make up around one-third of all the aquatic animals consumed and are thus second in importance for food supply after the fish. Frogs are caught predominantly in the rice fields, even in the dry season:

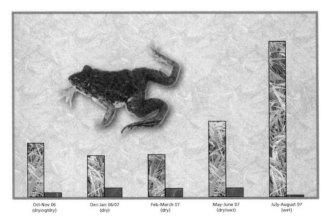

The study has impressively demonstrated that ricefield habitats including the rice fields themselves, natural ponds/trap ponds in rice fields and rice field streams/canals are important for aquatic animals which in turn are important as an everyday source of food for the people in rural areas.

Source: FAO/LARReC 2007

Valuing small fish and integrated production systems

Historically, fish were mostly captured and collected from the 'wild', including from agricultural production systems. Due to a combination of factors, and largely driven by a steady human population increase, these common resources have declined. Aquaculture can make up for the deficit but whether this will have the desired nutritional effects for local households will depend among others on the appropriate selection of aquatic species and the broader species composition in various production systems. Nutrient dense small sized fish species can be cultured alongside larger aquatic species to allow for both food-based and cash crop aquaculture and nutrition development strategies. Not enough attention has been paid so far to these small self-recruiting species and their potential in aquaculture development, particularly their potential to combat micronutrient deficiencies of vulnerable parts of the society such as pregnant and lactating women and small children. In addition, more attention should be paid to processing methods for dual reasons of improved fish availability during lean periods and reducing post-harvest losses.

Because of the multiple uses of inland waters, integration of such use becomes important and constitutes other hierarchies of biodiversity at the ecosystem and landscape levels. The requirements of fish and fisheries should be duly taken into consideration in planning and management. Where watersheds have been modified by hydro-electric development, mitigation measures need to be implemented, e.g. habitat rehabilitation, specific water-management programmes and fish-passage systems, to protect species that depend on longitudinal and lateral movements to complete their life cycle successfully.

Although rural people in developing countries may refer to themselves as farmers, the use of inland resources is often an integrated part of their livelihoods. The frequency and the ways in which they use aquatic organisms vary seasonally and with the cultural and geographic setting. Agricultural policies need to ensure that fishing or aquaculture which takes place in rice paddies are valued in economic as well as nutritional terms, taking into due account farmers' motivation to farm without the use of pesticides because the animals serve as natural predators and grazers. Animals in rice paddies can either be natural components of biodiversity that are 'trapped' in the paddies, or they can be purposefully stocked, such as many tilapia, barb and carp species. Especially in small-scale production systems, pond culture of larger fish intended for sale can be complemented by the concurrent culture of smaller nutrient-dense fish intended for household consumption. Agricultural policies should encourage such integrated use.

Agriculture and aquaculture can form integrated farming systems where nutrients are cycled between production components, where fish ponds can provide a source of water for irrigation, and where irrigation systems can be fished. Aquaculture is further used to support culture-based fisheries. There is also a trend for inland water biodiversity to be supplemented or even constructed to maximize benefits from the modified systems.

Clearly, enough attention has not been given to the aquatic diversity naturally found in agricultural ecosystems and its importance to rural livelihoods. Raising awareness and making this aquatic biodiversity in rice 'visible' is important and supported by relevant international codes and guidelines (FAO, 1995, 2005). As the first international forum, the International Rice Commission (IRC) has recognized the above results and recommended that 'Member countries should promote the sustainable development of aquatic biodiversity in rice-based ecosystems, and policy decisions and management measures should enhance the living aquatic resource base' (FAO, 2002). This was followed by a recommendation from the 21st IRC Session in 2006 stating that 'Member countries should, when appropriate, promote at all levels – particularly through national agriculture and rice development programmes and policies – the development and transfer of integrated rice–fish systems to enhance economic competitiveness of rice production, human nutrition, rural income and employment opportunities. Promotion should be based on identification of suitable areas, selection of nutrient-rich local aquatic species and appropriate farming practices. Under marginal rice-production conditions such as low-yield monsoon seasons new agro-enterprise such as aquaculture can lead to improved income and food security. An expert meeting to explore these options and to guide pilot development is recommended.'

Similarly, the Convention on Biological Diversity (CBD) at its 10th Conference of Parties welcomed Resolution X.31 of the tenth meeting of the Conference of the Parties to the Convention on Wetlands (Ramsar, Iran, 1971) on the subject 'Enhancing biodiversity in rice paddies as wetland systems', noting the culture of rice in 114 countries worldwide, that rice paddies (flooded and irrigated fields in which rice is grown) have provided large areas of open water for centuries and that they support a high level of rice associated biodiversity important for sustaining rice paddy ecosystems, as well as providing many other ecosystem services. The CBD adopted decision X/34 on Agricultural Biodiversity, recognizing the importance of agro-ecosystems for the conservation and sustainable use of biodiversity, and invited the Food and Agriculture Organization of the United Nations to undertake further studies on the valuation of the biodiversity and ecosystem services provided by agricultural ecosystems, in order to further support policy-relevant guidance to Parties for consideration by the Conference of the Parties at its eleventh meeting.

Various alternatives of integration of aquaculture have been examined and reviewed (e.g. Pullin and Shehadeh, 1980; Little and Muir, 1987; FAO et al., 2001; Halwart and Gupta, 2004; Morales et al., 2006) and show that this type of farming efficiently uses land, water and nutrients producing high-quality food. However, this has clearly not been a sufficient enough precondition for their wider acceptance and distribution. More recently, new approaches taking better into account the socio-economic circumstances of farming communities are being tried and supported through FAO and partners' work in countries such as Burkina Faso, Cambodia, Guyana, Lao PDR, Mali, or Suriname, following a Farmer Field School (FFS) approach which is a discovery based learning approach where small groups of farmers meet regularly facilitated by a specially trained technician, to explore new methods, through simple experimentation and group discussion and analysis, over the course of a growing season. This allows farmers to modify and adapt newly introduced methods to local contexts and knowledge, ultimately providing a higher likelihood of appropriate adaptation and adoption of improved technologies. It is only relatively recently that aquaculture has been integrated into an FFS-style curriculum (Halwart and Settle, 2008). The validation and dissemination of integrated fish farming in rice-based systems through Farmer Field Schools is currently being tested in field activities in Mali and Burkina Faso (Yamamoto et al., 2012), where considerable potential for the integration of irrigation and aquaculture exists (Halwart and Van Dam, 2006).

It is now important that countries mainstream successful experiences from farming communities and corresponding recommendations from international fora into their agricultural and nutritional development plans, policies and strategies, as is currently the case in Lao PDR (Vatthanatham et al., 2007). Ultimately, the understanding of the value of aquatic biodiversity from agricultural ecosystems for food and nutrition needs to be well integrated into national agricultural systems that embrace the concepts of an ecosystem approach and the role of agricultural biodiversity for people and the environment.

Acknowledgements

The author would like to thank colleagues and friends in FAO who have contributed to SOFIA and World Aquaculture 2010 which provided basic information for this chapter, and to FAO Aquaculture Statistician Xiaowei Zhou who ensured that accurate and most recent information is being reported. Jogeir Toppe provided valuable comments on an earlier draft. Claudia Aguado-Castillo assisted with the copy-editing of the chapter. This chapter was realized thanks to the encouragement of Danny Hunter of Bioversity which is also gratefully acknowledged.

Note

The views expressed in this publication are those of the author(s) and do not necessarily reflect the views of the Food and Agriculture Organization of the United Nations

References

Ainsworth, D., Aitken, S., Catling, P., Dang, P.T., Douglas, H., Fraleigh, B., Hall, P., Parker, D., Pratt, N., Small, E. (eds) (2008) 'The value of biodiversity to food and agriculture', *Biodiversity – Journal of life on earth*, vol 9, numbers 1&2, http://eusoils.jrc. ec.europa.eu/esdb_archive/eusoils_docs/Pub/Biodiversity.pdf

Alim, M.A., Wahab, M.A. and Milstein, A. (2004) 'Effects of adding different proportions of the small fish punti (*Puntius sophore*) and mola (*Amblypharyngodon mola*) to a polyculture of large carp', *Aquaculture Research,* vol 35, pp.124–133.

De Benoist, B., McLean, E., Egli, I., Cogswell, M. (eds) (2008) 'Worldwide prevalence of anaemia 1993–2005', *WHO Global Database on Anaemia*, WHO, Geneva. p.40.

Dey, M.M., Rab, M.A., Paraguas, F.J., Piumsombun, S., Bhatta, R., Alam, M.F., Ahmed, M. (2005) 'Fish consumption and food security: a disaggregated analysis by types of fish and classes of consumers in selected Asian countries', *Aquaculture Economics and Management,* vol 9 pp.89–111.

DFID (2001) 'Aquatic resources management for sustainable livelihoods of poor people', pp.11–16, in IIRR, IDRC, FAO, NACA and ICLARM, *Utilizing Different Aquatic Resources for Livelihoods in Asia: a resource book.* International Institute of Rural Reconstruction, International Development Research Centre, Food and Agriculture Organization of the United Nations, Network of Aquaculture Centers in Asia-Pacific and International Center for Living Aquatic Resources Management.

Elvevoll, E.O. and James, D.G. (2000) 'Potential benefits of fish for maternal, fetal and neonatal nutrition: a review of the literature', *Food, Nutrition and Agriculture*, vol 27, pp.28–39.

European Commission (2000) *Fisheries and Poverty Reduction*, Communication from the Commission to the Council and the European Parliament. Commission of the European Communities, Brussels, p.20, http://ec.europa.eu/development/icenter/repository/COM_2000_0724_en.pdf, accessed July 2012.

FAO (1995) *Code of Conduct for Responsible Fisheries*, Rome, FAO, p.41.

FAO (2002) Report of the 20th Session of the International Rice Commission held in Bangkok, Thailand from 23–26 July 2002, FAO, Rome, p.46.

FAO (2005) 'Voluntary guidelines to support the progressive realization of the right to adequate food in the context of national food security', adopted by the 127th Session of the FAO Council, November 2004.

FAO (2010) *The State of the World Fisheries and Aquaculture 2010,* FAO, Rome, p.197.

FAO (2011a) *The State of Food and Agriculture 2010–2011. Part II – World food and agriculture in review – Trends in undernourishment*, FAO, Rome, p.147.

FAO (2011b) *World aquaculture 2010,* FAO Fisheries and Aquaculture Department, Technical Paper, no 500/1, Rome, p.105.

FAO (2012a) *Aquaculture production statistics dataset (quantity and value) 1950–2010*, FAO, Rome.

FAO (2012b) 'FAO International Expert Workshop Improving the Information Base for Aquatic Genetic Resources for The State of the World's Aquatic Genetic Resources', Madrid, Spain, 1–4 March 2011, Rome, p.57.

FAO, IIRR and ICLARM (2001) 'Integrated agriculture-aquaculture: a primer', *FAO Fisheries Technical Paper*, no 407, Rome, p.149.

FAO/LARReC (2007) 'Aquatic biodiversity in rice-based ecosystems for Lao PDR', Technical Paper, FAO – Netherlands Partnership Programme (FNPP) 2006–2007 (unpublished).

FAO/MRC (2003) 'New approaches for the improvement of inland capture fishery statistics in the Mekong Basin', Report of the Ad Hoc Expert Consultation held in Udon Thani, Thailand, 2–5 September 2002, FAO/RAP Publication 2003/01, FAO/RAP, Bangkok, p.145.

FAO/NACA (2012) *Farming the Waters for People and Food*, R.P. Subasinghe, J.R. Arthur, D.M. Bartley, S.S. De Silva, M. Halwart, N. Hishamunda, C.V. Mohan and P. Sorgeloos (eds) Proceedings of the Global Conference on Aquaculture 2010, Phuket, Thailand, 22–25 September 2010, FAO, Rome and NACA, Bangkok, p.896.

FAO/WHO (2011) 'Report of the Joint FAO/WHO Expert Consultation on the Risks and Benefits of Fish Consumption', *FAO Fisheries and Aquaculture Report* no 978,

Rome, Food and Agriculture Organization of the United Nations; Geneva, World Health Organization, p.50.

Froese, R. and Pauly, D. (eds) (2012) *FishBase*, online, www.fishbase.org, accessed July 2012.

Gomna, A. and Rana, K. (2007) 'Inter-household and intra-household patterns of fish and meat consumption in fishing communities in two states in Nigeria', *British Journal of Nutrition*, vol 97, no 1, pp.145–152.

Greer, D. and B. Harvey (2004) *Blue Genes – sharing and conserving the world's aquatic biodiversity*, Earthscan and IDRC.

Halwart, M. (2003) 'Recent initiatives on the availability and use of aquatic organisms in rice-based farming', pp.195–205, in Dat van Tran (eds) *International Rice Commission – Sustainable rice production for food security*. Proceedings of the 20th Session of the International Rice Commission, Bangkok, Thailand, 23–26 July 2002.

Halwart, M. (2006) 'Biodiversity and nutrition in rice-based aquatic ecosystems', *Journal of Food Composition and Analysis,* vol 19, pp.747–751.

Halwart, M. (2008) 'Biodiversity, nutrition and livelihoods in aquatic rice-based systems', *Biodiversity: Journal of Life on Earth,* vol 9, no 1 and 2, *Special Biodiversity & Agriculture*, CBD & IDRC, pp.36–40.

Halwart, M. and Bartley, D. (eds) (2005) *Aquatic biodiversity in rice-based ecosystems. Studies and reports from Cambodia, China, Lao PDR and Viet Nam*. [CD-ROM], Rome, FAO, ftp://ftp.fao.org/FI/CDrom/AqBiodCD20Jul2005/Start.pdf, accessed July 2012.

Halwart, M. and Bartley, D. (2007) 'Aquatic biodiversity in rice-based ecosystems', pp.181–199, in D.I. Jarvis, C. Padoch and H.D. Cooper (eds) *Managing biodiversity in agricultural ecosystems*, Columbia University Press, p.492.

Halwart, M. and Gupta, M.V. (2004) *Culture of fish in rice fields*, FAO and the WorldFish Center, Penang Malaysia.

Halwart, M. and Settle, W. (eds) (2008) 'Participatory training and curriculum development for Farmer Field Schools in Guyana and Suriname', *A field guide on Integrated Pest Management and aquaculture in rice*. Rome, FAO, pp.116, http://www.fao.org/docrep/012/ba0031e/ba0031e.pdf, accessed July 2012.

Halwart, M. and Van Dam, A.A. (2006) 'Development of integrated irrigated and aquaculture in West Africa: the way forward', in M. Halwart and A.A. van Dam, (eds) *Integrated irrigation and aquaculture in West Africa: concepts, practices and potential*, pp.169–174, Rome, FAO, p.181.

Halwart, M., Bartley, D., Burlingame, B., Funge-Smith, S., James, D. (2006) 'FAO Regional Technical Expert Workshop on aquatic biodiversity, its nutritional composition, and human consumption in rice-based systems', *Journal of Food Composition and Analysis,* vol 19, pp.752–755.

Hansen, M., Thilsted, S.H., Sandström, B., Kongsbak, K., Larsen, T., Jensen, M. and Sorensen, S.S. (1998) 'Calcium absorption from small soft boned fish', *J. Trace Elements Med. Biol.,* vol 12: pp.148–154.

ICTSD (2006) *Fisheries, International Trade and Sustainable Development,* International Centre for Trade and Sustainable Development, Geneva, http://www.thew2o.net/events/highseas/docs/Fish_policypaper_exec.pdf, accessed July 2012.

Islam, F.U. (2007) *Self-recruiting species in aquaculture: Their role in rural livelihoods in two areas of Bangladesh*, https://dspace.stir.ac.uk/bitstream/1893/206/1/Islam%20AFU-PhD%20Thesis_2007.pdf, accessed July 2012.

James, D. (2006) 'The impact of aquatic biodiversity on the nutrition of rice farming households in the Mekong Basin: Consumption and composition of aquatic resources', *Journal of Food Composition and Analysis,* vol 19, pp.756–757.

Jarvis, D.I., Padoch, C., Cooper, H.D. (eds) (2007) *Managing biodiversity in agricultural ecosystems,* Columbia University Press, pp.492.

Jensen, I.J., Mæhre, H.K., Tømmerås, S., Eilertsen, K.E., Olsen, R.L. and Elvevoll, E.O. (2012) 'Farmed Atlantic salmon (*Salmo salar L.*) is a good source of long chain omega-3 fatty acids', *Nutrition Bulletin,* vol 37, no 25–29. doi: 10.1111/j.1467-3010.2011.01941.x.

Kawarazuka, N. and Béné, C. (2010). 'Linking small-scale fisheries and aquaculture to household nutritional security: an overview', *Food Security* 2: pp.343–357.

Kawarazuka, N. and Béné, C. (2011) 'The potential role of small fish species in improving micronutrient deficiencies in developing countries: building evidence', *Public Health Nutrition,* vol 14, no 11, pp.1927–1938.

Little, D. and Muir, J. (1987) 'A guide to integrated warm water aquaculture', *Institute of Aquaculture Publications,* University of Stirling, Scotland, UK.

MAF/FAO (2007) *Aquatic biodiversity and human nutrition – the contribution of rice-based ecosystems,* Ministry of Agriculture and Forestry Laos and FAO, Rome, ftp://ftp.fao.org/docrep/fao/010/ai759e/ai759e04.pdf, accessed July 2012.

Meusch, E., Yhoung-Aree, J., Friend, R. and Funge-Smith, S. (2003) *The role and nutritional value of aquatic resources in the livelihoods of rural people, A participatory assessment in Attapeu Province, Lao PDR.* FAO/LARReC/IUCN, Bangkok, Thailand, ftp://ftp.fao.org/docrep/Fao/004/AD454e/ad454e00.pdf, accessed July 2012.

Morales, E.J., Little, D.C., Immink, A., Demaine, H., Yakupitayage, A., Amilhat, E., Lorenzen, K. (2006) 'Project report: Contribution of self-recruiting species produced in farmer-managed aquatic systems in rural areas of Southeast Asia to food consumption', *Journal of Food Composition and Analysis,* vol 19: pp.759–760.

Nurhasan, M., Maehre, H.K., Malde, M.K., Stormo, S. K., Halwart, M., James, D., Elvevoll, E.O. (2010) 'Nutritional composition of aquatic species in Laotian rice field ecosystems', *Journal of Food Composition and Analysis,* vol 23, pp.205–213.

Prein, M. and Ahmed, M. (2000) 'Integration of aquaculture into smallholder farming systems for improved food security and household nutrition', *Food and Nutrition Bulletin,* vol 21, pp.466–471.

Pullin, R.S.V. and Shehadeh, Z.H. (1980) *Integrated agriculture–aquaculture farming systems,* International Center for Living Aquatic Resources Management (WorldFish Center), Penang, Malaysia.

Roos, N., Leth, T., Jakobsen, J., and Thilsted, S.H. (2002), 'High vitamin A content in some small indigenous fish species in Bangladesh: perspectives for food-based strategies to reduce vitamin A deficiency', *Int. J. Food Sci. Nutr.,* vol 53: pp.425–437.

Roos, N., Islam, M.M., Thilsted, S.H. (2003) 'Small indigenous fish species in Bangladesh: contribution to vitamin A, calcium and iron intakes', *Journal of Nutrition,* vol 133, pp.4021–4026.

Roos, N., Thorseng, H., Chamnan, C., Larsen, T., Gondolf, U., Bukhave, K., Thilsted, S.H. (2007) 'Iron content in common Cambodian fish species: Perspectives for dietary iron intake in poor, rural households', *Food Chemistry,* vol 104, pp.1226–1235.

Swaminathan, M.S. (2012) 'Aquaculture and sustainable nutrition security in a warming planet', Keynote Address 1, in R.P. Subasinghe, J.R. Arthur, D.M. Bartley, S.S. De Silva, M. Halwart, N. Hishamunda, C.V. Mohan and P. Sorgeloos (eds) *Farming the Waters for People and Food.* Proceedings of the Global Conference on Aquaculture

2010, Phuket, Thailand. 22–25 September 2010, pp.3–19, FAO, Rome and NACA, Bangkok.

Tetens, I., Thilsted, S.H., Choudhury, N.H., Hassan, N. (1998) 'The rice-based diet in Bangladesh in the context of food and nutrition security', *Scandinavian Journal of Nutrition,* vol 42, pp.77–80.

Thilsted, S.H. (2012) 'The potential of nutrient-rich small fish species in aquaculture to improve human nutrition and health', in R.P. Subasinghe, J.R. Arthur, D.M. Bartley, S.S. De Silva, M. Halwart, N. Hishamunda, C.V. Mohan and P. Sorgeloos (eds) *Farming the Waters for People and Food.* Proceedings of the Global Conference on Aquaculture 2010, Phuket, Thailand, 22–25 September 2010, pp.57–73. FAO, Rome and NACA, Bangkok.

Thorseng, H. (2006) 'Contribution of iron from *Esomus longimanus* to the Cambodian diet: studies on content and in vitro availability', MSc thesis. Frederiksberg, Denmark: Department of Human Nutrition, The Royal Veterinary and Agricultural University 2005 – data presented at the National Conference on Prioritizing Fisheries for Cambodia's National Development and Community Aspiration, organized by IFReDI/DoF, WorldFish Center and CDRI at Sihanoukville, Cambodia. 14–15 February 2006.

Tutwiler, A. (2012) *Global Forum on Food Security and Nutrition. Digest* no 947, 'Linking Agriculture, Food Systems and Nutrition: What's your perspective?' FSN Forum.

Vatthanatham, K., Phothitay, C., Roger, K., Khamsivilay, L., Garaway, C., Bamrungrach, P. and Halwart, M. (2007) 'Importance of aquatic biodiversity in rice-based ecosystems: policy impact in Lao PDR', in *Book of Abstracts, Fisheries and Aquaculture: Strategic outlook for Asia,* 8th Asian Fisheries Forum, 20–23 November 2007, Kochi, India, pp.244–245.

Welcomme, R. (2011a) 'Review of the state of the world fishery resources: Inland fisheries', *FAO Fisheries and Aquaculture Circular,* no 942, Rev. 2, Rome, FAO, pp.97.

Welcomme, R.L. (2011b) 'An overview of global inland fish-catch statistics: International', *Journal of Marine Science,* FDI special issue, no 3529.

WHO (2009) 'Global prevalence of vitamin A deficiency in populations at risk 1995–2005', WHO Global Database on Vitamin A Deficiency, World Health Organization, Geneva, pp.55.

Yamamoto, K., Halwart, M. and Hishamunda, N. (2012), 'FAO supports African rice farmers in their diversification efforts through aquaculture', *FAO Aquaculture Newsletter,* vol 48, pp. 42–3.

Part II

Creating an enabling environment

5   Lessons from sub-Saharan Africa

Delivery mechanisms for mobilizing
agricultural biodiversity for improved
food and nutrition security

Hervé B. D. Bisseleua and Amadou Ibra Niang

Introduction

Recent international fora have emphasized the importance of biodiversity for
food security and health. The World Summit on Sustainable Development
(WSSD) in Johannesburg, South Africa, 2002, emphasized the interconnections
among five focal areas (WEHAB) including health, agriculture and biodiversity
necessary for achieving long-term sustainability. A Decision (CBD Decision
VII/32) of the Conference of the Parties (COP7) of the Convention on
Biodiversity taken in Kuala Lumpur, 2004, specifically calls for a strengthened
focus on biodiversity for food and nutrition. A resolution accompanying the
adoption of the World Health Organization Global Strategy on Diet, Physical
Activity and Health (WHO, 2004), includes explicit reference to traditional and
indigenous diets.

The global struggle against poverty and hunger cannot be won without
increased collaboration in the conservation, and sustainable and fair use of
agricultural biodiversity. Diversity can also help improve productivity by
raising yield stability, contributing to pest and disease control, and improving
the environment (Flood, 2010). Meeting the Millennium Development Goals
(MDGs) will require political will, financial commitment and a readiness to
attempt innovative solutions. The very fact that 10 years after the adoption of
these goals, most African countries have been unable to make proportionate
progress in the elimination of hunger and poverty indicates the need for an
overall change in the manner in which we have addressed this challenge to date.
Without such a change we will not achieve the goal of a hunger-free world.

Agricultural biodiversity plays a central role in household food security and
income generation, and thus in achieving MDG1 of halving the proportion
of hungry and extremely poor people by 2015. However, its wider use to
address nutritional deficiencies and other aspects of poverty, all of paramount
importance, is yet to be fully realized. Today, undernutrition still persists
in the vast majority of African countries, affecting in particular, women and
children. This translates into a low consumption of essential micronutrients,
the result of which is a high prevalence of micronutrient deficiency related
diseases, and reduced capacity to fight the debilitating effects of diseases such

as malaria and HIV/AIDS (Underwood, 2000). Reducing undernutrition has therefore become a key objective of the MDGs and many African countries and international development organizations around the world are helping Africa to achieve this objective. This chapter outlines a cross-cutting approach to using agricultural biodiversity for food and nutrition in Africa with examples taken from the Millennium Villages Project.

Linking agricultural biodiversity conservation and nutrition in sub-Saharan Africa (SSA)

The world has made great strides in reducing hunger, yet the problem of malnutrition, particularly the 'hidden hunger' caused by missing micronutrients, constitutes a formidable challenge for the future. Biodiversity has a crucial role to play in mitigating the effects of micronutrient deficiencies, which are debilitating hundreds of thousands of people in sub-Saharan Africa, particularly children and women. In the developing world, people turned to fashionable 'modern' foods and abandoned the traditional diet as 'backward' and 'poor'. In the West, however, people are looking to some traditional diets, for example those of East Asia and the Mediterranean, as a source of inspiration about nutrition and health. Indeed, many of the epidemiological connections between diet and health have come from an observation of traditional peoples and the peculiarities of their food intake and health. The importance of plant sterols, omega-3 fatty acids, and other dietary components in reducing diseases has been established largely through the study of traditional diets that are associated with longevity and good health (Johns and Eyzaguirre, 2007).

Farmers and others, however, are well aware of these types of differences and often describe certain kinds of food, and indeed certain varieties or landraces, as having particular nutritional or therapeutic value. Ethiopian farmers, for example, recognized certain varieties of sorghum as having value for sick children and nursing mothers (NRC, 1996). The Luo people of western Kenya say that the leafy vegetables that form an important part of the traditional diet protect against gastro-intestinal helminthes and other disturbances (Johns et al., 1995).

A 2001 survey of household agricultural production in Mali revealed that the poorest rural household produces little more than cereals (rice, millet and maize) and spent almost 50 per cent of their total household expenditures on vegetable crops and legumes. Studies also revealed that the poorest families purchase food in the market often, resulting in a diet with very little diversity. Therefore, the likelihood of nutritional status being improved is tied to the improvement of diet diversity where nutritious food is available.

There is certainly some evidence that a varied diet is beneficial (Tucker, 2001). In Kenya, Onyango et al. (1998) demonstrated that diversity in the diet has clear beneficial effects on the development of young children up to three years old. However, the challenge is to collect this type of nutritional and health information using sound anthropometric methods and then to relate it to other kinds of analyses such as epidemiological and biochemical investigations.

Food composition provides an important link for biodiversity and nutrition, which are generally considered to be unrelated fields. Even though the terms genetic resources, ecosystems and biodiversity may not be part of the mainstream nutrition vocabulary, nutrition improvement activities have long embraced the concepts. In the nutrition science community, biodiversity has always been considered in the context of food and nutrients, with a focus on wild and gathered species or varieties, and underutilized and underexploited food resources. For instance throughout Africa, in the Millennium Villages Project (MVP)[1] areas of East and West Africa, hundreds of species of leafy vegetables – some cultivated, some gathered from the wild – find their way into people's diets. In many cases they contain considerably more minerals and vitamins than introduced crops such as cabbage (Bisseleua, personal communication). In addition, it leads us logically to one of the basic principles of nutrition/dietary diversity. Food composition is therefore a useful vehicle to explore certain synergies and develop common ground between biodiversity and nutrition.

Agricultural biodiversity in the wider context of the Millennium Development Goals

Livelihoods and economies in Africa depend critically on the ecosystem that land and its associated biodiversity provide. The populations of most African countries depend on agriculture for their livelihoods and still are barely able to feed themselves (Rouxel et al., 2005). Poverty and hunger are related and accelerated by food insecurity. The food security situation depends largely on domestic production which, in turn, depends on the amount of agricultural biodiversity available. However, this biodiversity is threatened by socio-economic and climatic determinants (Rouxel et al., 2005; Faye et al., 2010). Agriculture's contribution to fighting poverty in Africa goes beyond people simply having enough nutritious food to eat or sell.

The continent's economies still rely heavily on earnings from agriculture, and it is still the main source of livelihood for hundreds of millions of farmers. The success or failure of the national harvest has direct impacts on the fiscal performance of most countries across the continent. Despite this, agriculture has historically received low attention. As a result, farming in sub-Saharan Africa is characterized by a subsistence system of low inputs, low outputs and low investment.

Food production and vegetable and fruit consumption per capita in Africa has been declining in recent decades. Recent changes in lifestyle, particularly urbanization, have led to high consumption of fats and refined carbohydrates and relatively less consumption of fruit and vegetables. This has further complicated the nutrition problem in Africa with increased incidences of obesity, diabetes, cardiovascular disease, high blood pressure and cancer. Ironically, although the continent has to struggle with these nutrition problems, it is blessed with a high diversity of underutilized micronutrient-dense vegetables and fruits. In spite of the fact that the vegetables are easily accessible and adapted to local conditions, they have been neglected in research and extension and their consumption has been declining over the years, as has the range of vegetables consumed. The range has fallen from hundreds consumed regularly to only a few, and often mainly exotic species. Coupled with reduced consumption are parallel losses of local knowledge and landraces.

Recognizing these shortcomings and the potential of agricultural biodiversity to improve income and livelihoods and to fight against mineral and vitamin deficiencies, the MVP developed a field-based approach to enhance the role of these vegetables in improving the nutritional status and livelihoods of vulnerable groups, particularly women and children. This was to be achieved through promotion, increased production and consumption, improved processing, landrace improvement and sustainable management of the genetic resources. The project reported significant achievements, among them increasing agricultural production and enhancing ecosystem function by restoring and maintaining soil productivity, improving crop diversification and the diversification of farming systems; developing living genebanks to conserve genetic diversity; improving land productivity and land use diversity; providing high quality agricultural inputs, improving irrigation systems, training farmers and strengthening farmer cooperatives.

A series of activities were carried out to enhance agricultural biodiversity and commercialize agricultural production. These included diversifying crop production, introducing modern irrigation techniques, and adding value to agricultural products to increase their market value. Now, traditional staple foods grow alongside new high-value, nutritional crops and agro-forestry tree species, including groundnuts (*Arachis villosulicarpa*), soy beans (*Glycine max* L.), okra (*Abelmoschus esculentus, A. caillei*), green leafy vegetables such as amaranth (*Amaranth viridis*), jute mallow (*Corchorus olitorius*), black nightshade (*Solanum americanum*), cassava (*Manihot esculenta*) and pumpkin (*Cucurbita pepo*) leaves, and fruit trees such as jujube (*Ziziphus mauritiana*), tamarind (*Tamarindus indica*), baobab (*Adansonia digitata*), moringa (*Moringa oleifera*), citrus (*Citrus* sp), mango (*Mangifera indica*) and papaya (*Carica papaya*).

In Tiby, Mali, West Africa, activities aimed at providing diversified crops to farmers included the introduction of high value and nutritious crops and improved varieties of beans, groundnuts, cowpeas, melons, okra, shallots, and other garden vegetables, coupled with agricultural input distribution and training in farming methods and the management of diversity in crop lands. Training methods focused on seed bed preparation and planting, seed and germplasm production (Figure 5.1a), vegetable gardening, annual crop production, integrated pest and disease management, management of agro-forestry nurseries, post-harvest management and marketing. On-farm demonstration plots were established within the communities to demonstrate appropriate farming practices and to showcase positive effects of agro-forestry and horticultural technologies. The impacts of these combined initiatives on agricultural production have yielded considerable reductions in levels of chronic undernutrition among children under five (MDG annual report, 2010).

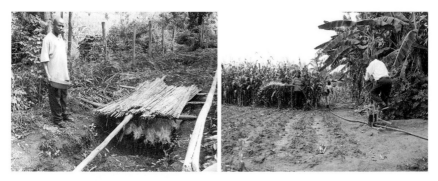

Figure 5.1 (a) Seed and germplasm production methods are part and parcel of the MVP diversity strategy (left); (b) pedal pumps are used to irrigate fields in Kenya (right). By Hervé Bisseleua

Four new high yielding varieties of rice (G4 of Wassa, Nionoka and Adny11 and R1 of Wat310) were introduced in Toya, Mali and farmers have devoted nearly two-thirds of the area under cultivation to rice (*Oryza* sp.), sorghum (*Sorghum* sp.) and millet (*Pennisetum glaucum*). In addition to that, to reverse desertification and provide a diversity of nutrients to the communities, the project introduced in the community gardens of Toya improved traditional vegetable varieties (onion, tomatoes, okra, potatoes, cucumber, melon, amaranths and black nightshade) and agro-forestry landraces (jujube, tamarind and moringa). Agro-forestry tree species were grown in community gardens in association with traditional vegetable species providing households with products having a diversity of nutrients and micronutrients.

In Bonsaaso, Ghana, West Africa, emphasis was placed on perennial crops. Nurseries and plantations of the cocoa tree (*Theobroma cacao*) were established in association with maize, cassava and banana (*Musa* sp.). The seedlings raised in these nurseries were also used to rehabilitate old cocoa plantations during the 2010 major planting season. Improved oil palm (*Elaeis guineensis*) plantations were established in place of poor yielding old plantations. During the cropping season 2009–2010 a total of 37.6 tons of oil palm fruits were harvested, generating an average annual income of GHS 3,205.50 to farmers. In addition, oil palm and cocoa farmers received training in the management of agricultural biodiversity in their cocoa and oil palm fields as well as information and development of cooperatives.

In Mayange, Rwanda, cassava farmers, whose entire plots had been wiped out by a virus, were given disease-resistant cuttings, and today more than 1,000 ha of land are cultivated with cassava. A new processing plant to mill raw produce into high-value flour has been built with an initial investment, which now also employs seven permanent staff and up to 50 casual weekly workers. The farmers' increased yields and their newly refined product have allowed them to expand their sales to Rwanda's capital, Kigali, and to neighbouring Burundi. The cooperative now regularly attends nationwide trade shows, and it was given an award by the District in recognition of its promotion of cassava production. However, the project proponents believe that there is still room for improvement – as a young organization, the cooperative needs help to boost its capacity to manage its newly-flourishing business in a more effective manner.

In Sauri, Kenya, 41 drip irrigation systems are now in operation, some of which have been paid for by private sector investors offering credit to farmers. The systems are expensive, however, and most farmers have opted to use pedal pumps (Figure 5.1b), which are cheap but effective enough to irrigate up to one hectare. Distribution of these pumps will be scaled up to benefit 990 farmers, who will be encouraged to grow mainly horticultural crops including tomatoes, onions, cabbages, African leafy vegetables and bananas that are propagated by tissue culture, to be marketed through their cooperatives. Women are given an equal chance to benefit, and all farmers received training on water management techniques, and accessing new markets for selling their produce.

Planting soy beans in Ruhiira, Uganda, has had a double benefit – the plant locks nitrogen into the soil, in an area where nutrients had been depleted, and it provides healthy food for people who have been affected by malnutrition. In 2010, the project proponents advised people about the benefits of soy bean, and encouraged them to plant it under integrated soil fertility management programmes, designed to boost productivity and diversify agriculture. At the same time, soy has a higher market value than maize, meaning that farmers earn more income by selling their harvests. More than 8,000 farmers in Ruhiira have been trained in soy bean cultivation, and most have been provided with improved, disease resistant seeds. Radio programmes and cooking demonstrations were used to alert the community to the plant's benefits, and a significant number of households now use part of their harvest in their own meals.

These combined interventions are perhaps best appreciated in Mwandama, Malawi. With hybrid maize seeds, fertilizer and topdressing provided to village farmers, Mwandama now boasts a record maize yield increase of up to 5.6 mt/ha, compared with Malawi's national average of 1.2 mt/ha. Drip irrigation schemes have been introduced to increase agricultural productivity for business, and to expand cultivation of high value crops, mostly vegetables and fruits. These allow farmers to earn enough profit through market sales to offset the extra irrigation cost. The initiative also teaches farmers how to produce the quality and quantity of these cash crops required year-round by nearby markets.

Taken together, the efforts made in the MVP's agriculture sector – improving harvests, diversifying diets and increasing business opportunities for farmers – have all contributed to the overall food security and health of the villagers.

Drylands, climate change, food security and the MDGs

The drylands region of the Sahel, one of the poorest areas in the world, has long been plagued by drought and desertification. These extremes of climatic variability have not only caused the deaths of many people but also hampered the production systems (Funk and Brown, 2009). Few climate change coping mechanisms are used currently by farmers in the Sahel. The most widely used strategies are the traditional agro-forestry parkland systems where trees, crops and livestock are combined in the same landscape (Rouxel et al., 2005; Faye et al., 2010). However, these systems are threatened by poor regeneration of the trees and the high pressure on the resources posed by rapidly growing human and animal populations (Garrity et al., 2010). While many response options have been developed in the Sahel by national and international research organizations, they are generally limited to specific sectors and have focused mostly on the biophysical aspects with very low technique adoption rates by rural communities (Reij et al., 2009).

Sahelian countries depend on agriculture to feed themselves to an even greater extent than many other countries in Africa. The food security situation in the Sahelian countries depends largely on domestic production which, in turn, depends on the amount of rainfall that these countries receive. The Sahel was struck by a devastating series of droughts in the 1970s and 1980s that affected most countries, causing immense human suffering due to a serious food shortage. These droughts demonstrated the fragility of food security, where the majority of food production is based on rainfall associated with climatic events. The region needs a multidimensional effort focused on poverty alleviation, with an integrated approach that both reverses soil depletion and preserves existing biodiversity as a means to overcome regional biophysical constraints and promotes income-generating, high-value agricultural products. Activities should aim to propose concrete solutions to reduce the risks farming households face due to climate change and its effects on drylands. To do so, rural communities should be helped to identify and invest in the most effective and sustainable coping mechanisms to reduce these risks and to invest in these mechanisms in a sustainable way.

However, over the past three decades, the Sahel has experienced an environmental renaissance, in terms of the development of vegetation and improvement of production systems. Experts link this phenomenon not only to an increase in rainfall but also to changes in land and tree use legislation which have incentivized farmers to plant and maintain trees in their farmlands (Garrity et al., 2010). Hundreds of thousands of farmers have transformed large swathes of the region's arid landscape into productive agricultural land, improving food and nutrition security and the livelihoods of millions of people. Sahelian farmers achieved their success by ingeniously modifying traditional agro-forestry, water, and soil management practices, specifically in Niger and Burkina Faso, primarily because of farmer-managed natural regeneration. Recent data has shown that more than 4.8 million hectares are greener today than 20 years ago in the regions of Zinder and Maradi in Niger, primarily because of farmer-managed natural regeneration of trees in densely populated and agriculturally overexploited areas (Reij et al., 2009).

This transformation resulted from a combination of incentive changes in government policy combined with village-level institutional innovations in managing land, along with successful changes in farmer practices. These experiences deserve careful attention as a basis for developing regional and national initiatives that could possibly result in a new era of transformative change across the Sahelian landscape. Lessons from success stories and case studies models in implementing the Sustainable Land Management practices have not been adequately synthesized to spearhead further expansion of the practices throughout the Sahel. The next section reviews these experiences, and their broader implications for sustainable food security in the Sahel, as manifestations of Climate SMART Agriculture, a fresh approach to achieving food security and environmental resilience through agricultural systems that increases productivity while enhancing adaptation and mitigation.

Fertilizer trees, conservation farming and the conservation of agricultural biodiversity

The challenge facing African agriculture is to produce more food while at the same time combating poverty and hunger. The risks that come with climate change make this task more daunting. However, hundreds of thousands of rain-fed smallholder farms in Zambia, Malawi, Niger, Mali and Burkina Faso have been shifting to farming systems that are restoring exhausted soils and are increasing food crop yields, household food security, and incomes using a type of conservation agriculture termed 'Evergreen Agriculture'.

Evergreen Agriculture is defined as combining agro-forestry with conservation agriculture through the integration of particular tree species into annual food crop systems (Figure 5.2). The intercropped trees sustain a green cover on the land throughout the year to maintain vegetative soil cover, bolster nutrient supply through nitrogen fixation and nutrient cycling, generate greater quantities of organic matter in soil surface residues, improve soil structure and water infiltration, increase greater direct production of food, fodder, fuel, fibre and income from products produced by the intercropped trees, enhance carbon storage both above and below ground, and induce more effective conservation of above- and below-ground biodiversity (Garrity et al., 2010; Reij et al., 2009).

In Zambia, maize and other food crops are intercropped within an agro-forest of the fertilizer tree *Faidherbia albida*. The Malawi Agro-forestry Food Security Programme (AFSP) integrates fertilizer, fodder, fruit, fuel wood, and timber tree production with food crops on small farms on a national scale. The agro-forestry trees include *F. albida*, *Gliricidia sepium*, *Tephrosia candida* and *Sesbania sesban* resulting in 100 to 400 per cent yield increase in food crops. It is estimated that currently about 500,000 Malawian farmers have *Faidherbia* trees on their farms (Phombeya, 1999). The majority of these stands were developed through assisted natural regeneration of seedlings that emerged in farmers' fields. Throughout Niger, studies have revealed a dramatic expansion of *Faidherbia albida* agro-forests in millet and sorghum production systems via assisted natural regeneration (Reij et al., 2009; Tougiani et al., 2009). Burkina Faso farmers developed a unique type of pit-planting technology (*zai*) along with farmer-managed natural regeneration of trees on a substantial scale resulting in

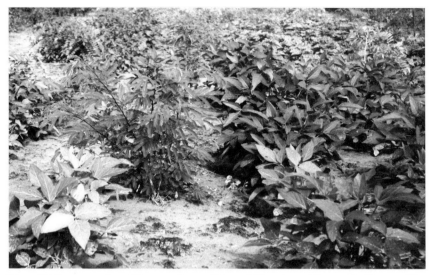

Figure 5.2 Intercropping of *Leucaena leucocephala* and *G. sepium* with green leafy vegetables in MVP farmer's field. By Hervé Bisseleua

a significant increase in cereal production by an average of at least 400 kg/ha, an increase of 40 per cent to more than 100 per cent (Reij et al., 2009).

Such complex landscapes characterized by highly connected crop–non-crop mosaics are best for long-term conservation, biological control and sustainable crop production and insure such landscapes from environmental perturbations (Tscharntke et al., 2007). They provide a number of important resources for pollinators, parasitoids and predatory arthropods such as permanent vegetation cover suitable as refuges from disturbance, as well as resources such as alternative prey, pollen and nectar (Bianchi et al., 2006). Such consideration of the landscape context ensures sustainable agricultural biodiversity conservation that is based on rich beneficial invertebrate communities and their capacity to reorganize after disturbances.

Conclusion

Africa is seriously threatened by food insecurity, land degradation and climate change. African farmers need science-based interventions. Special emphasis should be placed on measures to preserve local biodiversity using a farmer-centred approach of participatory action-research and development and based on coping strategies to climate change and desertification. Research programmes should analyse issues related to the desertification processes; look for ways to integrate crops of high nutritional value into existing farming systems; identify measures to further reduce climatic risks for each coping strategy while preserving biodiversity. This may include diversification of farming systems with trees and crops that are high-value and nutritious, and less susceptible to drought, and incorporate water and soil management and rehabilitation techniques, among others. In addition, new technological solutions should be tested using holistic, system-wide approaches that encompass socio-economic constraints of poor farming households and the need to improve their livelihoods; and finally, elements of sustainability and replicability should be analysed to ensure the long-term use and success of these methods and practices. For these technologies to be sustained over time, it will be important to identify, develop and promote higher market potential for the agricultural commodities that will strengthen farmers' management knowledge and skills. The Millennium Villages Project is tackling these critical issues head-on with a focus on achieving the MDGs: the world's commitment to end extreme poverty and ensure environmental sustainability by the year 2015.

Note

The Millennium Villages Project simultaneously addresses the challenges of extreme poverty in many overlapping areas: agriculture, education, health, infrastructure, gender equality, and business development and offers an innovative integrated approach to rural development.

Acknowledgements

We thank the MDG centres of West and East Africa and the respective Millennium Villages in East and West Africa; and two anonymous reviewers, whose comments helped to improve a previous version of the manuscript. This study was supported by the Prince Albert II Foundation and the Government of the Principality of Monaco grant to the MDG centre West and Central Africa.

References

Bianchi, F.J.J.A., Booij, C.J.H., Tscharntke, T. (2006) 'Sustainable pest regulation in agricultural landscapes: a review on landscape composition, biodiversity and natural pest control', *Proc. Roy. Soc. Lond.* B, vol 273, pp.1715–1727.

Faye, M.D., Weber, J.C., Mounkoro, B. and Dakouo, J.M. (2010) 'Contribution of parkland trees to farmers' livelihoods: a case study from Mali', *Development in Practice*, vol 20, no 3, pp.428–434.

Flood, J. (2010) 'The importance of plant health to food security', *Food Sec*, vol 2, pp.215–231.

Funk C. and Brown, M. (2009) *Declining Global Per Capita Agricultural Capacity Production and Warming Oceans Threaten Food Security*, Food Security. DOI 10.1007/s12571-009-0026-y

Garrity et al. (2010) 'Evergreen Agriculture: a robust approach to sustainable food security in Africa', *Food security*, vol 2, pp.197–214.

Johns, T. and Eyzaguirre, P.B. (2007) 'Biofortification, biodiversity and diet: a search for complementary applications against poverty and malnutrition', *Food Policy*, vol 32, pp.1–24.

Johns, T., Smith, I.F., Eyzaguirre, P.B. (2006) 'Understanding the links between agriculture and health', *IFPRI*, vol 13, no 16, p.2.

Johns T., Faubert, G. M., Kokwaro, J. O., Mahunnah, L. R. A. and Kimanani, E. K. (1995) 'Anti-giardial Activity of Gastrointestinal Remedies of the Luo of East Africa', *Journal of Ethnopharmacology*, vol 46, 17–23.

MDG West and Central Africa Annual report (2010) *Supporting, Planning and Implementing Millennium Development Goals at National and Local levels in West and Central Africa*, p. 71.

National Research Council (1996) *Lost Crops of Africa. Volume 1: Grains*. National Academy Press, Washington, DC. P 181.

Onyango, A., Koski, K. and Tucker, K. (1998) 'Food diversity versus breastfeeding choice in determining anthropometric status in rural Kenyan toddlers', *International Journal of Epidemiology*, vol 27, 484-489.

Phombeya, H.S.K. (1999) 'Nutrient sourcing and recycling by *Faidherbia albida* trees in Malawi', PhD Dissertation, Wye College, University of London, p.219.

Reij, C., Tappan, G., Smale, M. (2009) 'Agro-environmental Transformation in the Sahel: Another Kind of "Green Revolution,"' IFPRI Discussion Paper 00914, Washington DC: International Food Policy Research Institute.

Rouxel, C., Barbier, J., Niang, A., Kaya, B., Sibelet, N. (2005) 'Biodiversité spécifique ligneuse et terroirs: quelles relations? Le cas de trois villages de la région de Ségou (Mali)', *Bois et Forest des Tropiques*, vol 1, no 283, pp.33–49.

Tougiani, A., Guero, C., Rinaudo, T. (2009) 'Community mobilisation for improved livelihoods through tree crop management in Niger', *GeoJournal*, vol 74, pp.377–389.

Tscharntke, T., Bommarco, R., Clough, Y., Crist, T.O., Kleijn, D., Rand, T.A., Tylianakis, J.M., Nouhuys, S.V., Vidal, S. (2007) 'Conservation biological control and enemy diversity on a landscape scale', *Biological Control*, vol 43, pp.294–309.

Tucker, K.L. (2001) 'Eat a variety of healthful foods: old advice with new support', *Nutrition Reviews,* vol 59, pp.156–158.

Underwood, B.A. (2000) 'Overcoming micronutrient deficiencies in developing countries: Is there a role for agriculture', *Food Nutr Bull,* vol 21, no 4, pp.356–360.

WHO (2004) Global strategy on diet, physical activity and health. 57th World Health Assembly, Agenda Item 12.6.

6 Sustained and integrated promotion of local, traditional food systems for nutrition security

Ifeyironwa Francisca Smith

Introduction

The greatest biodiversity is found in developing countries where poor communities rely greatly upon agricultural biodiversity for their foods and livelihood (Hobblink, 2004). Thus maintaining the viability of developing countries' local food systems which contain immense agricultural biodiversity remains one sustainable way of ensuring food and nutrition security for resource-poor populations. Padulosi et al. (2009) furthermore highlighted that the larger the agricultural biodiversity basket available to farmers and value chain actors, the greater will be their capacity to effectively and sustainably meet the environmental challenges of climate change.

In sub-Saharan Africa (SSA), the agricultural biodiversity within traditional food systems contributes to food and livelihood security in very profound ways. Communities traditionally employ a wide range of locally available food resources in daily diets. However, across developing countries, socio-economic changes are contributing to changes in dietary patterns and food habits. These changes are believed to play significant roles in the many health problems faced by poor communities in particular. Sub-Saharan Africa continues to be overburdened by nutritional and diet related health problems, most of which can be traced to insufficient dietary intakes of micronutrients (vitamin A, iron and zinc in particular), and in the recent past, increases in the consumption of cheap, calorie-dense staple foods leading to increased incidences of obesity and other diet-related chronic diseases (Mendez et al., 2005).

Africa holds a rich and varied agricultural biodiversity that is part of local traditional food systems. Dykstra and colleagues (1996) observed that forest-based crops, root crops and cereal–root crop mixed farming constitute the main land use systems in West and Central Africa. In SSA and West Africa in particular, there are diverse agricultural ecosystems for the production of a wide range of indigenous/traditional foods which if effectively managed, mobilized, and their use in diets relentlessly promoted, can increase food availability, expand household food choices and ensure dietary diversity and better nutrition.

Using experiences from West Africa, this chapter examines the agro-ecology of the sub-region and the role played by the diversity within the local food systems in shaping the region's well known but now disappearing rich and healthy food culture. The chapter will also review changes in this food culture and dietary habits occasioned by globalization, urbanization and changes in food production practices, the evolution of the nutrition transition, and then discuss research and intervention programmes that have been put in place in the region to address and reverse, as much as possible, the deleterious effects of the nutrition transition on the population. These programme activities are expected to generate positive changes in the food choices of the population, eventually leading to increased diversification in household diets.

West Africa's physical geography presents a striking zonal arrangement – the Guinean zone where evergreen forest formations dominate, the Savannah zone that is still forested but with trees becoming smaller and rarer as one moves north, and a Sahelian zone that is semi-arid. These distinct ecosystems provide a wide range of indigenous and traditional foods, and to a large extent determine the food systems and food habits of communities in different parts of the sub-region. The rangeland food system of the Sahel and Savannah with its dominant cereals (millet – *Pennisetum typhoideum*; sorghum – *Sorghum vulgare*; hungry rice – *Digitaria exilis*) and cowpea staples contrasts with the forest and aquatic based systems dominated by roots, tubers, starchy fruits, and several traditional bean varieties such as the cowpea, bambara ground nut and African yam bean. Thus tubers, rhizomes, roots and starchy fruits were major staples that dominated the food habits of the southern Guinean zone, while cereals and grain legumes predominated in the northern Savannah and Sahelian zones (Figure 6.1). The respective major staples are supplemented with a diversity of indigenous minor food components such as oil seeds (the oil palm and shea butter in particular), fruit and leaf vegetables, a whole array of fruits, food condiments and spices, as well as uncultivated wild gathered tubers, fruits, seeds, twigs, leaves and flowers of some plants. Some of these minor food components are also used as adjuvants

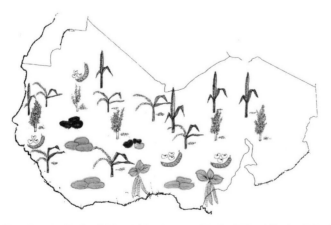

Figure 6.1 Pre-historic foods of West Africa (source: *Foods of West Africa* by F. Smith, 1998)

in traditional medicine. These indigenous foods defined the food habits of the populations in the Guinean, Savannah and Sahelian zones of West Africa.

Changes in dietary patterns

As has been reported for several developing countries (Shufa et al., 2002; Albala et al., 2002; Sodjinou et al., 2009; Delisle, 2010), West Africa has also undergone periods of changes in dietary habits and shifts in eating patterns in response to socio-economic and socio-political factors. However in West Africa the initial change was positive following the opening during the 8th century of the northern borders of the sub-region to Arab explorers, and the coastal borders to Portuguese and other colonial rulers between the 15th and 20th centuries (Smith, 1998). During these periods, the already diversified food base of communities was further expanded with the introductions of exotic food crops from North Africa, Asia and South America in particular.

These introduced foods included Asian rice, several species of beans, groundnuts, wheat, barley, taro, banana/plantain, cassava, maize, sweet potato, cocoyam, varieties of fruits, leafy greens such as Moringa, Jew's mallow, Indian spinach, quail grass, and such cash crops as sugar cane, cocoa, cotton, and rubber. Some of the foods introduced from the north of Africa became part of the food culture of the Sahelian zone while foods from South America and South Asia found more conducive environments in the Guinean zone and became part of the food habits of populations in the forest and coastal areas of the sub-region (Figure 6.2). As the introduced foods were selectively adopted by communities they became part of the traditional food systems of the region and were well established in community food habits. This influx of introduced foods, coupled with intra-regional movements of populations with their respective food cultures, created an expansion of the already diversified food base of communities all over the sub-region. During this period, and up to the mid-20th century, national and community food systems were extremely diversified (Figures 6.3 and 6.4), and this ensured some degree of food security and diversity in household diets of both rural and urban populations.

Evolution of the nutrition transition in West Africa

As the introduced food crops were adopted and cultivated, they initially complemented the indigenous food crops earlier described. More food varieties were available and the population of the region had a lot of foods to choose from. This food abundance and availability was aptly described by Schwab (1947) who reported that "the white man living in West Africa where ingredients are easily obtained, could use many of them with profit both to his health and his finances". Murdock (1959) also observed that the population of southern Nigerians catapulted in the presence of a new and abundant food supply. However during the second half of the 20th century, because of higher and better yields and perhaps low production costs, several of the introduced food

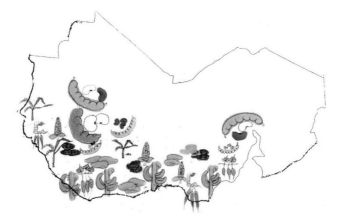

Figure 6.2 Foods introduced to West Africa (source: *Foods of West Africa* by F. Smith, 1998)

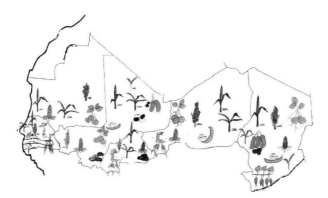

Figure 6.3 Common staples in the Sahelian north of the region (source: *Foods of West Africa* by F. Smith, 1998)

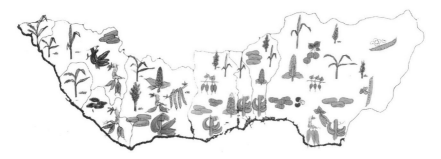

Figure 6.4 West African foods today – Guinea Bissau to Nigeria (source: *Foods of West Africa* by F. Smith, 1998)

crops displaced the indigenous varieties in the food systems and thus radically altered the dietary patterns and food habits of the population. This signalled the onset of the nutrition transition in the sub-region. Furthermore, following the adoption of the introduced food varieties in local food systems (Figures 6.3 and 6.4), and cash (export) crops, the scene was set for the exploitation of the now conducive crop production environment in the sub-region with the establishment of cash crop plantations during the early to mid-20th century. More emphasis was now placed on cash crop production to the detriment and marginalization of food crop production. Increases in the production of cash crops such as peanuts, benniseed (sesame), coffee beans, palm nuts, cocoa, and rubber in particular, defined national agricultural production policies and set the scene for the practice of single food crop agriculture (Read, 1938). The period 1950 to date could thus be described as a period of shrinking food supplies and increasing food shortages throughout the West African sub-region. Political and socio-economic factors played contributing roles in this shrinkage of food supplies (Delgado and Rearden, 1987; Lappia, 1987) but the net effect was a significant reduction not so much on the numbers of cultivated indigenous cereals, legumes, tubers and minor food components but in their level of production and thus their availability.

Nutrition transition in full bloom

As already mentioned, the mid-20th century witnessed the emergence of cash crop economies in West Africa. Forests were cleared to make way for cash-crop farming. These clearing and cultivating activities modified the existing ecosystems and eliminated some wild indigenous food trees as well as some wild uncultivated food crops which were part of the traditional food systems (Robson, 1976). The trend towards commercial farming and the attendant destruction and erosion of ecosystem diversity negatively affected and contributed to the decline in the cultivation and availability of indigenous food resources that hitherto defined regional food habits and contributed to ensuring the food and nutrition security of local populations. This decline and displacement of indigenous food resources from national and regional food systems coincided with the emergence of food shortages and the increased dependence of populations in the sub-region on introduced and food aid cereals. The reliance on food aid grains such as wheat, rice and maize in particular, combined with declining use of food resources from traditional food systems is associated with the gradual simplification of household diets in the sub-region.

Increasing urbanization and large movements of populations to urban centres with reduced access to traditional and indigenous food resources also exacerbated the nutrition transition phenomenon (Maire et al., 1992; Voster et al., 2000; Albala et al., 2002). This reduced access to indigenous food resources has resulted in the replacement in diets of the hitherto diversified food resources by energy dense and nutrient poor convenience foods. Fouere and colleagues (2000) also observed that urbanization and new socio-economic pressures on both rural and urban families, as well as lifestyle changes among the urban poor, force families to turn to high carbohydrate, high fat foods in order to meet their daily food needs. With increasing urbanization, the trend in dietary simplification continues as more and more women find employment outside the home, have less time for the preparation of family meals and so turn to high energy low nutritional value street foods, or easy to cook cereal foods and products like rice, wheat and maize. It is however interesting to note that in a study in Benin, West Africa, Sodjinou et al. (2009) found that many features of the "traditional diet" as defined by the study are maintained in the "transitional diet". These researchers reported that in the study context, they observed that the transitional diet is really not a shift from traditional to western foods, but rather a more diversified dietary pattern with some imported foods added to the traditional diet although this is associated with a significantly higher intake of energy from saturated fats and sugar.

Is this trend reversible?

There has been a resurgence of interest in agricultural biodiversity within traditional food systems and the possible role these resources could play in ongoing efforts to steer populations away from carbohydrate and energy rich foods that are typical of simplified diets to more diversified diets that engender household food and nutrition security. In spite of the ongoing nutrition transition trend, it is widely acknowledged that within the sub-region, the healthy components of West Africa's food traditions are still found in the lives and cooking pots of rural households in particular. This is confirmed by the study of dietary patterns of urban adults in Benin (Sodjinou et al., 2009). The investigators reported that many features of the traditional diet are maintained in the transitional diet patterns of the adults studied. This is indeed heartening because with the healthy components of the traditional food habits still playing a role in contemporary food habits in the sub-region, the possibility of reversing the trends in dietary simplification looks promising.

The author's experiences during the 1967–1970 Biafran war, and the war exigencies that compelled the population of the then south Eastern Nigeria (Biafra) to resort to the traditional food systems for food and health needs also provide evidence that the trend towards dietary simplification can be slowed down if not reversed. During the three-year period of the war, most of the population of former Biafra was crammed into a land space less than half the original size of the region. Gone were the exotic cereals and products (breads and other baked products, imported Asian rice, pastas), animal products (milk, butter, cheese, imported New Zealand beef, dry and salted stockfish from Scandinavia etc.), as well as several other food imports. The population turned to traditional food resources – indigenous roots and rhizomes, cereals, grain legumes, nuts and oilseeds, leaf and fruit vegetables, mushrooms, fruits, small game, edible snails and several molluscs and aquatic species. This experience was an "eye opener" to city dwellers (the author included) who were compelled to live among the villagers and discovered the rich agricultural biodiversity within family and community farms. The Biafran experience was enlightening and contributed to the interest of some local researchers on the nutrition, health and medicinal properties of some food resources from local traditional food systems (Smith, 1982; Achinewhu and Ryley, 1987; Achinewhu et al., 1995; Glew et al., 1997; Ighodalo et al., 1991; Nordiede et al., 1996; Jideani, 1990; Muhammad and Amusa, 2005; Achu et al., 2008; Ngondi et al., 2005; Dahiru et al., 2006; Baumer, 1995; Ladeji and Okoye, 1993; Eromosele et al., 1991; Johns et al., 1995). Data from these and other earlier studies have spurred further interest and continuing research into the nutrition and health attributes of foods from West African traditional food systems. Investigations during the past two decades on foods from these food systems have confirmed these earlier reports of their nutritional and health protecting properties. While these reports do not suggest an exclusive focus on local agricultural biodiversity as the sole way of addressing the urgent food and nutrition challenges faced by several developing countries, the body of evidence generated strongly suggests that the agricultural biodiversity within these food systems, if properly managed and mobilized, can engender dietary diversity and promote healthier diets.

Voster and colleagues (2011) also believe that the trend towards dietary simplification can be slowed down, and suggested some research and intervention approaches that are needed to move the nutrition transition in a more positive direction in Africa. Among the suggested public health promotion strategies, policies and intervention approaches are:

- Evidence-based interventions that address identified public health problems
- Holistic integrated food and nutrition interventions
- Addressing under- and overnutrition simultaneously
- Involving communities in planning interventions using a bottom-up rather than a top-down approach
- Involving relevant stakeholders at the planning stage to ensure their active participation in the implementation stage
- Focusing on diversification of diets rather than a reliance on fortified foods and supplementation where possible.

In West Africa, international organizations working in collaboration with regional research institutions as well as the West African Health Organization (WAHO) (Box 6.1) have, during the past decade, developed research and intervention programmes to address and ultimately slow down the trend towards dietary simplification and its deleterious effects on the population's nutrition and health. Key programmes developed target:

- The revitalization of traditional food systems
- Addressing important constraints to the production of traditional foods
- The development of public awareness products and tools to enable effective public awareness and education programmes on the nutrition and health benefits of consuming foods from traditional and local food systems.

Box 6.1 West African Health Organization (WAHO)

The West African Organization is a specialized Public Health Agency of the Economic Community of West African States (ECOWAS). WAHO coordinates the ECOWAS nutrition Forum and so is charged with facilitating effective food and nutrition policies and programmes, and ensuring food and nutrition security in the sub-region. Local foods from the region's traditional food systems play a fundamental role in meeting this objective. This explains WAHO's very active leadership role in initiatives aimed at enhancing the production, marketing and consumption by the population of nutrient-rich foods from the region's ecosystems in order to ensure adequate nutrition, improved health and livelihoods of populations within ECOWAS Member States.

During the past two decades several published reports (Delisle et al., 2003; Kennedy et al., 2005; McBurney et al., 2004; Barngana, 2004; Smith, 2000; VanHeerden and Schondeldt, 2004; Adegbooye et al., 2005; Frison et al., 2006) have echoed the need to mainstream the use of traditional food resources in the daily diets of resource poor communities and households in particular. However, these studies have also highlighted major bottlenecks and constraints that have over the years hampered such attempts. Important among these reported bottlenecks and constraints are:

- Very poor knowledge base on traditional food resources by the population at large including national and regional agricultural policy and decision makers who determine policies governing agricultural production
- Poorly developed seed systems for traditional food crops
- Lack of or low appreciation of local communities' indigenous knowledge of their traditional food systems and building on such knowledge when developing agricultural intervention programmes
- Lack of market access for traditional food resources
- Dearth of credible information on the nutrition and health attributes of a large number of traditional food resources, including information required for public awareness and education of the population
- Economic viability/market competitiveness of these food resources
- Ecological sustainability
- Productivity/weak agronomic knowledge
- Socio-cultural basis of decision making.

In countries and regions with rich agricultural biodiversity and food culture such as West Africa, use of locally available traditional food resources should be part of frontline strategies for nutrition interventions and so the revitalization of local traditional food systems is believed to be an imperative starting point.

Furthermore, addressing the aforementioned bottlenecks would to a significant extent pave the way for the successful development and execution of sustainable national and regional programmes aimed not only at revitalizing local traditional food systems but also at mobilizing and mainstreaming food resources from these systems in household diets of both rural and urban populations in the sub-region.

Within the sub-region, national and regional institutions as well as international organizations have been slow and perhaps ineffective in articulating appropriate programmes to address the social and human development challenges posed by these constraints. However, in recent years there have been encouraging successes in research and development programmes put in place within the sub-region specifically aimed at addressing and overcoming some of these identified constraints. Some of these programmes are presented in the following pages.

Addressing poor knowledge base on traditional foods by the population

The general ignorance of the nature and use of nutrient-rich indigenous and traditional food resources has over the years resulted in these foods being left out of most national strategies put in place to address food security and nutrition problems of the population. One of the earliest research for development programmes designed and put in place to enhance the knowledge base of local populations on traditional foods was a five-country (Botswana, Cameroon, Kenya, Senegal, Zimbabwe) multidisciplinary, community-based Bioversity International/National Agricultural Research Systems (NARS) collaborative study on the conservation through use of African traditional leafy vegetables (Chweya and Eyzaguirre, 1999).

In sub-Saharan Africa, leafy vegetables are vital dietary components and have been described as indispensable ingredients of soups or sauces that accompany carbohydrate staples (Smith and Eyzaguirre, 2007). This programme was therefore an appropriate start in the push to expand the knowledge base on traditional food resources. The five-country programme on promoting African leafy vegetables which started in 1996 significantly helped to change attitudes towards these hitherto underutilized nutrient-rich, health protecting food resources. In Kenya, which was one of the participating countries, the programme was instrumental in the development of entire leafy vegetable market chains (Gotor and Irungu, 2010). In Senegal, the introduced leafy vegetable *Moringa oleifera,* locally known as Nebeday (an adulteration of the plant's popular name Never die), is very commonly used in traditional dishes and is believed to contain healing properties. Nutritional analysis done during this programme (Ndong et al., 2007) confirmed reports (Sena et al., 1998; Oduro et al., 2008) that Moringa is a good source of several nutrients. The study by Ndong and colleagues (2007) however disputed the claim that Moringa is also a good source of dietary iron and provided evidence that points to poor bioavailability of iron from Moringa. These results are of particular importance in the Sahelian zone of West Africa where public awareness campaigns have encouraged the use of

Moringa in family meals, and where dried and ground Moringa leaves are very commonly consumed and also used to enrich weaning foods.

Addressing poorly developed seed systems for traditional food crops

A key issue that emerged from the leafy vegetable programme in Senegal and other participating countries is inadequate systems for germplasm management and seed production. Poorly developed seed systems have been cited by specialists as a major constraint in ongoing attempts to increase the production of several nutrient-rich traditional food crops (McGuirre, 2008; Sperling et al., 2008; Adegbooye et al., 2005). To address this challenge that confronts West African small-scale farmers, researchers from Bioversity International (formerly IPGRI), in collaboration with researchers from national agricultural research systems (NARS) in Burkina Faso, Mali and Niger, and national agricultural extension specialists, worked with small-scale farmers and farming communities in these countries to improve and increase farmers' capacities to select, produce and manage improved seeds of local food crop varieties. The capacity building programme which relied on the local farmers' indigenous knowledge of the food systems involved:

- Farmer participatory seed selection that eliminated through trials on demonstration plots low yield accessions with poor agronomic characteristics
- Quality seed production, maintenance and storage during which farmers acquired the ability to identify and maintain seed varietal characteristics during handling and storage
- Popularization of selected improved varieties through field demonstrations
- Improved cultivation practices
- Community-based *in situ* maintenance of local improved seed varieties.

Project activities (Vodouhe et al., 2008) resulted in participating farmers and their communities having access to quality seeds either through individual seed exchanges or through community seed fairs. This Sahelian farmers' project established a traditional seed system network in the three participating countries and has put in place an enabling structure in the form of seed fairs on which larger regional networks can be built. It is noteworthy that in executing project activities the farmers' knowledge of their traditional food systems was acknowledged and reflected in the participatory nature of project activities. Also, the capacity strengthening activities built on the existing indigenous knowledge of the participants.

Addressing market access for traditional food resources

One of the constraints to increased production of traditional food crops is a lack of market infrastructure and support for the marketing of local foods and products. Creating access to markets for West Africa's local traditional food resources, increasing their marketability and making them easily available in local markets has the potential to mainstream the food resources in household food choices and selection thereby increasing their use in family diets.

Realizing this vital role that markets can play in mainstreaming local foods in household diets, Bioversity is conducting a two-country (Benin and Kenya) study on the effects of market integration on the nutritional contributions of traditional food resources to the well-being of the rural poor. The ongoing project will characterize the level of integration and assess market potentials of key traditional food resources. The study also hopes to determine the potential of markets to foster a wider use of key nutrient-rich foods from the traditional food systems.

Addressing lack of information for public awareness and education on the nutrition and health attributes of local agricultural biodiversity

Information, education and communication strategies and social marketing of programmes and products have been found to be indispensable components of community mobilization for successful food and nutrition intervention programmes. Through information and culturally applicable nutrition education, community mobilization has the important effect of raising awareness on the links between local food diversity, nutrition and health of community members. In the sub-region, the lack of this vital tool – credible data and information on the compositional attributes of traditional food resources – has greatly hampered attempts to inform and educate the population on the healthful attributes of these foods. Beyond the food needs of the population, such a food composition database is also vital for the development of effective tools for advocacy and is critical for policy and programme development within the agriculture, food, nutrition and health sectors.

The West African Health Organization working in collaboration with Bioversity International, FAO, the University d'Abomey Calavi Benin, and the University of Ghana, Legon, trained local experts on the development, compilation and dissemination of food composition databases. Some of the trained experts were engaged to compile available published and unpublished data on the composition of local traditional foods from 7 of the 15 countries in the sub-region. The data compiled was used in the development of a new regional food composition database (Stadlmayr et al., 2010). This first edition of the regional food composition database (Composition of Selected Foods from West Africa) has since been expanded and updated with new published data (Stadlmayr et al., 2012).

Policy advocacy activities

In addition to the research-oriented activities which are expected to inform evidence-based interventions and programmes, advocacy was another area of thrust of the regional institutional collaboration. Also targeted in the attempts to enhance the knowledge base on traditional foods are national and regional policy and decision makers in the agriculture, food, and health public sectors in particular. These functionaries determine and develop policies that should ensure adequate food production, availability and use by all segments of the population. It is therefore appropriate that continuous policy advocacy activities in the form of workshops, round-table discussions and stakeholders' meetings are organized to inform and educate these groups of functionaries within the health, agriculture, education and rural development sectors in particular. Bioversity International, working in collaboration with the West African Health Organization and the United Nations Food and Agriculture Organization (FAO), organized two of these advocacy workshops between 2007 and 2009, as well as a stakeholders' consultation in 2010 involving participants from international and West African regional organizations operating in the food, agriculture and health sectors.

The first of these policy advocacy workshops involved director-level participants from the ECOWAS (Economic Community of West African States) national ministries of health, agriculture, representatives from private sector groups (farmers' associations, food processors and consumer organizations), representatives from universities and research institutions, international NGOs, regional and international organizations (Bioversity/WAHO/FAO, 2007). The workshop sought to inform, educate and convince the participants by way of topical presentations and group discussions of the need to re-assess existing food and nutrition related health and agriculture policies, harmonize such policies and develop cross-sectoral implementation strategies that would positively impact on food security, nutrition and health of the West African population. An indication of the relative impact of this first workshop was the request after the

---

Box 6.2 Reseau des Organisations Paysannes et des Producteurs Agricole de l'Afrique de l'Ouest (ROPPA)

The pillars of the initiative to promote the production and consumption of foods from traditional food systems are the small-scale farmers represented by ROPPA – a network organization of small-scale food producers that operates in 12 of the 15 ECOWAS member states, and implements activities at both national and regional levels. Since its restructuring in 2002, ROPPA has been actively involved in consultations for the development and implementation of West Africa's regional agricultural policies and programmes. It is also very active in advocacy on behalf of small-scale food producers and working to strengthen their capacities as well as implementing public awareness programmes. At national levels, ROPPA coordinates farmers' networks and activities, empowers farmer organizations by ensuring their credibility as well as the visibility of their network activities. ROPPA also provides additional support in the form of training and capacity development to women farmer cooperative groups.

Box 6.3 List of articulated constraints and challenges of West Africa's small-scale farmers

- Increasing lack of access to arable land with the ongoing decision of governments to allocate farm lands for the production of bio-fuels
- Land tenure problems hinder female farmers from farming in the same location for sufficiently long periods to improve and increase production.
- Preference of governments for cash crops discourages food crop production; small-scale farmers get very little help and support from governments
- No institutional/government support and/or protection from the effects of droughts, floods and invasions/destruction by locusts and crickets
- Very low use of inputs by farmers due to lack of operating funds which result in low production levels
- Inadequate systems for germplasm management and seed production
- Imposition of western-type farming in the form of new seed varieties
- Poor infrastructure for transportation needed to move foods from production areas to markets
- Lack of infrastructure for processing of fresh products to limit post-harvest losses
- Lack of financial support from governments and inability to obtain bank credits due to lack of or required adequate collateral
- Marketing difficulties due to absence of protection from competition from imports
- Little or no market infrastructure and lack of support for the marketing of local foods and products

workshop by the governing body of the regional small-scale farmers' associations (ROPPA, Box 6.2) to enter into a collaborative working relationship with WAHO. This relationship between WAHO and ROPPA, whose members are the producers of the traditional foods, is considered strategic for the development and implementation of regional programmes that aim to mainstream the use of traditional food resources for improved nutrition and health.

Another indication of a scaling up effect of this workshop was the decision by the ECOWAS Commission on Agriculture to join in the initiative for the promotion of foods from local traditional food systems. The Commission co-convened and hosted a 2010 stakeholders' consultation on national and regional programmes to promote foods from traditional food systems (WAHO/ROPPA/Bioversity/FAO/ECOWAS Agriculture Commission, 2010).

The second workshop was a three-day "listening workshop" (WAHO/ROPPA/Bioversity, 2009) which brought together representatives of 12 national farmers' associations, regional and international organizations, representatives from research institutions, private sector groups and organizations. The presentations and the group discussions that followed provided the ROPPA members with information that enabled them to better articulate the constraints and challenges they face and the types of support they require in order to improve and increase the production of traditional food crops in their farms. The list of constraints and challenges (Box 6.3) provided workshop organizers (WAHO and Bioversity) with greater insights into priority areas of intervention and support for ROPPA in order to enable this network of traditional food producers to achieve the mutual objective of increasing production, availability and easy accessibility of local traditional food resources.

Conclusion

The health consequences of the nutrition transition on developing country populations have been widely reported. While there are similarities in the determinants of the nutrition transition – shifts in eating patterns, dietary changes characterized by increased consumption of simplified high carbohydrate, high fat diets – countries differ in the strategies developed to address the resulting food security, nutrition and health challenges faced by governments. Dietary diversification is acknowledged as a vital component of any intervention strategy. Sub-Saharan Africa and West Africa in particular still have strong traditional food cultures and rich agricultural biodiversity within traditional food systems which can be mobilized and used in national strategies to encourage diversification in food systems and household diets.

Evidence presented from West Africa suggests that it is possible to reverse the trend of dietary simplification which is one of the defining characteristics of the nutrition transition, and according to Voster and colleagues (2011), steer the process into a more positive direction. The targeted programme activities that were presented in this chapter to revitalize local food systems, address key constraints to the production of traditional foods and provide public awareness of products and tools that can be adapted and applied to several developing country situations, particularly SSA countries. The policy advocacy workshops were organized to enable national policy makers make informed decisions on how best to tackle the issue of food and nutrition insecurity in the sub-region. The regional institutional cross-sectoral and multidisciplinary collaboration was developed over time but it remains vital to the successful implementation of the reported programme activities.

The active participation in the institutional collaboration of the network of small-scale food producers, who are considered the pillars of the initiative to increase production and availability of traditional foods, resulted in a synergistic partnership of food producers, government agencies, researchers and development agencies. This partnership provided the framework or "backbone" on which the reported programmes to increase food diversity within national food systems thereby engendering diversity in household diets were successfully developed and implemented.

References

Achinewhu, S.C., Ryley, J. (1987) 'Effect of fermentation on thiamine, riboflavin and niacin content of melon seed (*Citrullis vulgaris*) and African oil bean (*Pentaclethra macrophylla*)', *Food Chem.*, vol 20, pp.243–253.

Achinewhu, S.C., Ogbonna, C.C., Hart, A.D. (1995) 'Chemical composition of indigenous wild herbs, spices, fruits, nuts and leafy vegetables used as food', *Plant Foods Hum Nutr.*, vol 48, pp.341–348.

Achu, M.B., Fokou, E., Tchiegang, C., Fotso, M., Tchouanguep, F.M. (2008) 'Atherogenicity of *Cucumeropsis manii* and *Cucumis sativus* oils from Cameroon', *Afr. J. Food Sci*, vol 2, pp.21–25.

Adegbooye, O.C., Ajayi, S.A., Baidu-Forson, J.J., Opabode, J.T. (2005) 'Seed constraint to cultivation and productivity of African indigenous leaf vegetables', *Afr J. Biotech,* vol 4, no 13, pp.1480–1484.

Albala, C., Vio, F., Kain, J., Oauy, R. (2002), 'Nutrition transition in Chile: determinants and consequences', *Public Health Nutr.*, vol 5, no 1A, pp.123–128.

Barngana, R.K. (2004) 'The need for food composition data in Uganda', *J. Food Comp. Anal,* vol 17, pp.501–507.

Baumer, M. (1995) *Arbes, arbustes, et arbrisseaux nourrciers en Afrique occidentale*, Enda-Editions, Dakar Senegal.

Bioversity/WAHO/FAO (2007) 'Partnership for mobilizing the diversity in traditional food systems to ensure adequate nutrition and health within ECOWAS Member States', Workshop Report, Ouagadougou, Burkina Faso, http://www.bioversityinternational.org/fileadmin/bioversity/documents/news_and_events/Conferences%20and%20meetings/ecowas_workshop/Report_WAHO_Bioversity_workshop_Burkina_Faso_Sept_2007_web.pdf, accessed July 2012.

Chweya, J.A. and Eyzaguirre, P.B. (eds) (1999) *The biodiversity of traditional leafy vegetables*, International Plant Genetic Resources Institute, Rome, Italy.

Dahiru, D., Sini, J.M., John-Africa, L., (2006) 'Antidiarrhoeal activity of *Ziziphus mauritiana* root extract in rodents', *Afr J Biotech*, vol 5, no 10, pp.941–945.

Delgado, C.L., Rearden, T.A. (1987) 'Problemes pour les politiques alimentaire poses par la modification des habitude alimentaire dans le Sahel', Conference on the Dynamics of Cereal Consumption and Production Patterns in West Africa, Dakar, Senegal.

Delisle, H. (2010) 'Findings on dietary patterns in different groups of African origin undergoing nutrition transition', *Appl Physiol Nutr Metab,* vol 35, pp.224–228.

Delisle, H., Zagre, N., Bakari, S., Codjia, P., Zendong, R. (2003) 'Des solutions alimentaires a la carence en vitamin A', *Food Nutr Agric,* vol 32, pp.40–48.

Dykstra, D.P., Kowero, G.S., Ofosu-Asiedu, A., Kio, P. (1996) 'Promoting stewardship of forests in humid forest zone of Anglophone West and Central Africa', Final report of a collaborative UNEP/CIFOR Research Project.

Eromosele, I.C., Eromosele, C.O., Kuzhkuzha, D.M. (1991) 'Evaluation of mineral elements and ascorbic acid contents in fruits of some wild plants', *Plant Foods Hum Nutr*, vol 41, pp.151–154.

Fouere, T., Maire, B., Delpeuch, F., Martin-Prevel, Y., Tchibindat, F., Adoua-Oyila, G. (2000) 'Dietary changes in African urban households in response to currency devaluation: Foreseeable risks for health and nutrition', *Public Health Nutr*, vol 3, pp.293–301.

Frison, E.A., Smith, I.F., Johns, T., Cherfas, J., Eyzaguirre, P.B. (2006) 'Agricultural biodiversity, nutrition and health: making a difference to hunger and nutrition in the developing world', *Food Nutr Bull*, vol 27, no 2, pp.167–179.

Glew, R.H., VanderJagt, D.T., Lockett, C., Grivetti, L.E., Smith, G.C., Pastuszyn, A., Millson, M. (1997) 'Amino acid, fatty acid and mineral composition of 24 indigenous plants of Burkina Faso', *Food Comp Anal*, vol 10, pp.205–217.

Gotor, E., Irungu, C. (2010) 'The impact of Bioversity International's African leafy vegetables programme in Kenya', *Impact Assessment and Project Appraisal,* vol 28, no 1, pp.41–55.

Hobblink, H. (2004) 'Biodiversity. What's at Stake?' *Currents*, vol 35/36, pp.18–21.

Ighodalo, C.E., Catherine, O.E., Daniel, M.K. (1991) 'Evaluation of mineral elements and ascorbic acid contents in fruits of some wild plants', *Plant Foods Hum Nutr*, vol 41, pp. 151–154.

Jideani, I.A. (1990) 'Acha (*Digitaria exilis*) – The neglected cereal', *Agric Intern,* vol 42, pp.132–134.

Johns, T., Faubert, G.M., Kokwaro, J.O., Mahunnah, R.L., Kimanani, E.K. (1995) 'Antigiardial activity of gastrointestinal remedies of the Luo of East Africa', *J Ethnopharmacol,* vol 46, pp.17–23.

Kennedy, G., Islam, O., Eyzaguirre, P.B., Kennedy, S. (2005) 'Field testing of plant genetic diversity indicators for nutrition surveys: rice based diets of rural Bangladesh as a model', *J. Food Comp Anal*, vol 18, pp.255–268.

Ladeji, O., Okoye, Z.S.C. (1993) 'Chemical analysis of Sorrel leaf (*Rumex acetosa*)', *Food Chem.,* vol 48, pp.205–206.

Lappia, J.N. (1987) 'Maize as a priority in Sierra Leone: Competitiveness of production with imports and trade-offs with rice', Conference on the Dynamics of cereal consumption and Production patterns in West Africa, Dakar, Senegal.

Maire, B., Delpeuch, F., Cornu, A., Tchibindat, F., Simondon, F., Massamba, J.P., Salem, G., Chevassus-Agnes, S. (1992) 'Urbanization and nutritional transition in sub-Saharan Africa: exemplified by Congo and Senegal', *Rev Epidemiol Sante Publique*, vol 40, no 4, pp.252–258.

McBurney, R.P.H., Griffin, C., Paul, A.A., Greenberg, D.C. (2004) 'The nutritional composition of African wild food plants: from composition to utilization', *J Food Comp Anal,* vol 17, pp.277–289.

McGuirre, S.J. (2008) 'Securing access to seeds: social relations and sorghum exchange in Eastern Ethiopia', *Hum. Ecol.,* vol 36, pp.217–229.

Mendez, M.A., Monteiro, C.A., Popkin, B.M. (2005) 'Overweight exceeds underweight among women in most developing countries', *Am J Clin Nutr,* vol 81, pp.714–721.

Muhammad, S., Amusa, N.A. (2005) 'The important food crops and medicinal plants of north-western Nigeria', *J Agric Biol Sci*, vol 1, no 3, pp.254–260.

Murdock, G.P. (1959) *Africa, Its peoples and their culture history*, McGraw-Hill, New York.

Ndong, M., Wade, S., Dossou, N., Guiro, A.T., Gning, R.D. (2007) 'Valeur nutritionnelle du *Moringa oleifera,* etude de la biodisponibilite du fer, effet de l'enrichissement de divers plats traditionnels Senegalais avec la poudre des feuilles', *AJFAND-Online*, vol 7, no 3.

Ngondi, J.L., Oben, J.E., Minka, S.R. (2005) 'The effect of *Irvingia gabonensis* seeds on body weight and blood lipids of obese subjects in Cameroon', *Lipids Res Disease,* vol 4, no 3, pp.1–4 .

Nordiede, M.B., Hotloy, A., Folling, M., Lied, E., Oshaug, A. (1996) 'Nutrient composition and nutritional importance of green leaves and wild food resources in an agricultural district, Koutiala in southern Mali', *Intern J. Food Sci Nutr*, vol 47, pp.455–468.

Oduro, I., Ellis, W.O., Owusu, D. (2008) 'Nutritional potential of two leafy vegetables: *Moringa oleifera* and *Ipomoea batatas* leaves', *Scientific Res & Essay,* vol 3, no 2, pp.57–60.

Padulosi, S., Bhag Mal, S., Bala Ravi, J., Gowda, K.T.K., Gowda, G., Shanthakumar, N., Dutta, M. (2009) 'Food security and climate change: role of plant genetic resources of minor millets', *Indian J Plant Genet, Resources,* vol 22, no 1, pp.1–16.

Read, M. (1938) 'Native standards of living and African culture change', *Africa XI*, no 3 Supplement.

Robson, J.R.K. (1976) 'Changing food habits in developing countries', *Ecol Food Nutr.,* vol 4, pp.251–256.

Schwab, G. (1947) *Tribes of Liberian Hinterland*, The Museum, Cambridge Massachusetts USA.

Sena, L.P., Vanderjagt, D.J., Rivera, C., Tsin, A.T.C., Muhamadu, I., Mahamadu, O., Milson, M., Pastuszyn, A., Glew, R.H.(1998) 'Analysis of nutritional components of eight famine foods of the Republic of Niger', *Plant Foods Hum Nutr.,* vol 52, pp.17–30.

Shufa, D., Bing, L., Fengying, Z., Popkin, B.M. (2002) 'A new stage of nutrition transition in China', *Public Health Nutr.,* vol 5, no 1A, pp.169–174.

Smith, I.F. (1982) 'Leafy vegetables as sources of minerals in southern Nigerian diets', *Nutr. Rep Intern,* vol 26, pp.679–688.

Smith, I.F. (1995) *The Case for Indigenous West African Food Culture*, UNESCO BREDA Series, no 9. UNESCO Regional Office, Dakar, Senegal.

Smith, I.F. (1998) *Foods of West Africa, Their Origin and Use*, Ottawa, Canada.

Smith, I.F. (2000) 'Micronutrient interventions: options for Africa', *Food Nutr Bull,* vol 21, pp.532–537.

Smith, I.F., Eyzaguirre, P. (2007) 'African leafy vegetables: their role in the World Health Organization's global fruit and vegetables initiative', *AJFAND-Online*, vol 7.

Sodjinou, V., Agueh, V., Fayomi, B., Delisle, H. (2009) 'Dietary patterns of urban adults in Benin: relationship with overall diet quality and socio-demographic characteristics', *Eur J Clin Nutr.,* vol 63, pp.222–228.

Sperling, L., Cooper, H.D., Remington, T. (2008) 'Moving towards more effective seed aid', *J Dev Studies,* vol 44, pp.586–613.

Stadlmayr, B., Charrondiere, R., Addy, P., Samb, B., Enujiugha, V.N., Bayili, R.G., Fagbohoun, E.G., Smith, I.F., Thiam, I., Burlingame, B. (eds) (2010) *Composition of Selected Foods from West Africa*, FAO.

Stadlmayr, B., Charrondiere, U.R., Enujiugha, V.N., Bayili, R.G., Fagbohoun, E.G., Samb, B., Addy, P., Barikmo, I., Ouattara, F., Oshaug, A., Akinyele, I., Annor, G.A., Bomfeh, K., Ene-Obong, H., Smith, I.F., Thiam, I., Burlingame, B. (eds) (2012) *West African Food Composition Table*, FAO.

VanHeerden, S.M., Schondeldt, T. (2004) 'The need for food composition tables for southern Africa', *J. Food Comp Anal,* vol 17, pp.531–537.

Vodouhe, R., Avohou, T.H., Grum, M., Bellon, M., Obel-Lawson, E. (eds) (2008) Connaissances endogènes et gestion durable de l'agrobiodiversité à la ferme: expériences des paysans sahéliens. Actes d'un atelier regional, Bamako, Mali, 18–20 Février.

Voster, H.H., Wissing, M.P., Venter, C.S., Kruger, H.S., Kruger, A., Malan, N.T., De Ridder, J.H., Veldman, F.J., Steyn, H.S., Margetts, B.M., MacIntyre, U. (2000) 'The impact of urbanization on physical, physiological and mental health of Africans in North West Province of South Africa', *S Afr J Sci*, vol 96, pp.505–514.

Voster, H.H., Kruger, A., Margetts, B.M. (2011) 'The Nutrition Transition in Africa: Can it be steered into a more positive direction?' *Nutrients,* vol 3, pp.429–441.

WAHO/ROPPA/Bioversity (2009) 'Regional initiative for the promotion of local foods from the biodiversity of West Africa's traditional food systems', Workshop Report, Ouagadougou Burkina Faso. http://www.bioversityinternational.org/fileadmin/bioversity/publications/pdfs/1423_WAHO-ROPPA-BIOVERSITY%20INTERNATIONAL%20Regional%20initiative%20for%20the%20promotion%20of%20local%20foods%20from%20the%20biodiversity%20of-En.pdf?cache=1341711554, accessed July 2012.

WAHO/ROPPA/Bioversity/FAO/ECOWAS Agriculture Commission (2010) 'Stakeholders meeting on the regional initiative for the promotion of local foods from West Africa's traditional food systems', Workshop Report, Abuja, Nigeria. www.bioversityinternational.org/nc/publication/issue/stakeholders_meeting

7 Linking biodiversity and nutrition

Research methodologies

Roseline Remans and Sean Smukler

Introduction

- How do species, varieties and species compositions differ in nutritional function?
- What is the relationship between biodiversity and nutrition in various settings? Does this relationship change over time? How and why?
- How can we manage biodiversity and the ecosystem services it provides for human nutrition, while also managing for other components of human well-being?

In this chapter, a step is taken to explore research methodologies that can help address these questions as well as introduce how tools mostly used in ecology and agricultural sciences can be applied to integrate nutrition.

Although there have been important exceptions, much of the agricultural research conducted over the last decades has been focused on increasing productivity through improvements in crop genetics and the efficacy of inputs. Maximizing nutritional output of farming systems has never been a primary objective in modern agriculture, human health or public policy. Food-based interventions to tackle undernutrition in the past have been mostly single-nutrient oriented. From various recommendations for high-protein diets (Brock et al., 1955) and later for high-energy diets (McLaren, 1966, 1974), to more recent efforts directed at the elimination of micronutrient deficiencies (Ruel and Levin, 2002), the attention was generally concentrated on one single nutrient to improve nutritional outcomes. Literature reviews (Penafiel et al., 2011; Masset et al., 2011) further underline that although biodiversity could contribute to dietary diversification and quality, current research approaches are falling short to provide strong evidence.

Understanding and strengthening the link between biodiversity and nutrition requires a different approach (Figure 7.1; Fanzo et al., 2011). First, it calls for a dynamic systems approach in which the diversity of organisms and nutrients from production to consumption plays a central role. The first part of this chapter focuses on research frameworks and methodologies that allow such a systems approach at different spatial and time scales to link biodiversity

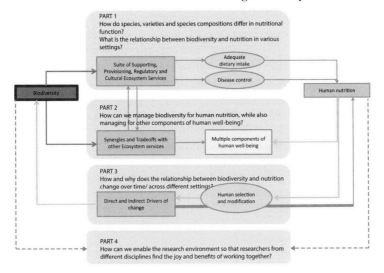

Figure 7.1 Schematic overview of the structure of the chapter. In this chapter, a step is taken to explore methodologies to address four sets of research questions linking biodiversity and nutrition: 1) How do species, varieties and species compositions differ in nutritional function? What is the relationship between biodiversity and nutrition in various settings? 2) How can we manage biodiversity for human nutrition, while also managing for other components of human well-being? 3) How and why does the relationship between biodiversity and nutrition change over time/ across different settings? 4) How can we enable the research environment so that researchers from different disciplines find the joy and benefits of working together?

with nutritional functions and outcomes. We provide an overview of existing methodologies and explore potential future paths.

Second, a basic challenge in investigating and describing the contributions that biodiversity can make to improving nutrition over the next few decades is one of relevance and realism. While there are many possible ways in which biodiversity can improve nutrition, they may not all be feasible in production systems or they may come with negative consequences for other ecosystem services (e.g. reduce fuelwood provisioning or water quality regulation) and components of human well-being (e.g. prove uneconomic or too labour intensive for adoption by farmers). Successful approaches are likely to bring together positive aspects of sustainable intensification and multi-functional agriculture, to reflect the realities and choices of farmers and ultimately improve not just human nutrition but also other components that contribute to human well-being. It is therefore important to investigate the linkages between nutrition and other functions of agro-ecological systems that influence human well-being and to adopt research approaches that can explore trade-offs and synergies in complex systems. Such methodologies are described and illustrated in the second part of the chapter.

Third, considering change over time, a strategy is explored that can help identify drivers of change, and unravel if, why and how the relationship between biodiversity and nutrition outcomes changes (or does not change) over time. Identifying what works in practice over time (see also other chapters), taking into account regional differences and different scales of farming, will be essential if diversity is to be used to improve nutrition in a sustainable way.

Finally, in order to efficiently link biodiversity and nutrition research, researchers from different disciplines must find the joy and benefits of working together. The chapter briefly introduces some tools that can facilitate cross-disciplinary communication (see also Chapter 10).

As new interest on the link between biodiversity and nutrition is emerging in the environment, agriculture and nutrition communities (e.g. the new cross-cutting initiative on biodiversity and nutrition of the Convention of Biological Diversity), this chapter will allow the reader to further enable holistic, cross-sectoral research approaches and help pave the way in developing tools that can guide sustainable decision-making on the ground.

Taking a systems approach to link biodiversity with nutritional functions and outcomes

This section explores approaches that address the questions: "How do species, varieties and species compositions differ in nutritional function?" and "What is the relationship between biodiversity and nutrition in various settings?"

The Millennium Ecosystem Assessment (MEA) provides a widely used framework that links biodiversity to human well-being through ecosystem functions and services (MEA, 2005). Ecosystem functions are the characteristic processes within an ecosystem that include energy and nutrient exchanges, as well as decomposition and production of biomass. The specific ecosystem functions that are apparently beneficial to human civilization are considered ecosystem services. Here, the MEA framework is applied to the relationship between biodiversity and human nutrition and identifies a suite of research methodologies or tools that provide ways to further unravel pieces of this framework (Figure 7.2). An overview of tools based on existing literature is provided in Table 7.1. While many tools are important, there will be a focus on a selection of methodologies highlighted in Figure 7.2 that are considered most relevant for this chapter. To illustrate these tools, data and examples are used from the literature and the Millennium Villages Project, a rural development project with research and implementation sites across all major agro-ecological zones in sub-Saharan Africa (Sanchez et al., 2007).

How do species, varieties and species compositions differ in nutritional function?

A human diet requires at least 51 nutrients in adequate amounts consistently (Graham et al., 2007). In food sciences, several methods have been developed to analyse the composition of food items for this diversity of nutrients and standardized nutrition indicators for biodiversity have been suggested (Kennedy and Burlingame, 2003; FAO, 2007, 2010a). While for many of the minor crops

How do species, varieties and species compositions differ in nutritional function | What is the relationship between biodiversity and nutrition in various settings

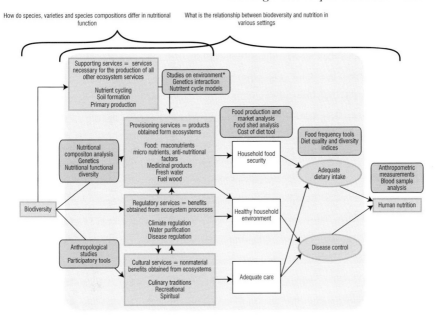

Figure 7.2 Application of the Millennium Ecosystem Framework in combination with the UNICEF Child and Maternal Nutrition Framework on the relationship between biodiversity and nutrition. Research methodologies and tools to investigate specific pieces of the framework are highlighted and a selection of these are further described in the text

the nutritional differences and possible advantages of one variety over another are not yet known, great progress is being made in extending food composition tables (e.g. the International Network of Food Data Systems, INFOODS; Stadlmayr et al., 2010) and in identifying the advantage of several minor crops in securing a healthy supply of specific nutrients (Penafiel et al., 2011; Golden et al., 2011; other chapters in this book). For example, nutritional composition analysis of African green leafy vegetables has clearly shown that these leafy greens (e.g. African spiderweed, black nightshade) provide higher levels of iron and vitamin A than several imported species (e.g. Chinese cabbage, Chweya and Eyzaguirre 1999; see also other chapters). This has helped promotion and adoption in local to regional markets (Shackleton et al., 2009).

Further, progress in genetics and genomics, for example the use of more advanced molecular markers such as microsatellites and the genome-wide screening of different varieties, now allow for more efficient identification of quantitative trait loci (QTL) and genes on the genome that contribute to specific nutritional functions (Galeano et al., 2011). For example, QTL explaining the higher iron and zinc variability in common bean varieties were recently identified (Blair et al., 2010). These tools thereby not only help to unravel the genetic base for differences in nutritional composition of varieties, but also provide means to improve the nutritional value of locally adopted varieties through cross-breeding.

Table 7.1 Overview of assessments and tools in the biodiversity–nutrition research framework

Assessment	Tools	References to examples/reviews/guidelines
Farming systems	Farming systems model	Dixon et al. 2001; Fanzo et al. 2011
Local biodiversity	Interviews (local names) and literature (scientific names) Observations / field and plant/animal identification	Penafiel et al. 2011; Fanzo et al. 2011
Genetics of nutritional traits	Quantitative Trait Loci (QTL) analysis Gene characterization and isolation	Vijay et al. 2009; Blair et al. 2010; Paine et al. 2005
Nutritional composition of food items	Chemical analysis Food composition tables and literature	FAO 2007; FAO-INFOODS: Engleberger et al. 2010; Penafiel et al. 2011; Kennedy and Burlingame 2003
Nutritional composition of agro-ecological systems	Nutritional functional diversity metric	Remans et al. 2011a; DeClerck et al. 2011
Impact of environment and agronomic practices on nutritional composition	Agronomic/environmental field trials combined with nutritional composition analysis Digital soil maps and GPS	Graham 2008; Graham et al. 2007; Bourn and Prescott 2002; Sanchez et al. 2009
Nutrient cycles, biodiversity and nutrition	Food web pathways Indicators: soil fertility and fauna indicators, diversity and cover of plants at the plot level, diversity of land use types in mosaics at landscape level	Elser and Urabe 1999; MEA 2005, Chapter 12

Assessment	Tools	References to examples/reviews/guidelines
Food consumption patterns and dietary intake	Food frequency questionnaires Dietary diversity scores 24-hour recalls Dietary reference intake tables Mean probability of adequacy (MPA) for macro and micronutrients	Willett 1998; Penafiel et al. 2011; FAO-FANTA 2008; FAO 2010a; Arimond and Ruel 2004; Arimond et al. 2010; Fanzo et al. 2011
Sources of food	Food shed analysis	Peters et al. 2008; Conard et al. 2011
Access to nutritious food	Cost of the diet tool Food security questionnaires Market analysis Value chain analysis	Perry 2008; Bilinsky and Swindale 2007; Coates et al. 2007; Remans et al. 2011a; Hawkes and Ruel 2011
Human nutrition outcomes	Anthropometric measurements Serum analysis	Cogill 2001; Massett et al. 2011; Golden et al. 2011; Fanzo et al. 2011
Trade-offs between multiple ecosystem services	Trade-off models: InVest, ARIES, EcoMetrix Life cycle analysis	Nelson and Daily 2010; Villa et al. 2009; Parametrix 2010; Bentrup et al. 2004

Recognizing the exciting progress made in methodologies to develop food composition tables and to identify the genetic base of nutritional differences between species and varieties (FAO, 2010b), there are still a couple of major gaps in current research approaches in order to address the question as to how do species, varieties and species compositions differ in nutritional function, in a more holistic way.

First, not much is known about the interaction between the nutritional composition of crop species or varieties, the agricultural management practices and environmental conditions. Food composition tables, for example, mostly do not include information about the management practices applied (e.g. fertilizer, irrigation) nor the environmental conditions in which a specific food item is grown. A number of studies (e.g. Remans et al., 2008; Graham et al., 2007; Graham, 2008; Weil et al., unpublished), however, clearly show that the nutritional composition, including protein, sulfur, iron, zinc content, of crops can vary significantly among different management and environmental conditions. For example, addition of zinc fertilizer to the soil can increase the concentration of trace elements in edible parts of common bean (Graham et al., 2007; Graham, 2008). Also, the concentration of sulfur containing amino acids in the grain of common bean increased as higher levels of sulfate were detected in the soil, while this was not the case for maize (Weil et al., unpublished).

To enhance our understanding as to how the nutritional function of species and varieties differ, there is a critical need to link food composition analyses to agricultural management, soil and environmental studies. There currently exist several opportunities that can strengthen this link in a systematic way. The African Soil Information Service (AfSIS) project is developing a digital soil map of Africa, collecting information not only on soil but also on vegetation, climate and the effects of agricultural management practices on soil fertility and crop productivity throughout the African sub-continent. Linking nutritional composition analyses to such Global Digital Soil Map initiatives could help unravel the interaction between management, environment and nutritional composition. In addition, methodologies such as infrared spectroscopy offer promising potential to analyse the nutritional composition of plant varieties in a relatively quick and cost-effective way in the field as compared with wet-lab analysis (Foley et al., 1998; Brown et al., 2006). These tools provide a way not only to speed up the analyses of plant nutritional composition, but also to directly link such results to soil characteristics if measured simultaneously in the field.

Further, Global Positioning Systems (GPS) tools provide a way to easily record the location where food items used for nutritional composition analysis are collected. This can enable integration of food composition data with spatially explicit environmental data, including soil, climate, land use/cover and water availability characteristics, and enable investigators to address questions such as "Can we identify 'nutritional deserts' where nutritional value of crops is lower than in other regions?" Or "Is the difference in nutritional value between certain varieties larger in conditions of optimal rainfall as compared with droughts?"

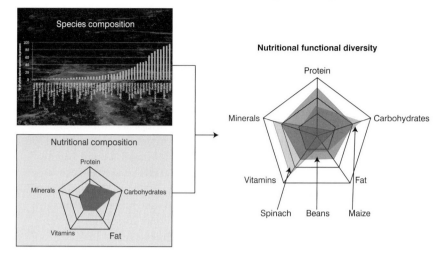

Figure 7.3 Schematic representation of the nutritional functional diversity metric, based on 1) species composition in a given farm or landscape and 2) nutritional composition of these species. Thereby the nutritional FD metric provides a way to assess complementarity between species for their nutritional function

In addition to enhancing our understanding of the interaction between environment and nutritional composition of species and varieties, there is need for research that enables greater consideration of the large diversity of species and varieties available in the system as a whole together with their nutritional composition. This brings us to the question, "How do different species *compositions* differ in nutritional function?" By using examples of rural villages in sub-Saharan Africa, this chapter illustrates how an ecological concept, the Functional Diversity (FD) metric, has potential to address this question.

FD is a metric used in ecology that reflects the trait distinctiveness of species in a community and the degree of complementarity in traits of species within a community. Though many ecologists have focused on the relationship between biodiversity and ecosystem functioning, there has been little focus on the role that ecosystems play in providing the essential nutrients of human diets.

Applying the FD metric to the nutritional traits of plants (and potentially animals) provides a novel metric, called nutritional functional diversity (nutritional FD, Figure 7.3, Remans et al., 2011a) that bridges agriculture, ecology and nutrition studies. The nutritional FD metric is based on plant species composition at the farm (or landscape scale) and the nutritional composition of these plants for a suite of nutrients (e.g., 17 different nutrients in the study by Remans et al., 2011a) that are key in human diets and for which reliable plant composition data are available. The nutritional FD value increases when a species or variety with a unique combination of nutrients is added to a community, and decreases when such a species is lost. The nutritional FD metric thereby reflects the diversity of nutrients provided by the farm and the complementarity

Box 7.1 Assessing nutritional diversity of cropping systems in African villages

Data on edible plant species diversity were collected for 170 farms in three Millennium Villages in sub-Saharan Africa. Nutritional FD metrics took into account 17 essential nutrients that were calculated for each of the 170 farms, based on farm species composition and species nutritional composition.

Figure 7.4 plots FD values against species richness for each of the 170 farms. Regression of FD against species richness reveals several patterns. First, there is a strong positive correlation ($p < 0.001$; $r^2 = 0.68$) between FD and species richness, independent of village. Thus, as the number of edible species increases, the diversity of nutritional functions that farm provides also increases. Second, at a level of around 25 species per farm, the relationship between FD and species richness starts levelling off, meaning that adding species to a farm with around 25 or more species, increases nutritional diversity very little. Third, although species richness and FD_{total} are correlated, farms with the same number of species can have very different nutritional FD scores. For example, two farms in Mwandama (indicated by arrows on Figure 7.4) both with 10 species show an FD of 23 and 64, respectively. The difference in FD is linked to a few differences in species nutritional traits. Both of these example farms grow maize, cassava, beans, banana, papaya, pigeon pea and mango. In addition, the farm with the higher FD score grows pumpkin, mulberry, and groundnut, while the farm with the lower FD score has avocado, peaches and black jack (*Bidens pilosa*). Trait analysis shows that pumpkin (including pumpkin leaves, fruits and seeds, which are all eaten) adds diversity to the system by its relatively high nutritional content in vitamin A, Zn, and S-containing amino acids (methionine and cysteine) compared with other species; mulberry by its levels of vitamin B complexes (thiamin, riboflavin) and groundnut by its nutritional content for fat, Mn, and S. The black jack, avocado and peaches found in the lower FD farm add less nutritional diversity to the system than pumpkin, mulberry, and groundnut since they do not contain the vitamin B or S complexes, and thus are less complementary to the other plants in the system for their nutritional content.

This example illustrates that by applying the FD metric on nutritional diversity, it is possible to identify differences in nutritional diversity as well as species that are critical for ensuring the provision of certain nutrients by the system (e.g., mulberry for vitamin B complexes). The results also emphasize that the species nutritional composition available in the system determine whether introduction or removal of certain species will contribute to the nutritional diversity of the farming or ecosystem. The quality and sensitivity of this type of metric will be enhanced if more data are available on the nutritional composition of species and varieties grown under different environmental and agronomic practices (see above).

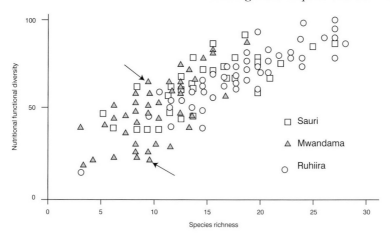

Figure 7.4 Nutritional functional diversity plotted against species richness for 170 farms in three Millennium Village project sites, Sauri in Kenya, Ruhiira in Uganda and Mwandama in Malawi

in nutrients among species on a farm or community. A concrete example of the application and interpretation of this metric is illustrated in Box 7.1 and Figure 7.4. One of the shortcomings of the metric is that it does not include a dimension of food consumption or food habits, e.g. ways in which foods are usually eaten locally. In addition, the current tool does not include abundance data, e.g. data on quantity of food produced or consumed. Current on-going research is exploring how these two dimensions can be incorporated in this tool.

While in the past, food-based interventions have focused mostly on single nutrients, the approach described by this metric can help guide agricultural interventions to provide a diversity of nutrients as well as to enhance nutrient redundancy or resilience of the system. In particular, this tool provides means to identify potential crops, varieties or groups of plants that add nutritional value (diversity or redundancy) to the system if introduced, promoted, or conserved.

What is the relationship between biodiversity and nutrition in various settings?

The methodologies described above provide ways to investigate and describe the nutritional function of species, varieties and species compositions. A suite of additional instruments is needed to unravel how biodiversity and ecosystem services relate to human nutrition outcomes (Figure 7.2; FAO, 2010a; Penafiel et al., 2011; Masset et al., 2011).

According to the UNICEF framework (UNICEF, 1990) that outlines the various direct and indirect determinants of child and maternal nutrition, biodiversity is in general considered part of the natural capital, which can have an impact on the level of poverty, household food security, dietary diversity and food habits (see also Chapter 6), child and maternal caring practices and access to a healthy (or unhealthy) household environment. These factors are determinants for dietary intake and disease control, the two direct determinants of nutrition health outcomes. The UNICEF framework illustrates the complexity of the pathway between biodiversity and nutritional outcomes as well as the many potential confounding factors, e.g. income, access to health services, and adequate care practices (e.g. breastfeeding), that can influence this pathway.

In the MEA framework, four types of ecosystem services provided by biodiversity are distinguished and can be linked to the UNICEF nutrition impact pathway (Figure 7.2): provisioning services (e.g. macro- and micronutrients, fresh water) that contribute to food security; regulatory services (e.g. disease regulation, climate regulation) that contribute to a healthy household environment; cultural services (e.g. culinary traditions, utilization of medicinal plants) that contribute to adequate care; and, as also mentioned above, supporting services (e.g. soil formation) that are critical to enable the other services.

Starting from this combined MEA and UNICEF framework, methodologies will be explored to investigate how biodiversity, food security, diet diversity and nutrition health outcomes are linked. This chapter will not go into depth on assessments of dietary diversity and food habits, but will emphasize that human selection, marketing and consumption habits are key drivers for biodiversity selection and promotion (feedback loop indicated by arrows in Figure 7.1). Critical for linking biodiversity and nutrition is the co-location of data in different scientific disciplines, i.e. ecology, agriculture, economics (e.g. food market prices and functioning, income data), nutrition (e.g. consumption, anthropometric measurements) and health, and a strong research design in order to push toward a firmer grasp of causal mechanisms to guide interventions (Barrett et al., 2011; Masset et al., 2011; Penafiel et al., 2011; Sachs et al., 2010; Golden et al., 2011). Most often, biodiversity studies do not include measurements of human well-being, such as food security, consumption and anthropometric measurements and operate at different time and spatial scales than agriculture or human health studies (e.g. at the landscape level versus at the individual or clinic level). Similarly, human health studies mostly do not include environmental or agricultural indicators. In order to better understand the relationship between biodiversity and nutrition, it is essential that future studies are designed for cross-sectoral hypothesis testing and for stronger integration of different datasets.

An example of co-location of data can be found in the Millennium Villages Project. In addition to the information on biodiversity described in Box 7.1, data were collected on the agro-ecological zones, the three pillars of food security including food availability, access and consumption, as well as anthropometric measurements of children under five years in age and blood samples of adult women and children (Remans et al., 2011a, 2011b).

Through multivariable regression functions, the integrated dataset allows exploring relationships between biodiversity and nutrition outcomes at different scales, i.e. at the household and village scale, as well as over time (MVP is a ten-year project), while controlling for a set of demographic and socio-economic variables. Preliminary findings show that no significant correlations at the household level could be found between species richness or nutritional FD and household food security or consumption indicators. However, certain trends between species richness, nutritional FD and human nutrition indicators are observed at the village or landscape level. For example, villages where biodiversity provides less mineral diversity as compared with other villages, face higher prevalence of iron deficiency among adult women. Also, higher species richness and nutritional FD at the village level corresponds with higher average levels of dietary diversity and food security (i.e. fewer months with inadequate food supply). These findings generate interesting hypotheses on the link between nutritional diversity and nutrition outcomes at the village or landscape level. Importantly, more research is needed to analyse the causal relationships and the role of markets and access to food (e.g. using the cost of the diet tool described by Perry, 2008). While most households in the studied villages are considered subsistence farmers, farm households are not closed systems. Food consumption and expenditure data show that the average proportion of food consumed that comes from own production is around 50 per cent. Also, a significant correlation was found between the number and value of food items bought and sold on local markets and the household food indicators at each of the three sites (Food Insecurity Score (FIS), Household Dietary Diversity Score (HHDDS), Months of Household Inadequate Food Supply (MHIFS)) (Lambrecht, 2009). These findings emphasize the importance of local markets and support the notion that these farm households are not closed systems. Therefore, the most appropriate scale to link nutritional FD metrics to food consumption and nutrition indicators would be the "foodshed", defined as the geographic area that supplies a population centre with food (Peters et al., 2008; Niles and Roff, 2008). Village level data show that for the Ruhiira Millennium Village site in Uganda, 82 per cent of food consumed is derived from production within the village. This indicates that in the case of this village, the foodshed currently largely overlaps with the village (Remans et al. 2011a). While the concept of foodshed seems most straightforward for settings where most of the food is from own production, the concept can and has also been applied at larger geographic scales, such as urban areas, and regional foodsheds, as well as for the global foodshed. For additional reading on this topic, please refer to Peters et al. (2008) and Conard et al. (2011) who describe foodshed analysis for urban areas. To further unravel the role of markets in the biodiversity–nutrition nexus and the dynamics of stocks and flows of nutrients in foodshed analysis, market and value chain analyses offer potential for future investigation (e.g. Hawkes and Ruel, 2011).

Trade-offs and synergies with other ecosystem services and components of human well-being

In addition to providing ecosystem services that directly contribute to human nutrition, biodiversity indirectly supports human nutrition by ensuring the availability of ecosystem services that contribute to other aspects of human well-being (MEA, 2005; Figure 7.1). This section explores methodologies that can help address the question as to how biodiversity and the ecosystem services it provides can be managed for improved nutrition, while also managing for other components of human well-being.

Improving human well-being necessitates managing agriculture for multiple services across geographic extents and through time

In an analysis of the state of the planet and its people, the MEA concluded that in order to address many of the threats to human well-being it is essential to learn to manage for multiple ecosystem services (MEA, 2005). Since the MEA came out much work has been done to develop strategies to assess multiple outcomes, including nutrition, related to biodiversity at various spatial and time scales. This has elucidated numerous challenges of such analysis, important to briefly outline here.

While ecosystem services are not all equally required to ensure human well-being some *combinations* of them are. Without an adequate supply of drinking water, caloric intake ensured by the provisioning of food cannot secure well-being. But the provisioning of drinking water does not suffice if it results in disease that compromises the ability to absorb nutrients, thus ecosystem services that regulate water quality are also required to improve nutrition. In addition, without the ability to cook food, using fuel from the provisioning of wood or fossil fuels, the nutrients might not be bio-available for human consumption. Beyond the need for multiple provisioning services (e.g. food, water, fuel) and regulating services (e.g. disease), well-being also requires a combination of cultural services. Having enough food, water and nutrients to be physically healthy does not ensure that one is mentally healthy.

It is clear that ensuring human well-being requires managing for multiple services but how much of which service is not clear. A clear understanding of how to manage for multiple services is currently elusive for a number of reasons. First, many ecosystem services are difficult to quantify (e.g. religious fulfilment), making it challenging to determine the *amount of each service* that is required to ensure well-being. When thinking about one service at a time, it may be fairly straightforward (as least for some services), to accurately quantify how much is needed to fulfil basic requirements to maintain human well-being. It is possible to see these amounts as thresholds for which, if the amount of the service falls below, a reduction in human well-being would be expected. For example, determining a threshold for food or water provisioning services can be based on our knowledge that humans require a basic amount of daily nutrient intake to prevent undernutrition or a certain number of litres of water to prevent dehydration. Determining thresholds for other services however, is much more difficult. For example, it may be possible to quantify how much one feels a sense of community but the amount required to maintain well-being may vary substantially from person to person. Or determining thresholds for supporting and regulating services that help ensure provisioning services is complicated because the relationship

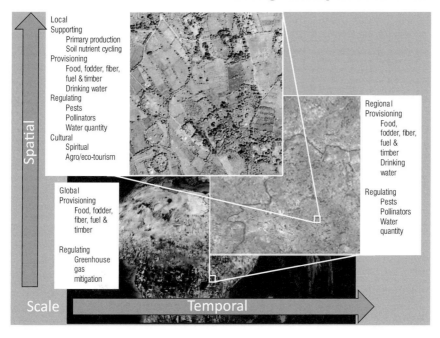

Figure 7.5 The availability of ecosystem services can vary by spatial and temporal scales, illustrated here for the local, regional, and global scales through time. How farmers manage their agrobiodiversity at the local scale not only impacts on quantities of multiple ecosystem services available to them; it can also impact the availability of a different suite of services for people in distant places or even people in the distant future

is indirect. How much soil regulation is required to ensure that crops can produce that daily intake of calories?

Further, there are inherently numerous *interactions among ecosystem services*. These interactions may be close dependencies, or loose associations. In some cases this means a number of ecosystem services will respond to the same driver of change similarly but in other cases they will not. If a storm causes severe soil erosion and reduces soil nutrient regulation, fuelwood and food provisioning are both likely to be negatively impacted. The provisioning of one service might actually be at a cost to the provisioning of another service. Growing enough food on a limited piece of land (food provisioning) may mean that there is no room to grow fuelwood trees (fuel provisioning). Being able to accurately quantify and/or predict changes in the availability of these services is key to understanding these trade-offs and managing for multiple ecosystem services. Equally as important, is the need to identify and understand possible synergies among ecosystem services, i.e. situations where multiple services are enhanced simultaneously by exogenous drivers such as particular management practices.

Beyond trade-offs and synergies among multiple services it is important to recognize that there may also be *trade-offs and synergies among locations and time periods* (Figure 7.5). The ecosystem services that humans rely on are often produced far from where they are consumed. Those that consume these services may have little or no relationship to those who manage the biodiversity that mediates their availability and there may be serious trade-offs between the types of services that are available to those that consume vs. those that manage the services. This holds true for those people who will consume services in the near future (i.e. future generations). There are likely large trade-offs in the availability of ecosystem services for the current generation as opposed to future generations. For example, while all humans need clean water very few people actually manage the areas of the landscape that regulate water quality. Watersheds are areas of a landscape that delineate the collection of water (e.g. rain, snow) and drainage, to streams, rivers and aquifers. Management of these watersheds can largely determine the fate of the quality of water that can be supplied far from the source. Managers of a watershed such as farmers, ranchers or foresters, can thus impact the availability and quality of the water for downstream users. This inherent disconnect between beneficiaries and managers for many ecosystem services poses one of the most important challenges to human well-being and illustrates a clear need for policy based on scientific guidance.

The more the trade-offs and synergies can be understood and predicted among ecosystem services in agricultural landscapes that dominate our terrestrial world, the more effective it will be to manage for improved human well-being (MEA, 2005).

Evaluating multiple services requires trade-off analysis

Methods to measure multiple ecosystem service outcomes and relate them to changes in human well-being have until recently been largely theoretical because of the challenges outlined above (Daily, 1997; Foley et al., 2005; Raudsepp-Hearne et al., 2010a, 2010b). Few studies have simultaneously measured ecosystem services (Chan et al., 2011; Nelson and Daily, 2010; Smukler et al., 2010) and fewer still have been able to also measure changes in well-being or nutrition (Raudsepp-Hearne et al., 2010b; Said et al., 2007). Some studies utilize spatially explicit ecosystem process models to predict future outcomes of particular management scenarios, while others have taken the approach of measuring and mapping actual outcomes (Figure 7.1). The evaluation of the trade-offs and synergies in the analyses in most of these studies is limited to graphically illustrating the multiple outcomes and how they have or might change based on different management practices (Figure 7.6).

Recent progress has been made in two key areas that will help with these types of efforts: the development of tools that can effectively model multiple outcomes and the collection of data that can be used to parameterize and validate these models (Nelson, 2011). What is noticeably missing from current analyses is an assessment of trade-offs and synergies of ecosystem services with nutritional outcomes as indicators of human well-being. In what follows, the

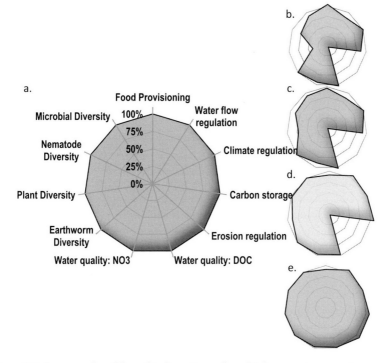

Figure 7.6 An example of how biodiversity and multiple ecosystem services may be graphically illustrated to assess potential trade-offs and synergies. In this case the quantities of six ecosystem services associated with four indicators of agricultural biodiversity are compared for different management scenarios in a case study of a tomato farm in California, USA (Smukler et al., 2010). The quantities of biodiversity and ecosystem services were considered to be 100 per cent for the measured baseline analysis of the current system (a.) and the values in modelled alternative scenarios are reported as percentages relative to this baseline. The scenarios include: (b.) tomato production only, (c.) tomatoes with native shrub hedgerows that provide habitat, (d.) tomatoes with native shrub hedgerows and riparian tree planting that also store carbon, (e.) tomatoes with native shrub hedgerows, riparian tree planting and a detention pond that purifies irrigation runoff

chapter describes these methodologies and discusses how key biodiversity–nutrition questions can be integrated to them.

There are numerous ecosystem process models, economic models, and bio-economic models that can simulate outcomes for one or two ecosystem services and a few outcomes of human well-being (Raudsepp-Hearne et al., 2010a). The MEA utilized a number of these individual models to predict outcomes for living space, food and energy for various land use / land cover change scenarios (MEA, 2005). There are however only a few integrated process models that can predict multiple outcomes simultaneously, yet these do not necessarily link services with well-being but rather predict associated changes in particular indicators.

Of the models currently employed for multiple ecosystem service analysis there are three examples that have recently demonstrated their capabilities and potential to model trade-offs and synergies. Two of these models are open source, the Integrated Valuation of Ecosystem Services and Trade-offs (InVEST) (Nelson and Daily, 2010) and Artificial Intelligence for Ecosystem Services (ARIES) (Villa et al., 2009), and one is a proprietary model, EcoMetrix (Parametrix, 2010). Although these models, and others like them, all attempt to quantify and valuate multiple ecosystem services and some aspects of human well-being their methodologies vary greatly (Nelson and Daily, 2010).

Both InVEST and ARIES were designed to provide a tool to assess ecosystem service trade-offs for various landscape management options to a wide range of stakeholders including international conservation organizations, government agencies, and businesses. EcoMetrix is a multi-resource tool designed for quantifying ecosystem services at a much smaller scale and is targeted at stakeholders who need to do site-specific evaluations to measure project impacts and benefits. InVEST and ARIES run a series of modules that simultaneously produce outcomes for ecosystem services ranging from carbon sequestration to water regulation and include analysis for biodiversity and economics. The EcoMetrix model is a compilation of over 50 biotic and abiotic (physical process) functions that are scored based on the percentage of optimal performance for the given site that allows the user to assess changes in the functional performance for a variety of ecosystem services such as water provisioning, water regulation, climate regulation and various cultural services. Using a percentage of optimal performance helps address the challenge of dealing with the various units of each ecosystem service and enables "stacking" of services into a single score. Because the value of ecosystem services depends on stakeholders preferences or site-specific conditions the model also allows for the "weighting of factors" and enables policy goals to be changed and tracked. Each of these models has been utilized in a number of environments and socio-economic situations including Tanzania, Oregon and China (Daily et al., 2009; Tallis and Polasky, 2009) but the number of studies remains small. Furthermore the extent that these models can demonstrate the relationship between ecosystem services and human well-being is limited mainly to economics and, to our knowledge, thus far neglects nutrition entirely.

What we need to do to effectively use trade-off analysis with biodiversity and nutrition questions

Although there is a strong theoretical framework for the relationship between various ecosystem services and nutritional outcomes, as described above, current ecosystem process models don't address this outcome. Developing modelling components that can integrate the various ecosystem services that are directly related to agro-biodiversity and nutrition (e.g. water regulation) is particularly critical for assessing various land management options in agricultural landscapes in impoverished regions, where substitution of services (e.g. buying bottled water) is not an option. Thus far modelling efforts have been largely focused on developing conservation strategies, which do not necessarily equate to sustainable development. It is argued that there is a critical need to modify such models so they can be used in agricultural landscapes to address near-term human well-being concerns such as nutrition and understand how agro-biodiversity may contribute to this goal. What is needed is to start measuring nutritional outcomes in the same locations as biodiversity and ecosystem services are measured. Using these data it is possible to then start to build additional modules into existing models and begin to assess correlations between these ecosystem services and nutrition outcomes.

Identifying drivers of change

In order to guide decision-making on future management of biodiversity for nutrition and other components of human well-being, it is not sufficient to understand the situation at this moment of time. Society and ecosystems change so fast that research methodologies that help to identify drivers of change are critical to enable forward-looking research and adaption to change. This section takes a step in exploring options to address the questions "How and why does the relationship between biodiversity and nutrition change over time? What are the major drivers of change?"

Several hypotheses already exist on these drivers of change. For example, it has been argued that changes in agricultural production systems from diversified cropping systems towards large-scale, industrial agriculture have contributed to ecologically more simple cereal based systems, poor diet diversity, micronutrient deficiencies and resulting malnutrition in the developed as well as the developing world (Welch and Graham, 1999; Frison et al., 2006; Graham et al., 2007). Historically, success of agricultural systems has been evaluated on and driven by metrics of crop yields, economic output and cost-benefit ratios (IAASTD, 2009).

There is, however, no systematic approach to identify trends and drivers of change for the relationship between biodiversity and nutrition. Identification of drivers of change is very complex because of the multiple interactions and feedback loops between factors (resulting in non-linear relationships) (Barrett et al., 2011), but lessons from other scientific disciplines, e.g. climate science, economics and anthropology, can help to pave the way.

Here we discuss a two-step approach as a minimum strategy. First, long-term time series of observational data on biodiversity, ecosystem services, and human well-being outcomes (including nutrition and other components) at different spatial scales need to be collected to enable the identification of trends and generate hypotheses on relationships. A global agricultural monitoring network as suggested by Sachs et al. (2010) could provide such data on biodiversity and nutrition. The network aims to collect data on the multiple dimensions (including biodiversity and nutrition) of agricultural landscapes across agro-ecological, climatic and anthropogenic gradients and over time (Sachs et al.,

2012). In addition, already existing time-series and geo-referenced data can be mobilized better to be integrated in cross-sectoral data-analysis and models; for example nutrition time series data are abundant (on anthropometry), as well as agricultural and environmental data (food production, food availability in FAOSTAT, land cover databases etc.).

Second, cross-disciplinary social and experimental research is needed to draw causal relationships on these interactions between social and ecological systems. For example anthropological studies, of which there are now a large number, help to understand why a community conserves certain species or varieties while ignoring others. Experimental research including randomized control trials can help unravel if and why certain species are more tolerant to changing environmental conditions.

It is beyond the scope of this chapter to extend on these approaches. But we do want to emphasize the importance and potential of research on drivers of change. Our science cannot afford to stand still at the snapshot of time that we currently live in. A better understanding of the scope of drivers of change will enable forward-looking research that can provide tools to enhance decision-making at the right time and the right place.

Tools for enhancing interdisciplinary communication

To address the complexity of the relationship between biodiversity and nutrition, it is widely recognized that collaboration between researchers and practitioners from different disciplines is needed. However, the barriers to

---

Box 7.2 Tools for enhancing interdisciplinary communication (Winowiecki et al., 2011)

- Interdisciplinary Toolbox – undertake structured dialogue about research assumptions.
- Integrated Timeline – brainstorm with all participants and disciplines about historic events that led to the current food-insecurity situation.
- Mind Mapping and Mini-Mind Mapping – brainstorm factors and drivers that influence food security.
- Cross-Impact Analysis – explore the relationships between each major theme identified in the mind-mapping exercises.
- Imagining the Ideal – create and share visions about the ideal outcome or solution to the research problem.
- Backcasting – undertake a scenario-building exercise that works backward from imagining the problem is solved (the world is food secure) and explores the paths to get there.
- Joint fieldwork and visits – undertake joint visits to the field to identify specific problems and related solutions.

efficient communication between different disciplines and enjoyment of the process are often underestimated. There are an increasing number of tools that can help enhance interdisciplinary thinking and communication and this topic is the focus of Chapter 10 of this book. To introduce the concept, we list a few examples in Box 7.2 of methods that we explored and found useful in the context of the research described in this chapter.

Conclusion

Addressing questions on the interaction between biodiversity and nutrition isn't easy. To provide effective science-based decision-making tools to improve human nutrition will require innovative research that utilizes a systems-approach and new thinking that begins to bridge the gaps between disciplines.

In this chapter, we have explored various frameworks and methodologies that can help address some of the key questions about the link between biodiversity and nutrition. We have also emphasized the importance of understanding possible synergies and trade-offs with other ecosystem services and components of human well-being as well as to identify drivers of change. Our objective was not to provide an exhaustive list of options but to trigger new thinking and to contribute to creating an enabling research environment for exploring this intriguing and critical interaction between biodiversity and human nutrition.

References

Arimond, M., Ruel, M.T. (2004) Dietary diversity is associated with child nutritional status: evidence from 11 demographic and health surveys, *J Nutr*, vol 134, pp.2579–2585.

Arimond, M., Wiesmann, D., Becquey, E., Carriquiry, A., Daniels, M.C., Deitchler, M., Fanou Fogny, N., Joseph, M.L., Kennedy, G., Martin-Prevel, Y., Torheim, L.E. (2010) Simple food group diversity indicators predict micronutrient adequacy of women's diets in 5 diverse, resource-poor settings, *J Nutr*, vol 140, pp.2059S–2069S.

Barrett, C.B., Travis, A.J., Dasgupta, P. (2011) On biodiversity conservation and poverty traps, *Proc Natl Acad Sci USA*, vol 108, pp.13907–13912.

Bentrup, F., Küsters, J., Kuhlmann, H., Lammel, J. (2004) Environmental impact assessment of agricultural production systems using the life cycle assessment methodology: I. Theoretical concept of a LCA method tailored to crop production, *Eur J Agronomy*, vol 20, pp.247–264.

Bilinsky, P., Swindale, A. (2007) *Months of Adequate Household Food Provisioning (MAHFP) for Measurement of Household Food Access: Indicator Guide*, Food and Nutrition Technical Assistance Project, Academy for Educational Development, Washington DC.

Blair, M.W., González, L.F., Kimani, P.M., Butare, L. (2010) Genetic diversity, inter-gene pool introgression and nutritional quality of common beans (Phaseolus vulgaris L.) from Central Africa, *Theoret Appl Genetics*, vol 121, pp.237–248.

Bourn, D., Prescott, J. (2002) A comparison of the nutritional value, sensory qualities, and food safety of organically and conventionally produced foods, *Crit Rev Food Sci Nutr*, vol 42, pp.1–34.

Brock, J.F., Hansen, J.D.L., Howe, E.E., Pretorius, P.D., Daval, J.G.A., Hendricks, R.G. (1955) Kwashiorkor and protein malnutrition. A dietary therapeutic trial, *Lancet*, vol 2, pp.355–360.

Brown, D.J., Shepherd, K.D., Walsh, M.G., Mays, D.M., Reinsh, T.G. (2006) Global soil characterization with VNIR diffuse reflectance spectroscopy, *Geoderma*, vol 132, pp.273–290.

Chan, K.M.A., Hoshizaki, L., Klinkenberg, B. (2011) Ecosystem Services in Conservation Planning: Targeted Benefits vs. Co-Benefits or Costs? *PLoS One* 6:e24378.

Chweya, J.A., Eyzaguirre, P.B. (eds) (1999) The biodiversity of traditional leafy vegetables, *Bioversity International*, Rome, p.181.

Coates, J., Swindale, A., Bilinsky, P. (2007) *Household Food Insecurity Access Scale (HFIAS) for measurement of Food Access: Indicator Guide (v. 3)*, Food and Nutrition Technical Assistance Project, Academy for Educational Development, Washington DC.

Cogill, B. (2001) *Anthropometric Indicators Measurement Guide*, Food and Nutrition Technical Assistance Project, Academy for Educational Development, Washington DC.

Conard, M., Ackerman, K., Gavrilaki, D. (2011) *Modeling Production, Processing and Distribution Infrastructure For A Resilient Regional Food System*, Urban Design Lab, The Earth Institute at Columbia University.

Daily, G. (1997) *Nature's services: societal dependence on natural ecosystems*, Island Press.

Daily, G., Polasky, S., Goldstein, J., Kareiva, P., Mooney, H., Pejchar, L., Ricketts, T., Salzman, J., Shallenberger, R. (2009) Ecosystem services in decision making: time to deliver, *Frontiers in Ecology and the Environment,* vol 7, pp.21–28.

Declerck, F., Fanzo, J., Palm, C. and Remans, R. (2011) Ecological approaches to human nutrition, *Food and Nutrition Bulletin*, vol 32, pp. S41–S50.

Dixon, J., Gulliver, A. and Gibbon, D. (2001) *Farming systems and poverty*, FAO and World Bank, Rome and Washington DC.

Elser, J.J., Urabe, J. (1999) The stoichiometry of consumer-driven nutrient recycling: theory, observations, and consequences, *Ecology*, vol 8, pp.745–751.

Engleberger, L., Lyons, G., Foley, W., Daniells, J., Aalbersberg, B., Dolodolotawake, U., Watoto, C., Iramu, E., Taki, B., Wehi, F., Warito, P., Taylor, M. (2010) Carotenoid and riboflavin content of banana cultivars from Makira, Solomon Islands, *Journal of Food Composition and Analysis*, vol 23, pp. 624–632 (DOI: 10.1016/j.jfca.2010.03.002).

Fanzo, J., Holmes, M., Junega, P., Musinguzi, E., Smith, I.F., Ekesa, B., Bergamini, N. (2011) *Improving nutrition with agricultural biodiversity*, Bioversity International, Rome, p.78.

FAO (2007) *Expert consultation on nutrition indicators for biodiversity 1, Food composition*, Food and Agriculture Organization, Rome, p.35.

FAO (2010a) *Expert Consultation on Nutrition Indicators for Biodiversity-2-Food Consumption,* Food and Agriculture Organization, Rome, Available at http://www.fao.org/infoods/ biodiversity/index_en.stm, accessed 18 July 2012.

FAO (2010b) *The second report on the State of the World's plant genetic resources for food and agriculture*, Commission on genetic resources for food and agriculture, Food and Agriculture Organization, Rome, p.370.

FAO and Food and Nutrition Technical Assistance Project (2008) *Guidelines for Measuring Household and Individual Dietary Diversity*, FAO, Rome.

Foley, W.J., McIlwee, A., Lawler, I., Aragones, L., Woolnough, A.P., Berding, N. (1998) Ecological applications of near infrared reflectance spectroscopy – a tool for rapid, cost-effective prediction of the composition of plant and animal tissues and aspects of animal performance, *Oecologia*, vol 116, pp.293–305.

Foley, J., DeFries, R., Asner, G., Barford, C., Bonan, G., Carpenter, S., Chapin, F., Coe, M., Daily, G., Gibbs, H., Helkowski, J., Holloway, T., Howard, E., Kucharik, C., Monfreda, C., Patz, J., Prentice, I., Ramankutty, N., Snyder, P. (2005) Global consequences of land use, *Science*, vol 309, pp.570–574.

Frison, E., Smith, I.F., Johns, T., Cherfas, J., Eyzaguirre, P.B. (2006) Agricultural biodiversity, nutrition, and health: Making a difference to hunger and nutrition in the developing world, *Food Nutr Bull*, vol 25, pp.143–155.

Galeano, C.H., Fernandez, A.C., Franco-Herrera, N., Cichy, K.A., McClean, P.E., Vanderleyden, J., Blair, M.W. (2011) Saturation of an Intra-Gene Pool Linkage Map: Towards a Unified Consensus Linkage Map for Fine Mapping and Synteny Analysis in Common Bean, *Plos ONE*, doi:10.1371/journalpone.0028135.

Golden, C.D., Fernald, L.C., Brashares, J.S., Rasolofoniaina, B.J., Kremen, C. (2011) Benefits of wildlife consumption to child nutrition in a biodiversity hotspot, *Proc Natl Acad Sci USA*, vol 108, pp 19653–19656.

Graham, R.D. (2008) Micronutrient Deficiencies in Crops and Their Global Significance, in B.J. Alloway (eds) *Micronutrient Deficiencies in Global Crop Production*, Springer, pp.41–62.

Graham, R.D., Welch, R.M., Saunders, D.A., Ortiz-Monasterio, I., Bouis, H.E. et al. (2007) Nutritious subsistence food systems, *Advances in Agronomy*, vol 92, pp.1–72.

Hawkes, C., Ruel, M. (2011) Value chains for nutrition. 2020 Conference Paper 4. Prepared for the IFPRI 2020 international conference "Leveraging Agriculture for Improving Nutrition and Health," February 10–12, 2011, New Delhi, India.

International Assessment of Agricultural Knowledge, Science and Technology for Development (IAASTD) (2009) Island Press, Washington DC.

Kennedy, G., Burlingame, B. (2003) Analysis of food composition data on rice from a plant genetic resources perspective, *Food Chemistry*, vol 80, pp.589–596.

Lambrecht, I. (2009) Linking agro-diversity and nutrition: A case study in two Millennium Villages. Master thesis, Katholieke Universiteit Leuven.

Masset, E., Haddad, L., Cornelius, A., Isaza-Castro, J. (2011) *A systematic review of agricultural interventions that aim to improve nutritional status of children*, London: EPPI-Centre, Social Science Research Unit, Institute of Education, University of London.

McLaren, D.S. (1966) A fresh look at protein calorie malnutrition, *Lancet*, vol 2, pp.485–488.

McLaren, D.S. (1974) The great protein fiasco, *Lancet*, vol 2, pp.93–96.

Millennium Ecosystem Assessment (MEA) (2005) *Ecosystems and Human Well-being*, Washington DC.

Nelson, E.J., Daily, G.C. (2010) Modelling ecosystem services in terrestrial systems, F1000 Biology Reports, vol 2, pp. 53–59 (doi: 10.3410/B2-53).

Nelson G.C. (2011) Untangling the environmentalist's paradox: Better data, better accounting, and better technology will help, *Bioscience*, vol 61, pp.9–10.

Niles, D., Roff, R.J. (2008) Shifting agrifood systems: the contemporary geography of food and agriculture; an introduction, *GeoJournal,* vol 73, pp.1–10.

Paine, J.A., Shipton, C.A., Chaggar, S., Howells, R.M., Kennedy, M.J., Vernon, G., Wright, S.Y., Hinchliffe, E., Adams, J.L., Silverstone, A.L., Drake, R. (2005) A new version of Golden Rice with increased pro-vitamin A content, *Nature Biotechnology*, vol 23, pp.482–487.

Parametrix (2010) *An introduction to EcoMetrix Measuring change in ecosystem performance at a site scale*, Parametrix Inc., pp.1–15.

Penafiel, D., Lachat, C., Espinel, R., Van Damme, P., Kolsteren, P. (2011) A systematic review on the contribution of edible plant and animal biodiversity to human diets, *EcoHealth* doi:10.1007/s10393-011-0700-3.

Perry, A. (2008) Cost of the Diet – novel approach to estimate affordability of a nutritious diet, Save the Children UK.

Peters, C.J., Nelson, L., Bills, N.L., Wilkins, J.L., Fick, G.W. (2008) Foodshed analysis and its relevance, *Ren Agr Food Syst* doi:10.1017/S1742170508002433.

Raudsepp-Hearne, C., Peterson, G.D., Bennett, E.M. (2010a) Ecosystem service bundles for analyzing trade-offs in diverse landscapes, *Proc Natl Acad Sci USA* vol 107, pp. 5242–5247.

Raudsepp-Hearne, C., Peterson, G.D., Tengö, M., Bennett, E.M., Holland, T., Benessaiah, K., MacDonald, G.K., Pfeifer, L. (2010b) Untangling the environmentalist's paradox: Why is human well-being increasing as ecosystem services degrade? *Bioscience* vol 60, pp. 576–589.

Remans, R., Ramaekers, L., Schelkens, S., Hernandez, G., Garcia, A., Reyes, J.L., Mendez, N., Toscano, V., Mulling, M., Galvez, L. (2008) Effect of Rhizobium – Azospirillum coinoculation on nitrogen fixation and yield of two contrasting Phaseolus vulgaris L. genotypes cultivated across different environments in Cuba, *Plant Soil* 312: 25–37.

Remans, R., Flynn, D.F.B., DeClerck, F., Diru, W., Fanzo, J., Gaynor, K., Lambrecht, I., Mudiope, J., Mutuo, P.K., Nkhoma, P., Siriri, D., Sullivan, C., Palm, C.A. (2011a) Assessing nutritional diversity of cropping systems in African villages, *PLoS ONE*, vol 6, no 6, e21235, doi:10.1371/journalpone.0021235.

Remans, R., Pronyk, P.M., Fanzo, J.C., Palm, C.A., Chen, J. et al. (2011b) Multisector intervention to accelerate reductions in child stunting: an observational study from 9 sub-Saharan African countries, *Am J Nutr* vol 94(6), pp. 1632–42 doi: 10.3945/ajcn.111.020099.

Ruel, M., Levin, C. (2002) Food based approaches for alleviating micronutrient malnutrition—an overview, *J. Crop Prod* vol 6, pp.31–35.

Sachs, J.D., Remans, R., Smukler, S.M., Winowiecki, L., Andelman, S.J., Cassman, K.G., Castle, D., DeFries, R., Denning, G., Fanzo, J., Jackson, L.E., Leemans, R., Lehmann, J., Milder, J.C., Naeem, S., Nziguheba, G., Palm, C.A., Pingali, P.L., Reganold, J.P., Richter, D.D., Scherr, S.J., Sircely, J., Sullivan, C., Tomich, T.P., Sanchez, P.A. (2010) Monitoring World's agriculture, *Nature*, vol 466, pp.558–560.

Sachs, J.D., Remans, R., Smukler, S.M., Winowiecki, L., Andelman, S., Cassman, K.G., Castle, D., DeFries, R., Denning, G., Fanzo, J., Jackson, L.E., Leemans, R., Lehmann, J., Milder, J.C., Naeem, S., Nziguheba, G., Palm, C.A., Pingali, P.L., Reganold, J.P., Richter, D.D., Scherr, S.J., Sircely, J., Sullivan, C., Tomich, T.P., Sanchez, P.A. (2012) Effective monitoring of agriculture: a response, *J. Environ Monitor*, vol 14, pp.738–742.

Said, M., Okwi, P., Ndeng'e, G., Agatsiva, J., Kilele, X. (2007) *Nature Benefits in Kenya: an Atlas of Ecosystem and Human Well-Being*, World Resource Institute (WRI); Department of Resource Surveys and Remote Sensing, Ministry of Environment and Natural Resources, Kenya; Central Bureau of Statistics, Ministry of Planning and National Development, Kenya; International Livestock Research Institute, May, 2007.

Sanchez, P.A., Palm, C., Sachs, J.D., Denning, G., Flor, R. (2007) The African Millennium Villages, *Proc Natl Acad Sci USA* 104: 16775–16780.

Sanchez, P.A., Ahamed, S., Carré, F., Hartemink, A.F., Hempel, J. et al. (2009) Digital Soil Map of the World, *Science*, vol 7, pp.680–681.

Shackleton, C.M., Pasquini, M.W., Drescher, A.W. (eds) (2009) African Indigenous Vegetables in Urban Agriculture, *Earthscan*, p.344.

Smukler, S.M., Sánchez-Moreno, S., Fonte, S.J., Ferris, H., Klonsky, K., O'Geen, A.T., Scow, K.M., Steenwerth, K.L., Jackson, L.E. (2010) Biodiversity and multiple ecosystem functions in an organic farmscape, *Agriculture Ecosystems and Environment*, vol 139, pp.80–97.

Stadlmayr, B., Charrondiere, U.R., Enujiugha, V.N., Bayili, R.G., Fagbohoun, E.G., Samb, B., Addy, P., Barikmo, I., Ouattara, F., Oshaug, O., Akinyele, I., Amponsah Annor, G., Bomfeh, K., Ene-Obong, H., Smith, I.F., Thiam, I., Burlingame, B. (2010) *Composition of selected foods from Africa*, Food and Agriculture Organization of the United Nations, Rome, pp.43.

Tallis, H., Polasky, S. (2009) Mapping and valuing ecosystem services as an approach for conservation and natural-resource management, *Ann N Y Acad Sci* vol 1162, pp. 265–283.

UNICEF (1990) *Strategy for improved nutrition of women and children in developing countries*, A UNICEF policy review, UNICEF: New York.

Vijay, K., Tiwari, V.K., Rawat, N., Chhuneja, P., Neelam, K., Aggarwal, R., Randhawa, G.S., Dhaliwal, H.S., Keller, B., Singh, K. (2009) Mapping of quantitative trait loci for grain iron and zinc concentration in diploid A genome wheat, *J Hered*, vol 100, pp.771–776.

Villa, F., Ceroni, M., Bagstad, K., Johnson, G. and Krivov, S. (2009) *ARIES (Artificial Intelligence for Ecosystem Services): a new tool for ecosystem services assessments, planning, and valuation*. Proceedings of the BioEcon conference, Venice, Italy.

Welch, R.D., Graham, R.D. (1999) A new paradigm for world agriculture: meeting human needs, Productive, sustainable, nutritious, *Field Crops Research,* vol 60, pp.1–10.

Willett, W. (1998) *Food frequency methods in: nutritional epidemiology*, 2nd edn. New York: Oxford University Press.

Winowiecki, L., Smukler, S., Shirley, K., Remans, R., Peltier, G., Lothes, E., King, E., Comita, L., Baptista, S., Alkema, L. (2011) Tools for enhancing interdisciplinary communication, *Sustainability: Science, Practice, & Policy*, vol 7, no 1, pp.1–7.

8 Successes and pitfalls of linking nutritionally promising Andean crops to markets

Michael Hermann

Introduction

This chapter focuses on three native plant species from South America that have provided food to native Amerindian populations since time immemorial (Table 8.1). They are all fully domesticated crops. Maca and yacon produce edible underground storage organs whereas quinoa is a chenopod grain. These plants represent the vast range of many thousands of species of local edible plants that have been used and/or domesticated since pre-history all over the world, but have lost ground in terms of production and dietary significance to a limited number of globally significant crops that nowadays dominate agriculture and food systems (Mayes et al., 2011). However, the three species covered in this chapter have seen in recent years a remarkable, in the case of maca and yacon even meteoric, rebound from nearly exclusive subsistence uses toward steeply increased commercial production, which in turn has generated the incentives for product development and scientific enquiry into the benefits of such previously "underutilized" species.

Key to this development has, in all three cases, been the discovery or substantiation and the growing consumer awareness of specific nutritional attributes. In striking contrast, those native edible species from the same geographic area that have not achieved as much "nutritional notoriety" because of unknown nutritional traits or lack of awareness thereof continue to linger in neglect. Examples include a range of Andean roots and tubers (mashua, mauka, ahipa) and a large number of New World fruits.

The approach taken in this chapter is to examine the three successful cases and tease out the factors that have shaped the re-emergence of these species from oblivion. This seems to be a more insightful and rewarding procedure than developing a "conceptual framework" for the promotion of such species on nutritional grounds.

The chapter will first narrate the recent re-emergence of the three species from neglect and underuse, and then it will examine the players and processes involved. While nutritional messages played a prominent role in raising awareness and the development of markets, the way these messages were brought to bear in the three cases are quite heterogeneous. As will be seen in

Table 8.1 Use attributes of quinoa, maca and yacon

Common and scientific name	Plant characteristics	Traditional use	Salient nutritional properties of commercial interest
Quinoa (*Chenopodium quinoa*, Chenopodiaceae)	Herbaceous annual crop (seed-propagated)	Edible seeds, cooked for a variety of dishes, Bolivia and Peru	Balanced protein, high iron content, gluten-free
Maca (*Lepidium meyenii*, Brassicaceae)	Herbaceous annual crop (seed-propagated)	Edible root, used as tonic at high altitudes, Peru	High in mustard oils, isothiocyanates, anti-oxidants
Yacon (*Smallanthus sonchifolius* Asteraceae)	Herbaceous annual crop (vegetatively propagated)	Edible root, eaten raw, Northern and Central Andes	High in fructans in roots, presence of hypoglycaemic principles in leaves

the following section, product characteristics, indigenous knowledge, crop dispersals outside the Andes, the opportunities afforded by export markets, food science research and food safety-inspired concerns of regulators intertwine to produce a complex picture. Based on these narratives commonalities will be determined and broader lessons will be determined for the promotion of nutritionally relevant agricultural biodiversity.

The transition from subsistence to commercial production

Quinoa

Quinoa is a small-grain staple of the Chenopodiaceae, which has been in cultivation for at least 5,000 years BP in its native range in the Andean highlands (Chepstow-Lusty, 2011; Oelke et al., 1992), predominantly around Lake Titicaca. Quinoa is adapted to the relatively cold conditions at high altitudes (3,500–4,000 masl) and this in combination with the plant's drought resistance and nutrient efficiency (facilitated by a deep root system) make quinoa production competitive vis-à-vis other starchy grains (mostly introduced Old World cereals) under the harsh climatic and poor soil quality of the Andean highlands (Aguilar and Jacobsen, 2003; Oelke et al., 1992). Although quinoa leaves are tasty and very similar in texture and flavour to amaranth leaves, they are rarely used in the Andes.

Recent archaeological work (Chepstow-Lusty, 2011) assessing ancient pollen abundance suggests that quinoa disappeared from mid-elevations in the Peruvian Andes after the introduction of maize – presumably from the Pacific lowlands to which maize had been introduced a few millennia earlier. This coincided with a relatively warm period and increased availability of animal dung, factors that appear to have boosted the evolution and productivity of locally adapted maize and possibly made it the preferred staple. The pollen record unveiled by Chepstow-Lusty (2011) suggests that quinoa's importance was much reduced by 2500 BP and that the crop found a refuge from maize competition at higher altitudes, in particular in the high Andean plains around Lake Titicaca, where the crop has remained unrivalled by other starchy grains to this day. It is here where nearly all quinoa in Bolivia and Peru is grown today.

Nutritional quality and importance of quinoa

Several sources stress the higher quantity and better quality of the quinoa protein versus other starchy foods (Repo-Carrasco et al., 2003), and this message has also been effectively communicated to consumers in both producer countries and export markets, where quinoa has acquired a reputation as a health food. The quinoa protein has indeed a desirable composition of essential amino acids, similar to the protein of milk (Oelke et al., 1992), and hence very good nutritional value as compared with other plant proteins, but total protein content in quinoa is not much higher than that of the cereals (Repo-Carrasco et al., 2003). In addition quinoa has good iron and calcium contents – for a plant food – further adding to the perception as a "superfood". To the best of my knowledge, there is no literature assessing the nutritional advantage arising from quinoa's superior protein. In any case, it is well known that proteins of lesser quality from different plant foods complement each other's nutritional value in that they mutually contribute limiting amino acids.

Authors frequently make misleading claims as to the high nutritional importance of quinoa to contemporary native communities, when indeed several lines of evidence suggest quite the opposite. For example, according to Rojas et al. (2004), Bolivia's production in 1999 of barley, wheat and rice exceeded that of quinoa by factors of three, six and nine, respectively. These ratios would be even more unfavourable for quinoa if the large quantities of cereals imported into Bolivia were taken into account, and the fact that a large proportion of quinoa is being exported to the USA, Europe and other health food markets. Field work undertaken by Astudillo (2007) shows that both the frequency and quantity of quinoa consumption in poor communities in Southern Bolivia is quite low, and seems to be further diminished in households producing quinoa for the market.

Quinoa production and demand constraints

In Bolivia, the most important quinoa-producing country, average quinoa yields were around 500 kg/ha in the 10 years to 2001 (Rojas et al., 2004), an average unlikely to have increased because of the predominant production for "organic" export markets and the concomitant avoidance of mineral fertilizers and resulting soil mining (see below). Recent data suggest that yields in many areas are actually declining (Rojas et al., 2004; Astudillo, 2007). Virtually all quinoa production is by manual labour and uses ancient technologies, including ploughing, sowing, harvesting, threshing and winnowing. What may appeal to the visitor as picturesque scenery in fact involves a lot of drudgery and production inefficiencies.

Quinoa grain as sold by farmers is still coated with saponin, which protects the plant from insect pests, but needs to be removed prior to consumption, either by washing or polishing the grain in machines specifically developed for that purpose (Fujisaka et al., 2006). Another inconvenience and additional post-harvest production cost of quinoa for urban or export consumption is the removal of black grains, which result from cross-pollination with wild *Chenopodium* species. Black grains are innocuous and account for less than 1 per cent of total grain but deter consumers, who perceive such grains as contamination. Grain separation technology could probably be adapted from high-accuracy cereal cleaning machines, but is prohibitively expensive in the context of the ubiquitous small-scale quinoa processing. Therefore, grains with undesirable colours are removed manually by workers, further adding to processing costs (2007, field observations).

The above-described constraints make the production, processing and marketing of quinoa quite inefficient, and result in production costs and quinoa prices that are much higher at wholesale and retail levels than for quinoa's starchy substitutes, such as wheat, rice, maize and derivatives from these grains. According to Astudillo (2007) quinoa in rural markets in Bolivia costs twice as much as rice. While a surprisingly large degree of awareness of quinoa's nutritional properties amongst the rural poor with little formal education was uncovered, Astudillo also found in the three communities in Southern Bolivia that price of food is the overriding criterion in food choice decisions, and much more important than nutritional properties and flavour. In 2011, press reports picked up by international media (Romero and Shahriari, 2011) suggested that soaring quinoa prices have made this ancient staple unaffordable for urban Bolivians as well, with the retail value of quinoa being five times that of noodles or rice, quinoa's main substitutes. Even before the recent price hikes, Iparuna, a La Paz-based processing firm specializing in native grain products, could not afford to include quinoa as an ingredient in products tendered for Bolivian school feeding programmes and relied entirely on imported raw materials in order to be able to offer an affordable product (Ms Martha Cordera, personal communication, 2007).

Quinoa enthusiasts often point to the nutritional qualities of quinoa and demand policies in producer countries to discourage the consumption of its main competitors, wheat and rice (see, for example, Jacobsen 2011). As Table 8.2 shows, quinoa is indeed superior to rice and wheat products for protein content and a number of other nutrients, although the raw grain of certain wheat varieties can have equally high protein content. Quinoa's nutritional superiority is partially attributable to the fact that its whole grain is consumed whereas the outer, nutrient-rich, layers of wheat and rice are typically removed (although some of the lost minerals are added in the customarily enriched derivatives such as flour, bread and noodles).

Table 8.2 Comparison of the content of selected nutrients in quinoa grain versus rice and wheat products (uncooked except for bread)

Nutrient	Quinoa grain (20035*)	Rice, white, short grain (20052)	Wheat grain, hard, spring (20071)	Wheat flour, white, unenriched (20481)	Wheat flour, white, enriched (20381)	Wheat noodles, enriched (20120)	Wheat bread (18064)
Water (g)	13.3	13.3	12.8	11.9	11.9	9.9	35
Protein (g)	14.1	6.5	15.4	10.3	10.3	13.0	10.4
Carbohydrates (g)	64	79	68	76	76	75	49
Energy (kcal)	368	358	329	364	364	371	270
Iron (mg)	4.6	4.2	3.6	1.2	4.6	3.3	3.5
Zinc (mg)	3.1	1.1	2.8	0.7	0.7	1.4	1.2
Calcium (mg)	47	3	25	15	252	21	138

Source: United States Department of Agriculture, National Nutrient Database, http://ndb.nal.usda.gov, rounded figures, per 100 g, *NDB number (USDA).

If we conservatively assume a price ratio of quinoa to wheat products of about three, which has been typical at the retail level prior to the current export boom, and if the approximate contents of key nutrients in quinoa versus wheat as shown in Table 8.2 are taken into account, it can easily be deduced that a dollar spent on unenriched (native) wheat flour buys three times as much food energy, twice as much protein and only slightly less calcium, iron and zinc than quinoa. For bread and noodles made from whole-wheat grain or enriched flour, the comparison is even more favourable for wheat. Even rice with its comparatively low protein content will provide 40 per cent more protein per food expenditure. As quinoa prices have climbed to new heights in 2010 and 2011, providing much opportunity for income generation, there will be increased incentives for quinoa producers to trade their precious commodity rather than consume it in pursuit of intangible benefits as proposed by a majority of authors that emphasize the importance of nutritional diversity and strengthened cultural identity.

Quinoa marketing

In light of the poor competitiveness and resulting high consumer prices for quinoa, it is no surprise that quinoa consumption has increased in the past 20 years predominantly amongst affluent consumers, a development that has initially been limited to the European health food scene, but has gained momentum in other export markets as well. Quinoa's fame as a "superfood" produced under "organic" conditions eventually also reached an affluent urban clientele in quinoa producer countries, although the consumption there is still dwarfed by export markets.

In addition to the celebrated nutritional qualities of quinoa (protein quality; high contents of calcium, magnesium, phosphorus, iron, zinc and vitamins B6 and E; low glycaemic index), it is its lack of gluten that is having the greatest impact on demand growth. Gluten is a storage protein of cereals causing allergy in many people in developed countries. In Germany alone an estimated 100,000 gluten intolerance sufferers are in need of substituting wheat, rice and maize with gluten-free starchy products such as quinoa.

Expansion of quinoa production and soil mining

Astudillo (2007) has described how the lure of high quinoa prices in the wake of the export boom has led to the growing investment in quinoa cropping by absentee landlords relying on hired labour and with little regard for communal action to maintain sustainability practices. In 2011, Bolivia had registered some 70,000 producers on an estimated total area of 50,000 ha. In the same year, the export FOB value was US$46 million, up from US$2 million in 2000,[1] translating into an average annual growth rate of 33 per cent.

Although there is a dearth of substantiating quantitative data, several sources report a tendency of declining quinoa area yields (Rojas et al., 2004; Astudillo, 2007). Based on production statistics from the Bolivian Ministry of Rural Development, Jacobsen (2011) calculated that average quinoa yields declined by 20 per cent in the 10 years to 2009. Local informants throughout the quinoa production zone consistently report reduced soil fertility, reduced fallow periods and the expansion of quinoa into steep and erosion-prone land to compensate for reduced area productivity (Medrano and Torrico, 2009; Jacobsen, 2011). Most of this expansion is on account of the demand for organically certified produce under various private and public labels, which invariably allow the application of locally available animal dung only. However, animal dung in the Altiplano is scarce, and there is circumstantial evidence for persistent net extraction of nutrients from the soil, a process also referred to as soil mining that leads to soil degradation.

Despite growing awareness for the decline in soil fertility (Ms Martha Cordera, personal communication, 2007; Medrano and Torrico, 2009) commercially motivated demands abound that the "purity" of quinoa production and organic quality standards be maintained.[2] Thus, the application of rational and science-based fertilization practices, including the use of mineral fertilizers to replenish nutrients removed by harvested produce, is being prevented and leads to the degradation of the resource base – all in the name of "organic" production methods so dear to distant quinoa consumers. Characteristically, Jacobsen (2011), in his discussion of sustainable soil management in quinoa cropping in the Southern Bolivian Altiplano, fails to even mention the option of using mineral fertilizers while giving much consideration to the improved use of animal dung and green manure, a proposal that seems of limited practical value in the context of the much needed "sustainable intensification", particularly in locations where "organic" sources of nutrients are either inaccessible or unaffordable.

Maca

Traditional uses

Maca (*Lepidium meyenii* Walpers) is a fully domesticated, seed-propagated root crop of the crucifer family. It is endemic to the high Andes around Lake Junín in Central Peru, a chilly plateau at 4,000 m altitude. In locations where temperatures range during the crop's growing season from 0°C to 12°C, maca presents one of the few cropping options, apart from other cold-adapted domesticates such as quinoa, and certain varieties of bitter potatoes (Tello et al., 1992).

Prior to the late 1980s, maca was estimated to be grown on no more than 15 ha, an area so small as to raise concerns that the crop might become extinct (IBPGR, 1982). The traditional cropping area is circumscribed by the shores of Lake Junín and adjacent slopes, with any two cropping sites not further apart than some 100 km as the crow flies. Such a restricted and "insular" distribution is remarkable for a crop plant, and all the more so when considering that suitable high altitude habitats extend for thousands of km south and north of the traditional distribution of the crop.

Claims about maca having been much more widely distributed across Peru and even other Andean countries in the past 500 years therefore seem plausible, and indeed abound in the maca literature. However, a thorough examination of historical production and trade records going back to the 16th century as well as the absence of archaeological evidence outside the crop's place of domestication – both in terms of plant remains and phytomorphic pottery – strongly suggest that maca, in pre-Hispanic and colonial times, never extended beyond the above-mentioned Lake Junín area (Hermann and Bernet, 2009).

Food value

Traditionally, maca roots are dried after harvest and remain edible for several years. Drying diminishes pungency owing to the significant reduction of the content of glucosinolates. Traditional drying, apart from reducing pungency, presumably converts some starch into free sugars and it also brings out the typical flavour of maca, which is peculiar and difficult to describe. Maca is typically rehydrated before being boiled and then blended into a range of dishes or potions to which the maca imparts a characteristic flavour.

One often-quoted botanist praised the maca aroma as reminiscent of butterscotch but according to Torres (1984) most maca novices find maca rather repulsive, and acceptance of maca was very low in a focus group recruited from Lima with no previous exposure to this food. Maca quite obviously is an acquired taste, and this must have been a major use constraint and is likely to be one of the reasons for the failure of this crop to expand beyond its narrow geographic distribution in the past.

In any case, traditional beliefs suggest that maca consumption improves human fertility, and physical stamina (Leon, 1964; Locher, 2006). Maca has high nutritional density (in root dry matter: 55–65 per cent highly digestible carbohydrates, 2.2 per cent lipids, 10–13 per cent protein) and it is particularly rich in iron, zinc and potassium. Maca protein is high in essential amino acids (Dini et al., 1994).

Maca contains high concentrations of isothiocyanates, which are the compounds responsible for the pungent flavour of raw maca (Johns, 1981), and other secondary metabolites, but it is not clear what their biological activity is and whether they are responsible for the reported pharmacological effects of maca in mammals (see below).

The transition from subsistence use to Internet notoriety

Beginning in the late 1980s maca experienced a meteoric rise from an obscure botanical curiosity to Internet notoriety with the total area cropped to maca extending across Peru and neighbouring countries and increasing in the 15 years to 2005 by a factor of at least 60 to some 3,000 ha. What had happened?

In the early 1980s, different local actors started to promote maca on the grounds of its locally perceived health benefits, with a small rural road-side restaurant playing a key role. Located on the heavily transited road between Lima and Huanuco, it marketed a "trade-mark", maca-fortified, hot drink to a clientele of truck drivers and travellers who conveyed a tale of increased sexual stamina and fertility to the nearby capital city of Lima. To this day, the little store serves the hot maca beverage to travellers, and numerous postcards on display thank the manager for restored marital lives and the arrival of desperately wanted children. The traditional beliefs of maca as a "strong food" had mutated into a more effective marketing message (Vilchez, 2001).

Emerging commercial interest on the part of local traders, and small Lima-based processors, was further stimulated by reports in national newspapers and TV channels of maca's miraculous properties, leading to supply shortages, higher prices and the expansion of production to satisfy an increasing demand from outside the crop's native highland range. It was also at that time that the first convenience products containing maca began to appear, using the root at lower concentrations or with ingredients that mask its strong flavour, thus improving its acceptance among urban consumers (Torres, 1984; Vilchez, 2001).

The 1990s saw an unprecedented expansion of the production of maca. Four factors were responsible for this:

1   Product development and diversification have been key in the expansion of maca demand, particularly the development of convenience products for urban consumption that mask the maca flavour, typically by limiting maca's share of total product weight to under 20 per cent (Figure 8.1).
2   Growing demand from export markets, particularly in Japan and the USA, based on Internet marketing stressing the purported aphrodisiac qualities of maca as the "natural alternative to Viagra", the "Peruvian ginseng", a rejuvenating tonic, or a "wellness" product.

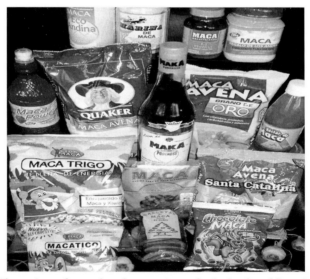

Figure 8.1 The variety of maca-based convenience foods developed have increased the demand for the root crop

3   A growing body of knowledge, as evidenced by the exponentially growing number of university theses and publications, was instrumental in the promotion of maca, particularly research dealing with maca food composition, nutritional studies with animal models, and product development. Private sector-funded research papers sought to substantiate traditional beliefs in the capacity of maca to increase fertility (Hermann and Bernet, 2009).

4   The intensification of maca production, notably through the use of mineral fertilizers, resulted in a significant increase of area yields (Hermann and Bernet, 2009).

Problematic maca marketing

The frivolous Internet marketing of maca as a libido booster quickly propelled it to international notoriety in the mid-1990s. Maca pills containing the crude flour became increasingly available in Europe by mail and over the counter, and were openly touted for their alleged pharmacological effects. The fact that none of these products had gone though internationally accepted registration procedures mandated for pharmacological products did not escape the attention of the regulatory entities in target markets. Particularly in the EU, an increasing number of maca shipments were confiscated in the 1990s and maca marketing became increasingly limited to informal distribution channels including sales through the Internet (Hermann and Bernet, 2009).

Peruvian exporters and their EU importer counterparts reacted by toning down advertisements and/or by removing health claims from their product labels, but this invariably resulted in reduced demand. It was also at this time that a sense of the need for scientific substantiation of maca's "invigorating" effects emerged, leading to research, which was eventually published in university theses and in peer-reviewed journals from 1999 onwards. However, the frequently reported enhanced sexual function following maca administration in rodents was observed at intake levels several orders higher than those recommended in commercial maca "nutraceuticals", casting doubt on the efficacy of commercial products. Also, authors of peer-reviewed articles reporting such effects mostly failed to disclose the private sources of funding for their research and the links of their work to commercial product development and promotion (Hermann and Bernet, 2009).

Specific market access barriers

Some maca suppliers, however, began to pursue a different marketing strategy aimed at the promotion of maca as a food or food ingredient consistent with the root's traditional use in its native area. This strategy was beset with two difficulties. One was the de facto positioning of maca as a drug in the Internet, which was further accentuated by the appearance of scientific papers suggesting the efficacy of maca's action on reproductive parameters in animals and humans. This necessarily led to concerns about possible toxicological effects at the much higher doses implied in consumption of maca as a food.

A second problem of this approach was that maca suppliers were unprepared to respond adequately to food safety concerns, particularly those embodied by the EU Novel Food Regulation (NFR). This regulation requires food safety assessments of traditional foods (viewed as novel from a European perspective) for pre-market approval. The NFR arbitrarily defines novel food as food or food ingredients that have not been used widely within the EU before 15 May 1997, an arbitrary cut-off date. If viewed as novel, market authorization needs to be preceded by a food safety assessment under the NFR that typically requires scientific data with regard to food composition, suggested intake levels, toxicological assessments and allergenic potential. Such a food safety assessment was not available and at any rate required resources, expertise and a degree of determination not possessed by the dispersed community of value chain stakeholders (Hermann, 2009).

The non-authorization of maca under the NFR resulted in the confiscation of numerous consignments and explicit prohibitions in several EU countries discouraged investment in export-oriented maca supply chains, and particularly in product and market development for the most attractive export market for natural products, the EU. This constraint in combination with the incoherent and even confusing use of product names, the widely varying product quality and frequent adulteration (especially at times of low supply) became a problem and compromised the reputation of maca (Hermann and Bernet, 2009).

Impact of the expansion of maca production on rural livelihoods and maca diversity

Despite marketing problems, maca remains an important local crop in a small area of Central Peru, because the roots can be stored and sold for cash, providing more income security to smallholders. With farm-gate prices over three Soles (ca. US$1) per kilogramme of dehydrated maca roots for several years, and conservatively estimating average dry matter yields of one tonne per hectare, the revenue from a two-hectare field of maca (typical of a smallholding), is likely to have exceeded US$2,000 in most years. This is by far more than farmers could expect from any other agricultural activity under the harsh conditions of the Puna, and significant income effects are evident from the display of greater wealth in terms of vehicles and new homes in production areas. Maca has become a source of self-employment and income for the rural poor, many of which have only recently started growing maca. Moreover, expanded maca production has triggered the development of a number of small-scale businesses related to maca processing and commercialization, which has allowed farmers to diversify activities and lower income risks (Locher, 2006).

Yacon

Origin and traditional uses

Yacon is another minor root crop domesticated in the Andes. It is a herbal species of the sunflower family with perennial rhizomes from which the edible storage roots emerge. In contrast to maca, the starch-free yacon roots are eaten raw and function as "fruits" in traditional diets. Farmers in the subtropical inter-Andean valleys and on the eastern slopes of the Andes, which descend toward the Amazon used to grow this plant more commonly in the past along field borders where the juicy roots provide a welcome source of refreshment during field work (Grau and Rea, 1997).

There is a dearth of information on indigenous knowledge surrounding the use of yacon. The extensive monograph of Grau and Rea (1997) based on a thorough review of the literature on the economic botany of this crop is silent on traditional beliefs as to its food qualities and uses. There is also no mention of medicinal properties in the limited number of early yacon publications that predate the fairly recent scientific discovery of yacon's dietary qualities. The apparent absence of significant indigenous knowledge and the use of yacon exclusively in the raw (uncooked) state, however, is consistent with the marginal significance of the crop in subsistence and trade throughout its traditional range in Ecuador, Peru, Bolivia and Argentina.

Until as late as in the early 2000s, yacon was mostly unheard of by the large majority of the people in the crop's native range, except for cultivators and occasional consumers in remote rural areas apt for its cultivation. Yacon was rarely offered in rural markets, and if so, mostly during the religious festival of "Corpus Christi", the celebration of which includes the serving of traditional foods rarely eaten during the non-festive season. This rather marginal use changed in a rather dramatic fashion in 2001, principally because of the crop's distribution outside the Andes, which will be examined in the following section.

International dispersal and discovery of food value

In 1979, Dick Endt, a renowned plant collector from New Zealand, while on a collecting mission to Ecuador, took yacon planting material from a "town garden" in Loja, Ecuador to New Zealand (D. Endt, personal communication). New Zealand has been successful with the introduction and development of Andean crops (such as tree tomato, babaco and oca), and yacon is still available from Endt's nursery, but yacon remained a garden curiosity in that country. However, yacon found much greater acceptance in Japan to which the first plants appear to have been introduced in the mid-1980s from material in Endt's collection. Within the space of some 20 years after its introduction in Japan, successful yacon cultivation and trade has been reported from a range of Asian countries. Various sources (Asami et al., 1989; Doo et al., 2000) suggest that the origin for the crop's dispersal in Asia, as shown in Figure 8.2, was indeed Japan. Incipient yacon cultivation has recently been observed in the Cameron highlands of Malaysia (Paul Quek, personal communication, 2011) suggesting that the crop's expansion in Asia continues in full swing.

It was in Japan in the 1980s where yacon food use, product development and its culinary discovery really "took off". In light of the many creative uses that the product has found in that country and elsewhere in Asia, we can surmise that yacon appeals much more to its new Asian consumers than to its original domesticators in the Andes. The succulent and crunchy texture of yacon roots

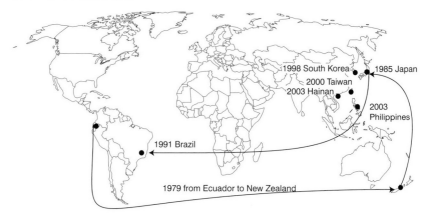

Figure 8.2 Origin and dispersion paths for yacon

is similar to radish or apple, and this as well as a mildly resinous but pleasantly sweet taste reminiscent of the peculiar texture and flavour of other plant foods popular in East Asia, probably explains its success there. Yacon also retains desired crunchiness after stir-frying, an added advantage for its use in Asia, but not exploited in the cuisine of Andean countries. Use of yacon in South Korea in a variety of dishes, including iced noodles, chopped noodles, fries, pancakes and dumplings (Doo et al., 2000) illustrates the versatility of yacon use in Asia.

With an estimated area of some 100 ha by the early 2000s (more recent data not available), yacon remained insignificant economically in Japan, but interest in the crop – as evidenced by the formation of a very active Japanese yacon association – led to research unravelling the plant's chemical composition. Most importantly, it was found that two-thirds of yacon carbohydrates, which account for about 90 per cent of the root dry matter, consist of fructo-oligosaccharides (FOS) (a polymer made up of fructose units) of a low degree of polymerization (Ohyama et al., 1990; Wei et al., 1991; Asami et al., 1992).

The nutritional significance of the sweet-tasting FOS is that the human small intestine has no enzyme to hydrolyse its glucosidic bonds. FOS are thus largely indigestible, but there is much literature suggesting benefits for gut health from the increased ingestion of FOS which stimulate the growth of bifidobacteria and suppress putrefactive pathogens in the human colon. They are thus increasingly added to pastry, confectionery, and dairy products (Geyer et al., 2008).

Apart from the content of FOS, the nutritional value of yacon is rather limited: the energy content ranges from 148 to 224 kcal/kg per root fresh matter and is several times lower than for comparable foods. Yacon is a reasonably good source of potassium (1.8–2.9 g/kg fresh matter), but low in protein (2.7–4.9 g/kg) and lipids (112–464 mg/kg) (Hermann et al., 1999).

First reports of additional hypoglycaemic properties of the leaves of yacon, which have only recently been confirmed in animal models (Genta et al., 2010), prompted the commercial development of yacon tea in Japan in the 1990s for use by type 2 diabetics. Recently, Habib et al. (2011) demonstrated lipid lowering principles of yacon roots in diabetes-associated hyperlipidemia, thus identifying another property to position yacon as a functional food.

In 1991, Mr Sergio Kakihara, a Japanese-Brazilian immigrant farmer, introduced yacon planting material from Japan to Capão Bonito, near Sao Paulo. Starting from a single propagule brought to Brazil more by chance than intent, he multiplied enough over the ensuing five years to comprise a total area of four hectares when the author of this chapter visited him in 1996. Initially marketed to Japanese-Brazilians at the Liberdade market in Sao Paulo (Kakihara et al., 1997), the crop eventually spread across Brazil, and has since become a standard item on offer in retail grocery stores, especially in Southern Brazil (Fenille et al., 2005).

The incipient use of yacon in Brazil and in Japan, the plant's salient attribute of being a prime source of short-chained FOS as well as anti-hyperglycaemic properties for innovative use as a product for diabetics, which has no parallel in traditional knowledge, remained unnoticed in the crop's native range throughout the 1990s. Ironically, a comprehensive priority-setting exercise led by the International Potato Center in Peru and relying on canvassing expert opinion, to assign priorities for research and development attention to a range of nine species of minor Andean root crops, was oblivious to yacon's potential, given the marginal use of this crop in traditional and modern food systems. A very large majority of urban people in the Andes had never heard of the product.

Yacon in the headlines

Yacon would probably have continued to linger in oblivion in the Andean countries for some more years, had it not been for Peruvian press reports that first appeared in August 2001, and eventually catapulted yacon into the limelight of markets and "put it on the map" of researchers and regulators. These reports referred to a 1999 incident, when Victor Aritomi, the former Peruvian ambassador to Japan and member of the meanwhile discredited Fujimori administration, on official diplomatic mission had carried yacon propagules to Japan, however without going through proper export procedures and the required material transfer agreement. Nothing could have more effectively enhanced public awareness for a hitherto underutilized crop than its name being brought into association with a much-despised former political regime. The apparent act of self-inflicted biopiracy fuelled national headlines for several weeks (Figure 8.3) and introduced a national audience to a genuine Peruvian crop which was highly appreciated on the opposite side of the world but unheard of in Peru itself. Once the scandal subsided, media reports – which Reuters and CNN eventually took up – began to cover the medicinal properties of yacon, as reported from Japan. These media reports tended to wildly exaggerate benefits, even suggesting yacon as a cure for diabetes, and were the basis for the emerging national interest in growing the crop, which has been sustained until the present day.

Ten years have passed since yacon was in the headlines. The "hype" surrounding yacon in Peru has subsided, but the fresh roots are now firmly established as a regular and year-round product in the fruit sections in urban markets and sought out by health-conscious consumers throughout the

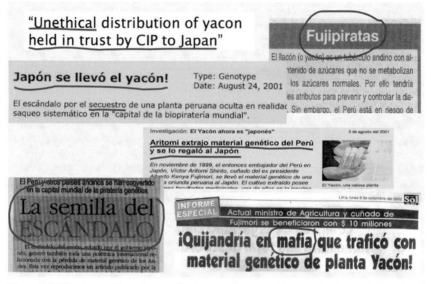

Figure 8.3 Biopiracy allegations referring to the use of yacon in Japan hit national headlines in Peru in 2001

country. Smallholder associations in some rural parts of Peru have established a reputation for growing yacon, but seed continues to be sourced through informal channels, and the lack of varietal performance guarantees, particularly in relation to the highly variable FOS content, has meant a constraint to large-scale cultivation for industrial processing (Seminario et al., 2003; Graefe et al., 2004; Manrique et al., 2005).

The last decade has also seen the development of a variety of convenience products motivated by the need to transform the perishable root into standardized products with export potential. According to statistics of PromPeru,[3] the value of total Peruvian yacon exports was US$1.1 million in 2011, up from US$0.2 in 2007, with the bulk of the produce going to Japan and the USA. In the EU, yacon requires authorization under the Novel Food Regulation, since it was not used as a food or food ingredient before 15 May 1997.[4] Therefore, an extensive food safety assessment under the Novel Food Regulation is required before it can be placed on the market in the EU as either a food or a food ingredient. Presumably, yacon sales in the EU, as evident from Internet marketing, are through informal and "under-the-counter" channels, which have not yet come under the scrutiny of EU regulators.

Discussion and conclusions

Re-emergence of underutilized food crops

A few dozen crops account for most of global food production, while the vast majority of food species are falling into disuse or reduced to subsistence systems. Much of the neglect of so many species is put down to the ongoing globalization of diets, the erosion of local food cultures, and the greater competitiveness of commodity crops ever more replacing traditional foods. However, the examination of the natural histories of the three food crops covered by this chapter reveals that the marginal or declining importance of food species – while being accentuated in the recent past – is not necessarily a modern phenomenon as often stated, but can have its roots in the very distant past.

Quinoa's importance began to erode in pre-Hispanic times. The pollen records unveiled by Chepstow-Lusty (2011) suggest that, as early as 2500 BP, quinoa was being replaced by maize in mid-elevation valleys in the Andes. It is reasonable to assume that quinoa retreated to the Altiplano, an ecologically narrowly circumscribed high-altitude plateau to which quinoa is supremely adapted, and where the crop is grown to this day. Based on a review of colonial and modern literature, Hermann and Bernet (2009) conclude that the production and consumption of maca never exceeded its very limited production area in a small mountainous region of central Peru. Maca was declared to be under threat of extinction in 1982. The early Spanish chroniclers, our only historical source on the economic botany of pre-Hispanic Andean civilizations, are either silent or provide only brief mention of yacon, suggesting that the crop was of much lesser use than other roots and tubers native to the Andes (Garcilazo de la Vega, 1609; Patiño, 1964; Antunez de Mayolo, 1981). As recently as 10 years ago, yacon's significance had declined to the status of a botanical rarity known only by a few specialists and occasional indigenous cultivators.

In conclusion, none of the three species have in the past been consumed by a large proportion of the population at substantial intake levels, and hence the often stated nutritional importance of these species is at odds with the marginal role of these crops in traditional food systems as evident from several sources. Moreover, restricted geographic distribution made these crops almost "invisible" to most Andean consumers and resulted in a lack of familiarity.

It was the discovery and communication of nutritional attributes that catapulted the three species into the minds of consumers in urban and export markets. The resulting demand expansion made all the difference. Seventy per cent of the Andean population is now urban, with a growing middle class and purchasing power. Importantly, the interest of export niche markets (fair trade, organic, health and ethnic food) provided key incentives for novel product development and diversification in order to overcome demand constraints.

Lessons for the development of minor food species

One often stated cliché is that minor food species are held back by the stigmata of "poor people's food" and "backwardness" associated with their rural producers. No evidence of this notion was found, and even if reputational problems existed, these would likely not be the cause of limited use but rather consequence and expression of objective demand constraints such as the inconvenience of use of (traditionally) unprocessed quinoa, and unappealing aspect and taste of maca and yacon. It is implausible how the promotion on nutritional grounds would be effective, unless accompanied with efforts to lessen or remove demand constraints as happened with the three crops of this study through the development of a diversity of appealing and novel products.

A variety of factors, however, made the products of the three species of this study prohibitively expensive for poorer sectors in producer countries. Growing consumer demand quickly exceeded supplies, and low productivity and predominantly manual production methods added to production costs and price pressures. For poorer people, whose food choices are strongly influenced by price, it would seem that costs have to come down to include these products in their diets. This can only be achieved by increasing area productivity, improved plant types and agronomic management as well as greater economies of scale through appropriate processing and more efficient value chain management.

Thus, this chapter provides a number of pointers for research investment in order to remove or lessen constraints that act on the supply (low productivity, narrow ecological adaptation) or the demand (lacking knowledge and consumer awareness of nutritional benefits, unavailability of convenience products, marketing inefficiencies) of these "neglected" crops. By comparison, globally established food crops have enjoyed vastly greater research and development efforts by both private and public entities. For example, many thousands of person-years must have been invested world-wide over past decades in the breeding of any of the major cereals. This has decisively contributed to their greater competitiveness vis-à-vis minor crops.

Communication of nutritional attributes to consumers

The communication of nutritional attributes was found to have been of key importance for the increased awareness of the food value of the three crops, although nutritional claims were often made in a sensationalist manner, exaggerating the significance of emerging scientific results, and in violation of Codex Alimentarius rules. However, it appears that focusing on key properties helped to position the products in the minds of consumers.

Access of quinoa to the EU market has not been a problem because of the long use tradition in some European countries; however, the lack of food safety documentation for maca and yacon has prevented the market authorization of these species under the EU Novel Food Regulation and discouraged investment in export value chains (Hermann, 2009). There is a need for authoritative species and food dossiers that substantiate the food value of traditional food products in new markets. These must provide details on food composition, traditional intake levels, and discuss potential hazards from processing or lack of familiarity of use. Recent EU market authorizations obtained for a range of traditional foods such as baobab and the Allanblackia tree provide models for the required procedures.

The role of indigenous knowledge

The importance generally attached to the role of indigenous knowledge in the continued use of agricultural biodiversity is clearly at odds with the findings of this chapter. Traditional beliefs about fertility-enhancing effects did indeed provide pointers for the modern use of maca, and recent research results appear to bear out certain pharmacological effects.

However, authentic indigenous knowledge surrounding the use of maca is very limited (Locher, 2006). As with other nearly forgotten foods subject to renewed commercial interest, what is described as "indigenous knowledge" actually has been enmeshed with attributions from press reports and contaminated with the hype associated with Internet claims. Genuine traditions are thus difficult to disentangle from modern product promotion, especially when they relate to the "immune system", better "concentration and memory", "lowered cholesterol" and other modern medical jargon (Hermann and Bernet, 2009).

None of the very limited traditional knowledge associated with the use of quinoa and yacon has had much bearing on the marketing and expansion of consumption of these products. Scientific research uncovered the previously unknown hypoglycaemic and bifidogenic properties of yacon, as well as the nutritional excellence of quinoa, particularly its potential as a starchy food for gluten intolerance sufferers. Moreover, awareness of the nutritional properties of quinoa and yacon as revealed by scientific methods has stimulated the interest of rural producers.

Likewise it has not been culinary traditions, but rather the ingenuity of modern product development and the versatility of food processing techniques that have helped overcome a number of use constraints, through the development of products that are more convenient to use, have longer shelf-life and better consumer acceptance.

The exaggeration and sensationalist use of indigenous knowledge in marketing maca paid quick dividends for some companies, but it eventually brought maca into ill repute, particularly in the EU, where regulators banned maca from the market for several years because of food safety concerns and the predominance of unsubstantiated product claims. Typically, indigenous knowledge on traditional food is silent on potential food hazards and even where it provides details on health and nutritional benefits, regulators will not allow its use in product claims, unless these are substantiated by scientific methods. This is often overlooked in discussions of the "complementarities" of "scientific" and "traditional knowledge". In recording indigenous knowledge greater emphasis needs to be placed on the documentation of traditional intake levels, frequency and distribution of use, data that are of great relevance to food safety assessments.

Multilateral access and benefit sharing of underutilized plant genetic resources

Current project funding and development priorities involving minor food species are posited on the widely held belief that these hold the greatest potential in their native range to benefit indigenous cultivators and consumers. On the surface, this appears to be a plausible proposition, but the lessons from this study suggest otherwise. All the three species have re-emerged from oblivion because of the discovery of nutritional properties outside the Andes following informal introductions[5] of germplasm to Brazil, Japan and a range of Asian countries. The case of yacon and quinoa is particularly interesting, as novel modes of preparations and the marketing in response to new demands outside the Andes (avoidance of gluten intolerance, interest in gut health, culinary interests) facilitated the diversification of crop uses. For instance, Japanese and Korean culinary techniques applied to yacon have hugely expanded its perceived food value and sparked scientific enquiry.

Unfortunately, myopic media opinion makers and misguided anti-biopiracy advocates have failed to realize that all three crops would most likely continue to be under-exploited had they not been taken out of the context of the demand constraints in their native agricultural and food systems.

Expansion of yacon and maca consumption in export markets has provided income opportunities for producer countries with benefits not only to poor farmers but also to processors and other value chain participants. Of course, increasing yacon production in Asia and Brazil is bound to curtail foreign currency revenues for Andean producers to some extent, but much of the understanding of yacon's and maca's nutritional properties have essentially been developed in these countries, and have hugely benefited product development, consumer interest and market development in the Andes as well.

The conclusion is that informal benefit-sharing mechanisms associated with the global dispersal of indigenous crops are still effective, although the time-scales involved exceed the short-term quid pro quo attitudes of post-CBD policy makers. The phenomena described are not applicable to every local food crop, but the number of crops being moved through informal seed systems across borders is substantial, and many more crop examples from the recent past support the chapter's conclusions. The implications are that the unfettered sharing of plant genetic resources for food within a multilateral access system not only benefits the use of global crops, but that the interdependence of countries with regard to minor species may be similarly high.

Notes

1   Unidad de estadísticas agropecuarias y rurales (MAGDER), Bolivia.
2   Associated Press, 10 January 2011. Quinoa's popularity boon to Bolivans. http://thedailynewsonline.com/lifestyles/article_10f5ef38-1d28-11e0-bf68-001cc4c002e0.html
3   http://www.siicex.gob.pe/siicex/apb/ReporteProducto.aspx?psector=1025&preporte=prodpres&pvalor=1953
4   http://ec.europa.eu/food/food/biotechnology/novelfood/novel_food_catalogue_en.htm
5   No evidence was found for negotiations or material transfer agreements related to these crop introductions as mandated by international agreements and recognized best practices.

References

Aguilar, P.C., Jacobsen, S. E (2003) 'Cultivation of quinoa on the Peruvian Altiplano', *Food Reviews International*, vol 19, no 1 and 2, pp.31–41.

Antunez de Mayolo, S.E. (1981) *La nutrición en el antiguo Perú*, Lima, Peru, Banco Central de Reserva del Peru, p.189.

Asami, T., Kubota, M., Minamisawa, K., Tsukihashi, T. (1989) 'Chemical composition of yacon, a new root crop from the Andean highlands', *Japanese Journal of Soil Science and Plant Nutrition*, vol 76, no 2, pp.121–126.

Asami, T., Minamisawa, K., Tsuchiya, T., Kano, K., Hori, I., Ohyama, T., Kubota, M., Tsukihashi, T. (1992) 'Oligofructans in the shoot, seed and tuber of yacon', *Japanese Journal of Soil Science and Plant Nutrition*, vol 63, no 1, pp.71–74.

Astudillo, D. (2007) 'An evaluation of the role of quinoa in the livelihoods of the households in the Southern Bolivian Altiplano: a case study in the municipalities of Salinas and Colcha K'. Project report, Mimeograph, p.77.

Chepstow-Lusty, A. (2011) 'Agro-pastoralism and social change in the Cuzco heartland of Peru: a brief history using environmental proxies', *Antiquity*, vol 85, pp.570–582.

Dini, A., Migliuolo, G., Rastrelli, L., Saturnino, P., Schettino, O. (1994) 'Chemical composition of *Lepidium meyenii*', *Food Chemistry*, vol 49, no 4, pp.347–349.

Doo, H.S., Li, H.L., Kwon, T.O., Ryu, J.H (2000) 'Changes in sugar content and storability of yacon under different storage conditions', *Korean Journal of Crop Science*, vol 5, no 5, pp.300–304.

Fenille, R.C., Campi, M.B., Souza, N.L., Nakatani, A.K., Kuramae, E.E. (2005) 'Binucleate Rhizoctonia *sp.* AG G causing root rot in yacon (*Smallanthus sonchifolius*) in Brazil', *Plant Pathology*, doi: 10.1111/j.1365-3059.2005.01161.x.

Fujisaka, S., Hermann, M., Jarvis, A., Cock, J., Douthwaite, B., Gonzalez, A., Hoeschle-Zeledon, I. (2006) 'Determining CGIAR priorities to improve benefits to the poor from under-utilized plant genetic resources', Report to the System-wide Genetic Resources Programme (SGRP), CIAT, IPGRI, California, p.76.

Garcilazo de la Vega (1609) *Los comentarios reales de los Incas*, Lisboa.

Genta, S.B., Cabreraa, W.M., Mercado, M.I., Grau, A., Catalán, C.A., Sánchez, S.S. (2010) 'Hypoglycemic activity of leaf organic extracts from Smallanthus sonchifolius: Constituents of the most active fractions', *Chemico-Biological Interactions,* vol 185, pp.143–152.

Geyer, M., Manrique, I., Degen, L., Beglinger, C. (2008) 'Effect of yacon (*Smallanthus sonchifolius*) on colonic transit time in healthy volunteers', *Digestion*, vol 78, pp.30–33.

Graefe, S., Hermann, M., Manrique, I., Golombek, S. and Bürkert, A. (2004) 'Effects of post-harvest treatments on the carbohydrate composition of yacon roots in the Peruvian Andes', *Field Crops Research*, vol 86, no 2–3, pp.157–165.

Grau, A., Rea, J. (1997) 'Yacon. *Smallanthus sonchifolius* (Poepp. & Endl.) H. Robinson', in: M. Hermann and J. Heller (eds): *Andean roots and tubers: Ahipa, arracacha, maca, yacon. Promoting the conservation and use of underutilized and neglected crops. 21*, Institute of Plant Genetics and Crop Plant Research, Gatersleben/International Plant Genetic Resources Institute, Rome, Italy, pp.199–242.

Habib, N.C., Honoré, S.M., Genta, S.B., Sánchez, S.S. (2011) 'Hypolipidemic effect of *Smallanthus sonchifolius* (yacon) roots on diabetic rats: biochemical approach', *Chemico-Biological Interactions*, vol 194, pp.31–39.

Hermann, M. (2009) 'The impact of the European Novel Food Regulation on trade and food innovation based on traditional plant foods from developing countries'. *Food Policy*, vol 34, pp.499–507.

Hermann, M., Bernet, T. (2009) 'The transition of maca from neglect to market prominence: Lessons for improving use strategies and market chains of minor crops', Agricultural Biodiversity and Livelihoods Discussion Papers 1. Bioversity International, Rome, Italy, p.101 .

Hermann, M., Freire, I., Pazos, C. (1999) 'Compositional diversity of the yacon storage root', in: *Impact on a changing world, Program Report 1997–1998*, International Potato Centre (CIP), Lima, Peru, pp.425–432.

IBPGR (1982) 'Plant genetic resources of the Andean region', Proceedings of a meeting of IBPGR, IICA, and JUNAC, Lima, Peru.

Jacobsen, S.E. (2011) 'The situation for quinoa and its production in Southern Bolivia: from economic success to environmental disaster', *Journal of Agronomy and Crop Science,* vol 197, pp.390–399.

Johns, T.A. (1981) 'The añu and the maca', *Journal of Ethnobiology*, vol 1, no 2, pp.208–212.

Kakihara, T.S., Câmara, F.L.A., Vilhena, S.M.C. (1997) 'Cultivo e industrialização de yacon: uma experiência brasileira'. I workshop de yacon, 31 October 1997, Botucatú (SP), Brazil.

Leon, J. (1964) 'The maca (*Lepidium meyenii*), "a little known food plant of Peru"', *Economic Botany*, vol 18, no 2, pp.122–127.

Locher, N.M. (2006) 'Screening of maca ecotypes, review of potential standardization procedures and testing of maca to be used as fertility enhancer in breeding bulls', Thesis Dipl. Ing. Institut für Nutztierwissenschaften, ETH Zürich, Switzerland.

Manrique, I., Párraga, A., Hermann, M. (2005) 'Yacon syrup: Principles and Processing', Series: Conservación y uso de la biodiversidad de raíces y tubérculos andinos: Una década de investigación para el desarrollo (1993–2003), no 8B. Centro Internacional de la Papa, Universidad Nacional Daniel Alcides Carrión, Fundación Erbacher, Agencia Suiza para el Desarrollo y la Cooperación. Lima, Peru, p.31.

Mayes, S., Massawe, F.J., Alderson, P.G., Roberts, J.A., Azam-Ali, S.N., Hermann, M. (2011) 'The potential for underutilized crops to improve security of food production', *Journal of Experimental Botany,* vol 2011, no 1–5, doi: 10.1093/jxb/err396.

Medrano, A.M., Torrico, J.C. (2009) 'Consecuencias del incremento de la producción de quinua (*Chenopodium quinoa* Willd.) en el altiplano sur de Bolivia', *CienciAgro*, vol 1, no 4, pp.117–123.

Oelke, E.A., Putnam, D.H., Teynor, T.M., Oplinger, E.S. (1992) *Quinoa. Alternative Field Crops Manual*, University of Wisconsin, http://www.hort.purdue.edu/newcrop/afcm/quinoa.html, accessed August 2012.

Ohyama, T., Ito, O., Yasuyoshi, S., Ikarashi, T., Minamisawa, K., Kubota, M., Tsukihashi, T., Asami, T. (1990) 'Composition of storage carbohydrate in tubers of yacon (*Polymnia sonchifolia*)', *Soil Science and Plant Nutrition*, vol 36, no 1, pp.167–171.

Patiño, V.M. (1964) Plantas cultivadas y animales domésticos en América Equinoccial, Tomo II, Plantas alimenticias. Cali, Imprenta Departamental, Colombia.

Repo-Carrasco, R., Espinoza, C., Jacobsen, S. E. (2003) 'Nutritional value and use of the Andean crops quinoa (*Chenopodium quinoa*) and kañiwa (*Chenopodium pallidicaule*)', *Food Reviews International*, vol 19, no 1 and 2, pp.179–189.

Romero, S., Shahriari, S. (2011) 'Quinoa's global success creates quandary at home', *New York Times*, 19 March, http://www.nytimes.com/2011/03/20/world/americas/20bolivia.html?_r=1&hp, accessed July 2012.

Rojas, W., Soto, J.L., Carrasco, E. (2004) 'Estudio de los impactos sociales, ambientales y económicos de la promoción de la quinua en Bolivia', Mimeograph, PROINPA, La Paz, Bolivia, p.86.

Seminario, J., Valderrama, M., Manrique, I. (2003) 'El yacón: fundamentos para el aprovechamiento de un recurso promisorio', Centro Internacional de la Papa (CIP), Universidad Nacional de Cajamarca, Agencia Suiza para el Desarrollo y la Cooperación (COSUDE), Lima, Peru, p.60.

Tello, J., Hermann, M., Calderón, A. (1992) 'La maca (*Lepidium meyenii* Walp): cultivo alimenticio potencial para las zonas altoandinas', *Boletín de Lima*, vol 14, no 81, pp.59–66.

Torres, R.C. (1984) 'Estudio nutricional de la maca (Lepidium meyenii Walp) y su aplicación en la elaboración de una bebida base', Thesis Ing., Universidad Nacional Agraria La Molina, Lima, Peru.

Vilchez, J.P. (2001) 'El cultivo de la maca y su consumo', Mimeograph, CONCYTEC, Lima, Peru.

Wei, B., Hara, M., Yamauchi, R., Ueno, Y., Kato, K. (1991) 'Fructo-oligosaccharides in the tubers of Jerusalem artichoke and yacon', *Research Bulletin of the Faculty of Agriculture, Gifu University*, vol 56, pp.133–138.

9 Biodiversity's contribution to dietary diversity

Magnitude, meaning and measurement

Peter R. Berti and Andrew D. Jones

Introduction

> Biodiversity refers to the variability among living organisms from all sources, including terrestrial, marine and other aquatic ecosystems and the ecological complexes of which they are part. This includes diversity within species (genetic diversity), between species and of ecosystems.
>
> (United Nations Environment Programme, 2002)

Recent publications (Frison et al., 2011; Bélanger and Johns, 2008; Burlingame et al., 2009a), and chapters within this book are increasing the focus upon biodiversity and its role in improving nutrition. At times a relationship between higher biodiversity and improved nutrition is assumed, without explanation of the type of biodiversity in question, documentation of supporting research, or a theoretical framework for expecting such a relationship. In this chapter, the basis for a potential relationship between biodiversity and nutrition is described, and the basis for biodiversity's nutrition benefits is elaborated.

Three links between biodiversity and nutrition

Biodiversity may be linked to nutrition in three different ways: at a macro level, at a farm level, and at a dietary level. At a macro level, biodiversity plays a role in "environmental services" that have a positive influence in agriculture and food production, including adaptation to climate change, soil protection, crop pollination, and pest control (Snapp et al., 2010; Frison et al., 2011). All the services contribute to longer term farm well-being, food supply stability, food security, and ultimately nutrition.

At the farm level, biodiversity (as crop diversity) can lead to greater production (Myers, 1996), sustainability (Brussaard et al., 2007; Frison et al., 2011) and stability (Zhu et al., 2000). Factors increasing production include niche differentiation (different crops taking advantage of favourable temporal and spatial on-farm niches); reduced loss to pests and diseases and weed competition and more efficient use of natural resources (e.g., different crops access different soil nutrients, and in the case of legumes, increased nitrogen available in the soil for other crops to use) (Frison et al., 2011). Stability in production results from greater disease suppression in mixed crops (Zhu et al., 2000). Biodiversity in production systems minimizes vulnerability to existing and emerging stresses that is experienced in monocultures (Frison et al., 2011), allowing for longer term sustainability in production.

The focus of this chapter is on the role of biodiversity at the dietary level. Biodiversity has been proposed to be a prerequisite or correlate for dietary diversity and the health benefits that follow from having a diverse diet (Penafiel et al., 2011; Bélanger and Johns, 2008), and, depending on how biodiversity is defined, such a relationship is automatic – many different plants or animals must be cultivated or gathered to produce diversity on the plate – but whether multiple varieties of single plant or animal species are required for a diverse diet is not usually discussed in the biodiversity literature.

The following section reviews what dietary diversity means, how it is measured, and summarizes dietary diversity at a global scale. We then review the arguments made and the evidence for a relationship between biodiversity and dietary diversity. The next section considers the magnitude of biodiversity from a nutrition perspective, and presents the case for how biodiversity and dietary diversity could be considered in nutrition programming in a rural Bolivian population. The conclusion integrates the information from across the sections to generate a series of questions that should be considered prior to embarking on a biodiversity-based nutrition intervention.

Dietary diversity

Meanings and measurement

Dietary diversity is defined as the variety of foods in a diet over a given period of time (Ruel, 2003). National dietary guidelines consistently recognize and promote the importance of diverse diets (Health Canada, 2007; US Department of Agriculture and US Department of Health and Human Services, 2010; World Health Organization, 1996; German Nutrition Society, 2005). The basic diversity concept is simple, relatively easy to explain, and therefore intrinsically desirable for programme managers developing nutrition education messages. However, there is no consensus among the nutrition community as to what precisely constitutes a diverse diet or how to measure it.

Dietary diversity is typically measured by counting the number of different foods or food groups in a diet. A variety of scores have been developed for this purpose. Research in low-income settings has tended to emphasize simple food variety and diet diversity scores measuring the number of different foods and food groups, respectively, in the diet (Onyango et al., 1998; Arimond and Ruel, 2004; Rao et al., 2001) while research in wealthier countries has similarly relied on these types of count measures, but has also employed scales with scores based on meeting goals for recommended intakes of specific nutrients (e.g., energy, saturated fat, dietary cholesterol, calcium, sufficient servings of fruits and vegetables) (Drescher et al., 2007; Kant, 2004; Kennedy et al., 1995). A multivariate approach has been used in a newly developed method for calculating "nutritional functional diversity" (Remans et al., 2011). The differences in the emphasis and levels of simplicity of the measurement tools employed speaks to the diverse nutrition challenges (i.e., undernutrition, overnutrition, and the overlapping of the two) facing different population groups and the variation in the nutritional significance of diversity across contexts.

Sensitivity and specificity analyses can be conducted to determine the relevant cut-off points for the number of individual foods or food groups necessary for an individual to achieve an adequate dietary intake (Food and Nutrition Technical Assistance Project, 2006). However, these cut-offs points are difficult to generalize outside the specific contexts within which data are collected.[1] Fundamental decisions regarding even the selection of foods and food groups to include in diversity measures are highly dependent on the local availability of different foods, the nutritional content of these foods and the frequency of their consumption by different population groups (Ruel, 2003). Furthermore, emphasizing only foods or food groups in diversity indicators may fail to account for important nutritional variation within species (i.e., subspecies, varieties, cultivars, breeds) (Burlingame et al., 2009b).

Despite the multiple approaches used to measure dietary diversity and the varied determinants of diversity across locales, findings from multiple contexts consistently confirm the importance of including a diverse selection of foods in diets. Adult and child diets containing a greater number of different foods or food groups are associated with greater energy and nutrient intakes (Kant, 2004; Rose et al., 2002; Ogle et al., 2001; Tarini et al., 1999; Onyango et al., 1998) as well as more adequate nutrient intakes (Torheim et al., 2004; Steyn et al., 2006; Hatløy et al., 1998).[2] Furthermore, it is positively associated with adult and child nutritional status (Savy et al., 2005; Rah et al., 2010; Arimond and Ruel, 2004), birth weight (Rao et al., 2001), and further "downstream" health outcomes, including better cognitive function (Wengreen et al., 2009; Clausen et al., 2005), improved haemoglobin concentrations (Bhargava et al., 2001; Siegel et al., 2006), a reduced incidence of cancer (Jansen et al., 2004) and decreased mortality (Kant et al., 1993).

These improved health outcomes likely result in part from the greater likelihood that an individual will attain his or her energy and nutrient requirements from a more diverse diet, but the reason that these are achieved may not be obvious. First, there is some evidence of a "buffet effect" (i.e., when there is more food variety available, people will eat more) (Herforth, 2010). Secondly, there are nutrient density differences (mg of vitamins and minerals per gram of food, or per joule of food) at different levels of dietary diversity. Individuals with very low diversity diets (usually the very poor, very food insecure) have diets dominated by staple foods, which in most settings are starchy cereals, roots or tubers and are of relatively low nutrient density. At slightly higher levels of diversity in the slightly less poor, a few fruits and vegetables are added, and these bring nutrients not present or in low concentration in the staple food. At still higher levels of diversity, there are more fruits and vegetables bringing in more nutrients, and at the higher levels still, nutrient-dense animal-source foods (e.g., meat, eggs, milk) are eaten, increasing the likelihood that the consumer will meet her nutrient requirements. So while adding rice to a corn-based diet will make it more diverse, it would not greatly increase nutrient intake as is usually intended and expected as dietary diversity increases. In fact, higher dietary diversity is more strongly associated with increased consumption of non-staple foods (e.g., animal-source foods, fruits and vegetables) compared with increased variety within a staple food group (Hoddinott and Yohannes, 2002). However, diverse diets convey benefits beyond just enhanced nutrient intakes.

Foods are not merely nutrient delivery devices, but complex mixtures of chemical compounds and elements anchored in cultural contexts whose many constituents act as agonists and antagonists to digestion and absorption in the gut and may have beneficial health effects independent of their nutrient content (Liu, 2003). Notwithstanding advances in nutritional biochemistry, a comprehensive understanding of human biochemistry, particularly with regards to the dynamics of "food synergy", or the interactions between the various components of the food matrix, is a distant goal (Jacobs and Tapsell, 2007). Research on the relationships between single foods and nutrients is important in advancing nutritional science, but there may be greater public health significance of elucidating relationships between dietary patterns and health outcomes (Mozaffarian and Ludwig, 2010). These patterns, in fact, exhibit more consistent relationships to health outcomes than foods and nutrients alone (Slatterly, 2008).

Global landscape of dietary diversity

Food variety and food group diversity scores vary widely between countries (Ruel, 2003). Across all world regions, grains, roots and tubers contribute the largest percentage of energy to diets with all other food groups contributing less than 10 per cent (with the exception of meat and fish) (Figure 9.1) although on a weight basis (i.e., grams per person per day) consumption of fruits and vegetables is similar to grains, roots and tubers in the Americas, Mediterranean and Europe (Figure 9.2). But the regions are not homogenous, and Figure 9.3 demonstrates intra-regional differences in dietary diversity. Consumption of animal-source foods in most countries of the Americas is greater than that of African countries; however, large disparities exist even within the Americas, with the per capita consumption of animal-source foods in the United States quadruple that of Bolivia and more than 12 times that of Haiti.[3] Several studies have found significant positive associations between dietary diversity and household socioeconomic status within countries (Thorne-Lyman et al., 2010; Rashid et al., 2006; Rah et al., 2010; Hoddinott and Yohannes, 2002; Hatløy et al., 2000; Anzid et al., 2009). Differences in socioeconomic status likely account for some of the variance between countries as well.

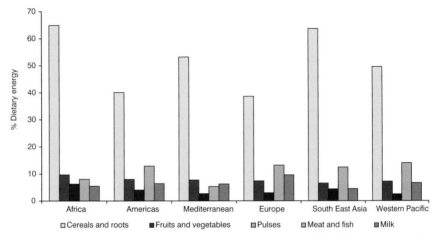

Figure 9.1 Consumption of select food groups as a percentage of total dietary energy by world region

Note: Data from FAOSTAT 2005–2007. The consumption amounts are the quantity of food estimated to be available for human consumption, but actual consumption may be lower due to wastage and losses during storage, preparation, thrown out or given to animals (http://faostat.fao. org/, accessed July 2012). Countries classified according to WHO regions.

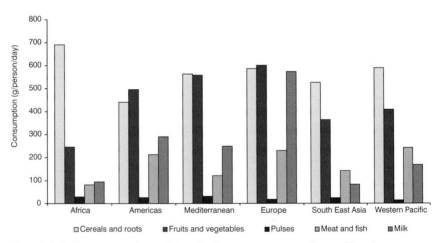

Figure 9.2 Daily consumption of select food groups per person by world region

Note: see footnote to Figure 9.1.

Biodiversity and dietary diversity

At the heart of the biodiversity-for-health position, it is assumed that there is a positive relationship between biodiversity, as manifested in on-farm crop and animal diversity, and dietary diversity. Certainly at some scale, this must be true (if all farmers grew only corn or only rice then there would be little dietary

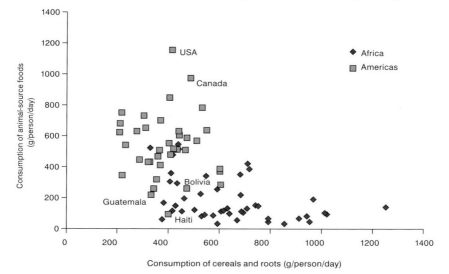

Figure 9.3 Daily consumption of animal-source foods and grains/roots/tubers per person in Africa and the Americas

diversity), but in practice, little evidence exists to support the relationship between biodiversity and household dietary diversity. Evidence from Kenya and Tanzania indicates a positive relationship (Herforth, 2010); however, contradictory evidence from Ecuador shows dietary diversity related to farm size, but not farm diversity (Oyarzun et al., submitted), and a study in Peru showed no relationship between number of varieties grown and child growth or household food security (Scurrah et al., 2011).

Despite the limited evidence, it is posited that biodiversity, in the form of crop diversity and domesticated animal diversity, is a necessary if not sufficient condition for dietary diversity. Presumably there could be increased dietary diversity as more food species and varieties of species are grown, but the magnitude of increased dietary diversity that followed would be a function of the species and varieties introduced. Some varieties of individual crops may be so different from one another as to be considered different foods (Herforth, 2010), such as white- and orange-fleshed sweet potatoes, and therefore variation may be nutritionally meaningful. For other crop varieties, variation may be agronomically meaningful, but nutritionally irrelevant.

If the assumption of a positive relationship between biodiversity and dietary diversity is valid then there are two key (and nuanced) implications for agriculture and nutrition interventions:

1   If the distributions of nutrient contents among varieties of most foods are lognormal (or even just positively skewed – see next section) then varieties chosen at random from the distribution of varieties are likely to have nutrient content less than the average, and far less than the maximum.

Likewise, a food chosen at random from the food system (whose distribution is also positively skewed) would exhibit the same pattern. While foods are not chosen at random from food systems, varieties are chosen at random with respect to nutrient content. Varieties may be planted for agronomic, economic, taste, storage or other reasons, but in the absence of a specific nutrition intervention (e.g., a biofortification programme or any intervention that screens and selects varieties based on compositional analysis or traditional knowledge), it is unlikely that the nutrient content of the different varieties will influence cropping decisions. In other words, a highly informed selection process would be required to select a variety with higher-than-average nutrient content. A critical difference, however, is that the high-end of the distribution of foods can be relatively easily selected by a local nutritionist (e.g., most orange-coloured foods have significant quantities of vitamin A activity and most animal-source foods have high levels of iron), whereas such easily applied shortcuts are not available to identify the high-end varieties of a crop (with the exception of the depth of orange colouring indicating vitamin A levels in some foods like orange-fleshed sweet potatoes; Takahata et al., 1993).

2   Figure 9.4 shows a scatterplot of quantities of individual food items consumed (g/day) on one day of observation of 20- to 40-year old women in the rural Bolivian Andes by the vitamin A content of the food (μg/100g) (data set described in Berti et al., 2010b).[4] Five hundred micrograms of

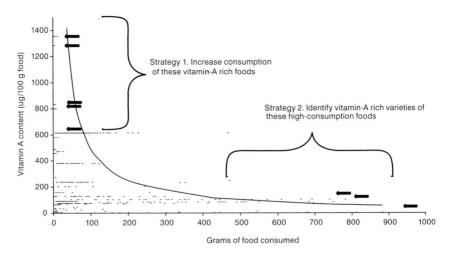

Figure 9.4 Consumption of vitamin A containing foods in women (20–40 yrs) in a rural Bolivian population (3,454 points from 360 women consuming 92 different foods).

Notes: Each point on the graph represents the intersection of the amount of a single food item consumed by a woman on one day and the level of vitamin A in that food. The curved line represents the function of grams of food and vitamin A levels that would provide an intake of 500 μg of vitamin A. 500 μg is the recommended safe intake for adult women (World Health Organization and Food and Agriculture Organization of the United Nations, 2004).

vitamin A is the recommended safe intake for adult women and can serve as a target (daily vitamin A intake will often come from more than one food and so this serves as a guideline, not a prescription). To put more points "above the line", a strategy may be (1) to increase the consumption of the vitamin A-rich foods (i.e., foods with greater than 600 μg/100g of vitamin A, of which there are five in this food system) – a conventional "dietary modification" strategy, although also used within biodiversity programmes to promote nutrient-dense, underutilized species within the food system; or (2) to introduce into production varieties of foods that have higher vitamin A levels and are consumed frequently in substantial quantities (e.g., greater than 400 g/day, of which potato is the only example in this population) – a "biodiversity strategy".

Whether a dietary modification strategy or biodiversity strategy would be appropriate will be situation specific – in this Bolivian setting, dietary modification would be preferred as there are no available vitamin A-rich potato varieties, and even if there were, there are many strong agronomic and cultural reasons for choosing the varieties they do, which would create resistance to changing the varietal mix currently in use. The best candidates for promotion as a vitamin A-rich food already in the diets are carrots and a couple of types of indigenous dark green leafy vegetables – increasing their production is considered feasible by local agronomists and they would be welcomed into their daily meals. There may be other relatively unknown native species and types that would be nutritious and also well suited for cultivation in this environment.

Nutrition and biodiversity

There are many proposed and existing ways to measure biodiversity (Reiss et al., 2009). To quantify the level of biodiversity in a way that is meaningful to human nutrition, there is consideration in the variation in nutrient content of food varieties and within food systems. Many commonly consumed crops have hundreds or thousands of varieties (e.g., more than 100,000 varieties of rice (Sackville Hamilton, 2006) and 4,000 varieties of potato (Burlingame et al., 2009b)), and there are many breeds of domesticated animals (e.g., over 1,000 breeds of sheep and 600 breeds of goats; Jensen, 2009), but only a small fraction of these varieties have nutrient content data available. Additionally there are many underutilized indigenous and wild plants (e.g., Maroyi, 2011; Jeambey et al., 2009; Herforth, 2010), totalling some unknown number of distinct food species, varieties, or breeds. For the vast majority of these there are no nutrient composition data. Therefore, for this chapter, available data are collected on levels of iron and vitamin A (two micronutrients of global public health significance) for specific varieties of various food crops. A similar analysis of less common foods would be desirable but is not currently possible.

Variation in nutrient content between food varieties

Data were available for a number of staple foods (e.g., potato, beans, rice) as well as some less commonly consumed foods (e.g., choysum, strawberries). For some foods, there were many varieties tested (123 varieties of potato, 67 of common bean), and for other foods only a few (four varieties of lentils, six of peas). The minimum and maximum values of vitamin A and iron are shown in Table 9.1. The table includes a variety of food types, including globally important staple foods, common and regional fruits and vegetables. The range in vitamin A is marked, with an over 10,000-fold difference in vitamin A levels between banana varieties, and 100-fold difference for other foods. There is a much lower range in iron levels, with a maximum of a 23-fold difference in iron content between sweet potato varieties, and most of the foods having less than a 5-fold difference between varieties. But even for those foods with small differences (e.g., cassava with 2.5 versus 0.9 mg iron per 100 g) there could still be the difference between sufficiency and insufficiency of the diet (e.g., 400 g of high-iron cassava would meet a five-year-old's iron requirements, but low-iron cassava would supply only one-third of the requirement).[5]

The distribution-fitting function of Crystal Ball (version 11.1, Oracle, Redwood Shores, CA) was used to find the best fitting distributions for those foods with data on ten varieties or more. In general, the data had lognormal distributions, or similar to lognormal distributions (positively skewed, with the mean greater than the median), with SD between one-tenth and three-quarters of the mean (although the strength of the fit to a lognormal distribution was variable, and for some foods, other distributions (normal, gamma, etc.) fit the data more closely). The distribution of iron in 123 potato varieties is shown in Figure 9.5.

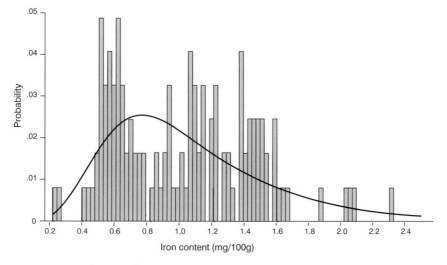

Figure 9.5 Distribution of iron in 123 potato varieties. The bars represent the number of observations at each level. The curve represents a lognormal function fit to the data.

Variation between varieties compared with variation in food systems

To capture the magnitude of interspecies variation within a given food system, there is an evaluation of the iron and vitamin A content in foods in USDA food composition tables (US Department of Agriculture, 2010) – representing perhaps the most variety of any food system in the world – and 92 foods appearing in the diet of a population in rural Bolivia (Berti et al., 2010a; Ministerio de Salud y Deportes, 2005), a diet that is limited in variety and is perhaps typical of diets in low-income countries. Figure 9.6 shows the plotted distribution of iron in the two food systems over the minimum and maximum values from food varieties in Table 9.1. Thus there are two types of distributions with overlapping plots. The bars represent the range of iron content (in mg per 100 g) found in the foods listed on the left vertical axis. The lines represent the distribution of the relative frequency (plotted against the right vertical axis) of iron content in foods in the US and Bolivian food systems. Thus the most common iron content in the USDA and Bolivian food systems is about 1.5 mg per 100 g, but there are some foods with more than 10-fold as much iron per 100 g. The variation in the iron levels is different between crops, with an especially high level of variation in beans and sweet potato. However, this level of variation is less than that found even in the simple Bolivian food system, where 10 per cent of the foods have above 10 mg/100g.

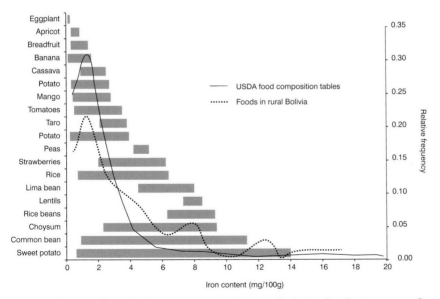

Figure 9.6 Range of iron levels among crop varieties, and relative distribution curves for USDA and rural Bolivian food systems.

Notes: The graph is truncated at 20 mg. USDA foods continue at low frequency to 120 mg. Bolivian foods also include two items > 20 mg: lentils (38 mg) and beef blood (61 mg).

Table 9.1 Minimum and maximum iron levels (mg/100 g raw) and vitamin A levels (retinol equivalents/100 g raw) in selected foods. All vitamin A data are as compiled by Burlingame et al. (2009a), except for pumpkin which is from Murkovic et al. (2002).

Food type	Vitamin A Minimum	Vitamin A Maximum	Iron n varieties tested[a]	Iron Minimum	Iron Maximum	Reference
Apricot	33	1157		0.3	0.85	Burlingame et al. 2009a
Banana	<1	14167		0.1	1.6	Burlingame et al. 2009a
Breadfruit	1	157		0.29	1.4	Burlingame et al. 2009a
Cassava	1	132		0.9	2.5	Burlingame et al. 2009a
Choysum			22	2.31	9.4	Hanson et al. 2011
Common bean			67	0.89	11.29	de Araújo et al. 2003, Talukder et al. 2010, Barampama and Simard, 1993
Eggplant			32	0.102	0.247	Raigón et al. 2008
Lentils			4	7.3	8.5	Wang and Dean, 2006
Lima bean			18	4.5	8	Ologhobo and Fetuga, 1983
Mango	3	720		0.4	2.8	Burlingame et al. 2009a
Pandanus	2	150				
Peas			6	4.21	5.19	Wang et al. 2008
Potato	<1	1	123	0.22	3.94	Andre et al. 2007, Burgos et al. 2007, Burlingame et al. 2009a
Pumpkin	60	1660				

Rice			15	0.7	6.4	Pereira et al. 2009, Burlingame et al. 2009a
Rice beans			7	6.3	9.3	Kaura and Kapoor, 1992
Strawberries			13	2.01	6.23	Hakala et al. 2003
Sweet potato	17	3850		0.6	14	Burlingame et al. 2009a
Taro	1	340		2.1	3.8	Burlingame et al. 2009a
Tomatoes			8	0.49	3.5	Guil-Guerrero and Rebolloso-Fuentes, 2009

Note
a Number of varieties tested not listed in Burlingame et al. (2009a).

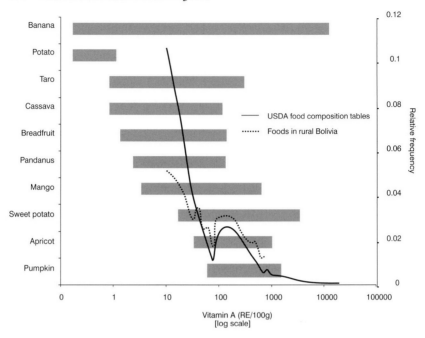

Figure 9.7 Range of vitamin A levels among crop varieties, and relative distribution curves for USDA and rural Bolivian food systems.

Note: 41 per cent of USDA foods have 0 vitamin A and 15 per cent have < 5 RAE. 52 per cent of Bolivian foods have 0 vitamin A and 4 per cent have < 5 RAE. These figures are not shown in the graph.

Figure 9.7 is similar to Figure 9.6, summarizing the levels of vitamin A in varieties of different crops, as well as in the food systems of the US and rural Bolivian population. As with the example of iron, the USDA data represents a food system with great variety, and the Bolivian food system has minimal variety.

Conclusion

Drawing from various data sources, we have considered biodiversity from a nutrition perspective, particularly regarding its link to dietary diversity. If an agricultural intervention aims to introduce a new food crop or animal to increase dietary diversity and nutrient intake, then the analyses summarized in Figures 9.6 and 9.7 suggest that there are more potential foods to be found through considering the entire food system rather than just varieties of a single food (Strategy 1 of Figure 9.4). As summarized in the discussion of Figure 9.4, however, this will be context specific. Another important advantage of prioritizing the diversity of food systems is that high-nutrient content foods can be identified by any locally trained nutritionist (e.g., carrots, mangos and papayas are all high in ß-carotene; lentils, soybeans and all meats are high in iron)

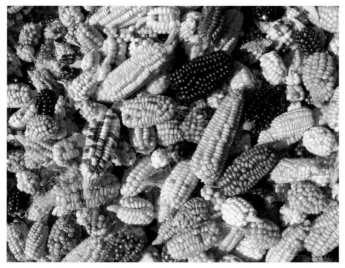

Figure 9.8 Harvested maize stored at a local homestead in northern Potosí, Bolivia. Photograph by Andrew Jones

without difficult analysis of varieties. However, in some settings, it may be easier to identify or develop varieties of staples that are rich in micronutrients than it would be to increase consumption of non-staple, micronutrient-rich crops (Strategy 2 of Figure 9.4). This strategy has not been explicitly tested though and trials comparing the effectiveness of "Strategy 1" and "Strategy 2" are needed.

This chapter concludes with a series of questions that should be considered, regardless of the strategy envisioned. These questions have direct nutrition consequences for participating farming households, but may not normally be asked prior to an agriculture–nutrition intervention.

1 What is the problem that needs to be addressed? Are there specific nutrient deficiencies?
2 Are there priority nutrition problems that have been identified that justify carrying out any sort of intervention? Could these problems possibly be addressed through food-based interventions? Whose needs will be met through the intervention?
3 How will a new variety ultimately be used? And who controls decisions of use and the benefits of that end use?
4 Will the crop be consumed by the farming household? If it is sold, will it be sold locally, benefiting other local families or will it supply the export market? If sold, who will control the earned income?[6]
5 Will the variety displace micronutrient-dense crops, be introduced on pastureland that is used to raise animals and provide meat, milk or eggs for the family, or displace other plants or animals with biodiversity importance? Or will it replace less desirable crops?

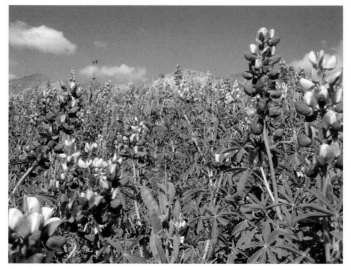

Figure 9.9 A field of Andean lupine, known locally as "tarwi", in northern Potosí, Bolivia. Photograph by Andrew Jones

6 It is possible that a crop is introduced for biodiversity reasons, but then the market for it expands and the acreage for this introduced crop increases and ultimately reduces on-farm biodiversity.

7 Will the new variety fill gaps in seasonal food supplies?

8 Will it be late maturing, early maturing, could it be harvested at multiple times throughout the year? Will it store well?

9 What is the pattern of food distribution within the household? Will the new variety be a preferred food among all family members? Will specific efforts be required to promote consumption by children?

10 How will the new variety affect time allocation, particularly for women?

11 If the new variety leads to more work for women and this is not managed properly, it could lead to less time for child feeding (especially breastfeeding), child care and ultimately poorer health outcomes.

12 Are there any safety issues associated with the new species or variety?

13 Are there disease vectors associated with the species? Is pesticide use expected? Does the culture have a practice of safely preparing the species or variety for consumption?

These questions are not new, but there is a different dimension when they are addressed from biodiversity and dietary diversity points of view. As programmes in biodiversity and dietary diversity increasingly overlap and, hopefully, mutually reinforce each other, the experiences of the practitioners and their answers to these questions should be documented and disseminated to improve future efforts.

Notes

1　For example, 15 different foods had high sensitivity to identify nutritionally inadequate diets as inadequate among preschool-aged children in urban Mali (Hatløy et al., 1998), but only six different foods were required to achieve both high sensitivity and specificity for dietary adequacy among a nationally representative sample of South African children (Steyn et al., 2006). Likewise, dietary diversity indices that appropriately select cut off points based on the internal distribution of the diversity indicator within their sample (Moursi et al., 2009; Ruel and Menon, 2002) are not able to generalize those cut offs to populations outside those from which data were collected.

2　One study did fail to show a positive association between dietary diversity and nutrient intakes (Ferguson et al., 1993). In one study that compared individual foods and food groups, though both were associated with dietary adequacy, consumption of a greater diversity of food groups was a stronger determinant of dietary adequacy than consuming a larger diversity of individual foods (Hatløy et al., 1998). In two other studies that measured both indicators, the relative strength of individual foods versus food groups in predicting dietary adequacy was less clear (Steyn et al., 2006; Torheim et al., 2004), though Torheim and others found that a food variety score contributed more significantly to regression model variation than a food group score.

3　Though diets high in fat and dietary cholesterol are associated with higher risk of chronic disease (American Heart Association, 1996; Oh et al., 2005) animal-source foods are an excellent source of bioavailable micronutrients, such as iron, zinc and vitamin A, that are often lacking in diets in low-income countries, and are particularly important for proper child growth (Penny et al., 2005).

4　Note that the data collection and analysis tools used tended to group foods together (e.g., perhaps five to ten types of potatoes were all commonly eaten, but all were grouped as one general type, "potato"). This reduces the apparent variation that exists in the diet, and in Figure 9.4, and so the figure should be considered for illustration of the concept, but as a simplified presentation of the real situation.

5　400 g ´ 2.5 mg/100g = 10 mg, which is the EAR (estimated average requirement) of iron, for a low bioavailability diet.

6　Control of new income within households will no doubt determine in part the extent to which increased incomes lead to more diverse diets and improved health outcomes for family members. Strong evidence from many different regions suggests that income controlled by women benefits child nutrition and household food security to a greater extent than income controlled by men (Quisumbing et al., 1995; Kennedy and Cogill, 1987).

References

American Heart Association (1996) Dietary guidelines for healthy American adults, *Circulation,* vol 94, pp.1795–1800.

Andre, C.M., Ghislain, M., Bertin, P., Oufir, M., Herrra Mdel, R., Hoffmann, L., Hausman, J.F., Larondelle, Y. and Evers, D. (2007) Andean potato cultivars (Solanum tuberosum L.) as a source of antioxidant and mineral micronutrients, *J Agric Food Chem,* vol 55, pp.366–378.

Anzid, K., Zahra Elhamndani, F., Baali, A., Boetsch, G., Levy-Desroches, S., Montero Lopez, P. and Cherkaoui, M.T. (2009) The effect of socio-economic status and area of residence on household food variety in Morocco, *Annals of Human Biology,* vol 36, pp.727–749.

Arimond, M. and Ruel, M.T. (2004) Dietary diversity is associated with child nutritional status: evidence from 11 demographic and health surveys, *Journal of Nutrition*, vol 134, pp.2579–2585.

Barampama, Z. and Simard, R.E. (1993) Nutrient composition, protein quality and antinutritional factors of some varieties of dry beans (*Phaseolus vulgaris*) grown in Burundi, *Food Chemistry*, vol 47, pp.159–167.

Bélanger, J. and Johns, T. (2008) Biological diversity, dietary diversity, and eye health in developing country populations: establishing the evidence-base, *EcoHealth*, vol 5, pp.244–256.

Berti, P.R., Jones, A.D., Cruz Agudo, Y., Larrea Macias, S., Borja, R. and Sherwood, S.G. (2010a) Dietary assessment in an isolated Andean population: Current inadequacies and scope for improvement using locally available resources, *American Journal of Human Biology*, 22, pp.741–749.

Berti, P.R., Jones, A.D., Cruz, Y., Larrea, S., Borja, R. and Sherwood, S. (2010b) Assessment and characterization of the diet of an isolated population in the Bolivian Andes, *Am J Hum Biol*, vol 22, pp.741–749.

Bhargava, A., Bouis, H.E. and Scrimshaw, N.S. (2001) Dietary intakes and socioeconomic factors are associated with the hemoglobin concentration of Bangladeshi women, *Journal of Nutrition*, vol 131, pp.758–764.

Brussaard, L., De Ruiter, P.C. and Brown, G.G. (2007) Soil biodiversity for agricultural sustainability, *Agriculture, Ecosystems and Environment*, vol 121, pp.233–244.

Burgos, G., Amoros, W., Morote, M., Stangoulis, J. and Bonierbale, M. (2007) Iron and zinc concentration of native Andean potato cultivars from a human nutrition perspective, *Journal of Science of Food and Agriculture*, vol 87, pp.668–675.

Burlingame, B., Charrondiere, R. and Mouille, B. (2009a) Food composition is fundamental to the cross-cutting initiative on biodiversity for food and nutrition, *Journal of Food Composition and Analysis*, vol 22, pp.361–365.

Burlingame, B., Mouille, B. and Charrondière, R. (2009b) Nutrients, bioactive non-nutrients and anti-nutrients in potatoes, *Journal of Food Composition and Analysis*, p.22.

Clausen, T., Charlton, K.E., Gobotswang, K. and Holmboe-Ottesen, G. (2005) Predictors of food variety and dietary diversity among older persons in Botswana, *Applied Nutritional Investigation*, p.21.

De Araújo, R., Miglioranza, E., Montalvan, R., Destro, D., Goncalves-Vidigal, M.C. and Moda-Cirino, V. (2003) Genotype x environment interaction effects on the iron content of common bean grains, *Crop Breeding and Applied Biotechnology*, vol 3, pp.269–274.

Drescher, L.S., Thiele, S. and Mensink, G.B.M. (2007) A new index to measure healthy food diversity better reflects a healthy diet than traditional measures, *Journal of Nutrition*, vol 137, pp.647–651.

Ferguson, E., Gibson, R., Opare-Obisaw, C., Osei-Opare, C., Lamba, C. and Ounpuu, S.S. (1993) Seasonal food consumption patterns and dietary diversity of rural preschool Ghanaian and Malawian children, *Ecol Food Nutr*, vol 29, pp.219–234.

Food and Nutrition Technical Assistance Project (2006) *Developing and Validating Simple Indicators of Dietary Quality and Energy Intake of Infants and Young Children in Developing Countries: Summary of findings from analysis of 10 data sets*, Washington DC: Academy for Educational Development.

Frison, E.A., Cherfas, J. and Hodgkin, T. (2011) Agricultural biodiversity is essential for a sustainable improvement in food and nutrition security, *Sustainability*, vol 3, pp.238–253.

German Nutrition Society (2005) *10 guidelines of the German Nutrition Society (DGE) for a wholesome diet*, German Nutrition Society.

Guil-Guerrero, J.L. and Rebolloso-Fuentes, M.M. (2009) Nutrient composition and antioxidant activity of eight tomato (Lycopersicon esculentum) varieties, *Journal of Food Composition and Analysis,* vol 22, pp.123–129.

Hakala, M., Lapvetelainen, A., Huopalahti, R., Kallio, H. and Tahvonen, R. (2003) Effects of varieties and cultivation conditions on the composition of strawberries, *Journal of Food Composition and Analysis,* vol 16, pp.67–80.

Hanson, P., Yang, R.Y., Chang, L.C., Ledesma, L. and Ledesma, D. (2011) Carotenoids, ascorbic acid, minerals, and total glucosinolates in choysum (Brassica rapa cvg. parachinensis) and kailaan (B. oleraceae Alboglabra group) as affected by variety and wet and dry season production, *Journal of Food Composition and Analysis,* vol 24, pp. 950–962.

Hatløy, A., Torheim, L.E. and Oshaug, A. (1998) Food variety – a good indicator of nutritional adequacy of the diet? A case study from an urban area in Mali, West Africa, *Eur J ClinNutr,* vol 52, pp.891–898.

Hatløy, A., Hallund, J., Diarra, M.M. and Oshaug, A. (2000) Food variety, socioeconomic status and nutritional status in urban and rural areas in Koutiala (Mali), *Public Health Nutrition,* vol 3, pp.57–65.

Health Canada (2007) *Canada's Food Guide*, Ministry of Health.

Herforth, A. (2010) *Promotion of Traditional African Vegetables in Kenya and Tanzania: A Case Study of an Intervention Representing Emerging Imperatives in Global Nutrition,* PhD thesis, Cornell University.

Hoddinott, J. and Yohannes, Y. (2002) *Discussion Paper No. 136: Dietary diversity as a food security indicator*, Washington: International Food Policy Research Institute, Food Consumption and Nutrition Division.

Jacobs, D.R. and Tapsell, L.C. (2007) Food, not nutrients, is the fundamental unit in nutrition, *Nutrition Reviews,* vol 65, pp.439–450.

Jansen, M.C.J.F., Bas Bueno-De-Mesquita, H., Feskens, E.J.M., Streppel, M.T., Kok, F.J. and Kromhout, D. (2004) Quantity and variety of fruit and vegetable consumption and cancer risk, *Nut. Cancer,* vol 48, pp.142–148.

Jeambey, Z., Johns, T., Talhouk, S. and Batal, M. (2009) Perceived health and medicinal properties of six species of wild edible plants in north-east Lebanon, *Public Health Nutrition,* vol 12, pp.1902–1911.

Jensen, P. (eds) (2009) *The ethology of domestic animals,* Cambridge, MA: CABI.

Kant, A.K. (2004) Dietary patterns and health outcomes, *J Am Diet Assoc.,* vol 104, pp.615–635.

Kant, A.K., Schatzkin, A., Harris, T.B., Ziegler, R.G. and Bloc, G. (1993) Dietary diversity and subsequent mortality in the First National Health and Nutrition Examination Survey Epidemiologic Follow-up Study, *Am J ClinNutr,* vol 57, pp.434–440.

Kaura, D. and Kapoor, A.C. (1992) Nutrient composition and antinutritional factors of rice bean (Vigna umbellata), *Food Chemistry,* vol 43, pp.119–124.

Kennedy, E.T. and Cogill, B. (1987) *Income and Nutritional Effects of the Commercialization of Agriculture in Southwestern Kenya*, Research Report 63, Washington DC: IFPRI.

Kennedy, E.T., Ohls, J., Carlson, S. and Fleming, K. (1995) The healthy eating index: design and applications, *Journal of the American Dietetic Association,* vol 95, pp.1103–1108.

Liu, R.H. (2003) Health benefits of fruit and vegetables are from additive and synergistic combinations of phytochemicals, *American Journal of Clinical Nutrition* 78, pp.517S– 520S.

Maroyi, A. (2011) The gathering and consumption of wild edible plants in Nhema communal area, Midlands Province, Zimbabwe. *Ecol Food Nutr,* vol 50, pp.506–525.

Ministerio de Salud y Deportes, Gobierno DE Bolivia (2005) *Tabla Boliviana de Composicion de Alimentos,* 4th edn, La Paz, Bolivia.

Moursi, M.M., Treche, S., Martin-Prevel, Y., Maire, B. and Delpeuch, F. (2009) Association of a summary index of child feeding with diet quality and growth of 6–23 months children in urban Madagascar, *European Journal of Clinical Nutrition,* vol 63, pp.718–724.

Mozaffarian, D. and Ludwig, D.S. (2010) Dietary guidelines in the 21st century – a time for food, *JAMA,* vol 304, pp.681–682.

Murkovic, M., Mulleder, U. and Neunteufl, H. (2002) Carotenoid content in different varieties of pumpkins, *Journal of Food Composition and Analysis,* vol 15, pp.633–638.

Myers, N. (1996) Environmental services of biodiversity, *Proceedings of the National Academy of Sciences of the United States of America,* vol 93, pp.2764–2749.

Ogle, B.M., Hung, P.H. and Tuyet, H.T. (2001) Significance of wild vegetables in micronutrient intakes of women in Vietnam: an analysis of food variety, *Asia Pac J ClinNutr,* vol 10, pp.21–30.

Oh, K., Hu, F.B., Manson, J.E., Stampfer, M.J. and Willett, W.C. (2005) Dietary fat intake and risk of coronary heart disease in women: 20 years of follow-up of the Nurses' Health Study, *Am J Epidemiol,* vol 161, pp.672–679.

Ologhobo, A.D. and Fetuga, B.L. (1983) Compositional differences in some limabean (Phaseolus lunatus) varieties, *Food Chemistry,* vol 10, pp.297–307.

Onyango, A., Koski, K. and Tucker, K.L. (1998) Food diversity versus breastfeeding choice in determining anthropometric status in rural Kenyan toddlers, *Int J Epidemiol,* vol 27, pp.484–489.

Oyarzun, P.J., Borja, R., Sherwood, S. and Parra, V. (submitted), Much we assume, little we know: agro biodiversity and peasant family diets in the Andes, *Ecology of Food and Nutrition.*

Penafiel, D., Lachat, C., Espinel, R., Van Damme, P. and Kolsteren, P. (2011) A systematic review on the contributions of edible plant and animal biodiversity to human diets, *EcoHealth*, vol 8, pp. 381–399.

Penny, M.E., Creed-Kanashiro, H.M., Robert, R.C., Narro, M.R., Caulfield, L.E. and Black, R.E. (2005) Effectiveness of an educational intervention delivered through the health services to improve nutrition in young children: a cluster-randomised controlled trial, *Lancet,* vol 365, pp.1863–1872.

Pereira, J.A., Bassinello, P.Z., Cutrim, V.D.A. and Ribeiro, V.Q. (2009) Comparação entre características agronômicas, culinárias e nutricionais em variedades de arroz branco e vermelho, *Caatinga,* vol 22, pp.243–348.

Quisumbing, A.R., Brown, L., Feldstein, H., Haddad, L. and Pena, C. (1995) Women: the key to food security, *Food Policy Report*, Washington DC: International Food Policy Research Institute.

Rah, J.H., Akhter N., Sembra, R.D., De Pee, S., Bloem, M.W., Campbell, A.A., Moench-Pfanner, R., Sun, K., Badham, J. and Kraemer, K. (2010) Low dietary diversity is a predictor of child stunting in rural Bangladesh, *European Journal of Clinical Nutrition,* vol 64, pp.1393–1398.

Raigón A.M.D., Prohens, J., Muñoz-Falcón, J.E. and Nuez, F. (2008) Comparison of eggplant landraces and commercial varieties for fruit content of phenolics, minerals, dry matter and protein, *Journal of Food Composition and Analysis,* vol 21, pp.370–376.

Rao, S., Yajnik, C.S., Kanade, A., Fall, C.H., Margetts, B.M., Jackson, A.A., Shier, R., Joshi, S., Rege, S., Lubree, H. and Desai, B. (2001) Intake of micronutrient-rich foods in rural Indian mothers is associated with the size of their babies at birth: Pune Maternal Nutrition Study, *Journal of Nutrition,* vol 131, pp.1217–1224.

Rashid, D.A., Smith, L. and Rahman, T. (2006) Determinants of dietary quality: evidence from Bangladesh, *American Agricultural Economics Association Annual Meeting,* Long Beach, CA.

Reiss, J., Briddle, J.R., Montoya, J.M. and Woodward, G. (2009) Emerging horizons in biodiversity and ecosystem functioning research, *Trends Ecol Evol,* vol 24, pp.505–514.

Remans, R., Flynn, D.F., Declerck, F., Diru, W., Fanzo, J., Gaynor, K., Lambrecht, I., Mudiope, J., Mutuo, P.K., Nkhoma, P., Siriri, D., Sullivan, C. and Palm, C.A. (2011) Assessing nutritional diversity of cropping systems in African villages, *PLoS One,* 6, e21235.

Rose, D., Meershoek, S., Ismael, C. and McEwan, M. (2002) Evaluation of a rapid field tool for assessing household diet quality in Mozambique, *Food and Nutrition Bulletin,* vol 23, pp.181–189.

Ruel, M.T. (2003) Operationalizing dietary diversity: a review of measurement issues and research priorities, *Journal of Nutrition,* vol 133, pp.3911S–3926S.

Ruel, M.T. and Menon, P. (2002) Child feeding practices are associated with Child Nutritional Status in Latin America: innovative uses of the Demographic and Health Surveys, *Journal of Nutrition,* vol 132, pp.1180–1187.

Sackville Hamilton, R. (2006), *How many rice varieties are there?* [Online]. International Rice Research Institute, http://beta.irri.org/news/index.php/rice-today/how-many-rice-varieties-are-out-there.html, accessed July 2011.

Savy, M., Martin-Prevel, Y., Sawadogo, P., Kameli, Y. and Delpeuch, F. (2005) Use of variety/diversity scores for diet quality measurement: relation with nutritional status of women in a rural area in Burkina Faso, *European Journal of Clinical Nutrition,* vol 59, pp.703–716.

Scurrah, M., de Haan, S., Olivera, E., Canto, R., Creed, H., Carrasco, M., Veres, E. and Barahona, C. (2011) Ricos en Agrobiodiversidad pero Pobres en Nutrición: Desafíos De La Mejora De La Seguridad Alimentaria En Comunidades Chopcca, Huancavelica (forthcoming), *SEPIA XIV.* PIura, Peru, 23–26 August 2011.

Siegel, E.H., Stoltzfus, R.J., Khatry, S.K., Leclerq, S.C., Katz, J. and Tielsch, J.M. (2006) Epidemiology of anaemia among 4- to 17-month-old children living in south central Nepal, *European Journal of Clinical Nutrition,* vol 60, pp.228–235.

Slatterly, M.L. (2008) Defining dietary consumption: is the sum greater than its parts? *American Journal of Clinical Nutrition,* 2008, pp.14–15.

Snapp, S.S., Blackie, M.J., Gilbert, R.A., Bezner-Kerr, R. and Kanyama-Phiri, G.Y. (2010) Biodiversity can support a greener revolution in Africa, *Proceedings of the National Academy of Sciences of the United States of America,* vol 107, pp.20840–20845.

Steyn, N.P., Nel, J.H., Nantel, G., Kennedy, G. and Labadarios, D. (2006) Food variety and dietary diversity scores in children: are they good indicators of dietary adequacy? *Public Health Nutrition,* 2006, p.5.

Takahata, Y., Noda, T. and Nagata, T. (1993) HPLC determination of carotene content of sweet potato cultivars and its relationship with color values, *Japan J Breed,* vol 43, pp.421–427.

Talukder, Z.I., Anderson, E., Miklas, P.N., Blair, M.W., Osorno, J., Dilawari, M., Hossain, K.G. and USDA ARS (2010) Genetic diversity and selection of genotypes to enhance Zn and Fe content in common bean, *Canadian Journal of Plant Science,* vol 90, pp.49–60.

Tarini, A., Bakari, S. and Delisle, H. (1999) The overall nutritional quality of the diet is reflected in the growth of Nigerian children, *Sante,* vol 9, pp.23–31.

Thorne-Lyman, A.L., Valpiani, N., Sun, K., Sembra, R.D., Klotz, C.L., Kraemer, K., Akhter, N., de Pee, S., Moench-Pfanner, R., Sari, M. and Bloem, M.W. (2010) Household dietary diversity and food expenditures are closely linked in rural Bangladesh, increasing the risk of malnutrition due to the financial crisis, *Journal of Nutrition,* vol 140, pp.82S–188S.

Torheim, L.E., Ouattara, F., Diarra, M.M., Thiam, F.D., Barikmo, I., Hatloy, A. and Oshaug, A. (2004) Nutrient adequacy and dietary diversity in rural Mali: association and determinants, *European Journal of Clinical Nutrition,* vol 58, pp.594–604.

United Nations Environment Programme (2002) *GEO: Global Environmental Outlook – 3: Past, present, and future perspectives,* London: Earthscan.

US Department of Agriculture, A.R.S. (2010), USDA National Nutrient Database for Standard Reference, Release 23.

US Department of Agriculture and US Department of Health and Human Services (2010) *Dietary Guidelines for Americans, 2010,* Washington DC, US Government Printing Office.

Wang, N. and Dean, J.K. (2006) Effects of variety and crude protein content on nutrients and anti-nutrients in lentils (*Lens culinaris*), *Food Chemistry,* vol 95, pp.493–502.

Wang, N., Hatcher, D.W. and Gawalko, E.J. (2008) Effect of variety and processing on nutrients and certain anti-nutrients in field peas (*Pisum sativum*), *Food Chemistry,* vol 111, pp.132–138.

Wengreen, H.J., Neilson, C., Munger, R. and Corcoran, C. (2009) Diet quality is associated with better cognitive test performance among aging men and women, *Journal of Nutrition,* vol 139, pp.1944–1949.

World Health Organization (1996) *World Health Organization. Preparation and Use of Food-Based Dietary Guidelines, WHO Technical Report, Series 880. Report of a Joint FAO/WHO Consultation,* Geneva, World Health Organization.

World Health Organization and Food and Agriculture Organization of the United Nations (2004) *Vitamin and Mineral Requirements in Human Nutrition.*

Zhu, Y., Chen, H., Fan, J., Wang, Y., Li, Y., Chen, J., Yang, S., Hu, L., Leung, H., Mew, T.W., Teng, P.S., Wang, Z. and Mundt, C.C. (2000) Genetic diversity and disease control in rice, *Nature,* vol 406, pp.718–722.

10 Opening a can of mopane worms[1]

Can cross-sectoral partnerships leverage agricultural biodiversity for better quality diets?

Margaret McEwan, Gordon Prain and Danny Hunter

Introduction

Previous chapters have highlighted the multi-faceted nature of nutrition problems and provided examples of how agricultural biodiversity can contribute to dietary diversity and quality. They have illustrated the convergence of two streams of thinking which has taken place over the last three decades. Firstly, the agricultural and biodiversity community has a greater appreciation of the environmental benefits from more highly diverse systems (e.g. ecosystem services such as nutrient cycling, pest and disease regulation, pollination, hydrology etc., and climate regulation and carbon sequestration) (McNeely and Scherr, 2003; Pretty, 1995; Scherr and McNeely, 2007). Secondly, within the nutrition community there has been a growing consensus around the limitations of single nutrient interventions to address nutrition problems and the importance of food-based approaches to sustain nutritional well-being (Berti et al., 2004; DeClerck et al., 2011; Remans and Smukler – this volume). This convergence has helped to increase the understanding of the interdependence between human and ecosystem health, and how agricultural biodiversity plays a role in maintaining both (Blasbalg et al., 2011; Johns et al., 2006; Collette et al., 2011; Frison et al., 2011; Jackson et al., 2007; WHO, 2005).

Some of the case studies described in this book have shown the need and value of bringing an inter-disciplinary[2] bearing to the analysis of nutrition problems, and a cross-sectoral[3] approach to the design and implementation of interventions. However, while this kind of cooperation may seem obvious, it has until recently happened for the most part at the theoretical level rather than as action on the ground (Garrett et al., 2011). This chapter will explore some of the factors which have limited practical responses to previous calls for cross-sectoral collaboration between the environment, agriculture and health sectors to address nutrition concerns. The chapter begins with a brief examination of pre-World War II efforts to implement multi-sectoral and collaborative approaches between agriculture and health in Malawi. This is followed by an overview of the evolution of disciplinary perspectives in the agriculture, environment and nutrition sectors. This shows that these sectors have occasionally demonstrated some meeting of concepts and approaches; yet this never seems to have been translated into practical, effective cross-sectoral and inter-disciplinary collaboration required to address current nutrition problems.

Given renewed calls for greater leveraging of agriculture for improving nutrition and health and greater synergies among relevant sectors, the chapter briefly reviews how new findings from research on partnerships could contribute to more effective cross-sectoral partnerships. The chapter concludes with an example of how a national model such as *Fome Zero* in Brazil has successfully linked strengthening agricultural biodiversity and improved nutrition; and an examination of what current reforms in the CGIAR and UNSCN might have to offer for greater mobilization of agricultural biodiversity. Finally the chapter poses the question as to what is different now that may make our current efforts more successful.

A glimpse backwards

Stretching back to the early 1930s, the need for multi-sectoral analysis and collaboration to address food and nutrition concerns has been recognized. During a special session of the League of Nations Health Commission in 1935 there was a plea for a "marriage of health and agriculture" (Berry and Petty, 1992). The call reflected an appreciation that malnutrition was a multi-sectoral problem, demanding a multi-sectoral, multi-disciplinary solution involving politicians, economists, agriculturalists, social workers as well as the medical profession. This was the time when the Colonial Nutrition Committee was established in Britain and multi-disciplinary field research into local food systems was commissioned. An example of this was the Nyasaland Nutrition Survey carried out in 1938–39 in Southern Africa by a team composed of a medical officer, an agriculturalist, a food investigator, an anthropologist and a botanist, each using their own disciplinary approaches and methods. The Nyasaland Survey and other field work (e.g. Richards, 1939) undertaken during the 1930s and early 1940s conducted nutrient analysis of local foods, and surveyed their use in different agro-ecological zones and among different wealth groups. These studies recorded the roles of women and men in collecting or hunting for wild foods such as leaves and spinaches, fruits, small birds, rodents and insects, tubers, fungi, and honey, as well as collecting medicinal plants. They also documented the cultural rights and customs associated with these practices and the significance of these foods in contributing to dietary diversity, and in particular to fill seasonal shortfall periods. In Nyasaland, the findings from the survey were the basis for the establishment in 1939–40 of the Nutrition Development Unit (NDU) with the mandate to continue investigations and to introduce improved practices for fisheries, agriculture, livestock, forestry, soil degradation, in addition to medical interventions focusing on women and children (Berry and Petty, 1992). Investments in improved nutrition were seen by the Colonial Office as leading to greater well-being and greater efficiency in production (Quinn, 1994). However, the initial intervention approach used by the Nutrition Development Unit was top-down. While this was quickly recognized by the team as being unrealistic and ineffective, the Second World War intervened, political support and funding dwindled, and the NDU was closed in 1943.

After Nyasaland declared Independence in 1964 to become Malawi, the emphasis of national development planning was on achieving macro-economic growth. This was the era of "the stages of economic growth", a theory of economic development which preached the inevitability of emerging societies such as Malawi achieving high mass-consumption as part of modernization (Rist, 1997). With the shift to a macro-economic perspective, nutrition reverted to its traditional home within the health sector, with malnutrition regarded as a technical issue (lack of animal protein) within the context of disease and ignorance. Issues related to poverty were down-played and theories of planning were based on a single-sector approach (Quinn, 1994).

Shifting disciplines and paradigm shifts

Shifts in ideology and the global context have influenced not only change in national policies related to food and nutrition, but also the evolution of related disciplines and specializations (Maxwell, 2001a). As individual practitioners, policy makers or scientists, we bring to any collaborative effort different disciplinary perspectives and paradigms. These paradigms change in response to the advancement of theoretical and empirical understanding within our own disciplines, but also reflect changes in broader development theories and in the global setting. Often, one particular conceptual framework dominates the causal explanation of interrelated phenomena – in this case the causes of inadequate nutrition and poor health. The dominant explanation then strongly influences the choices around the most appropriate approaches and types of interventions for "solving" the problem. The following section briefly describes key shifts in conceptual and planning approaches in the agriculture, environment and nutrition disciplines over the last 50 years. These shifts have in turn influenced the types of institutional arrangements for cross-sectoral efforts to address nutrition problems.

Agriculture, biodiversity and diets

Recurrent famines during the 1960s in different parts of the "underdeveloped regions" as they were then called were interpreted by science policy makers and philanthropists in the West as a problem of food availability and led to the major agricultural research and development effort that became known as the Green Revolution. The philosophical underpinnings of the Green Revolution were themselves part of a post-war "development paradigm" involving a belief in the power of science and technology to carry the whole world towards an ideal state of high mass-consumption (Rostow, 1960). The "transfer of technology" was the specific mechanism through which "advanced countries" could enable poorer countries to achieve economic take off (Biggs, 1990; Rist, 1997). The focus of the Green Revolution was on the increased production of macro-nutrients and this global and national preoccupation with the staple production and supply of calories intensified with the dramatic oil price increases of the early 1970s. This period witnessed the first high-yielding rice and wheat varieties of the Green Revolution becoming more widely available. This was also the time when the political preoccupation with urban food supplies came under attack as "urban bias" (Lipton, 1977).

Although radical critiques of the "transfer of technology" paradigm were relatively common during the 1970s (e.g. Bernstein, 1973), these were still on the margins. From the beginning of the 1980s two currents of criticism gathered force and led to major changes in thinking about development, even if actual development during at least the 1980s was on hold, pending "structural adjustment" (Rist, 1997). Firstly, economists such as Amartya Sen (1981) offered a new analysis of food crises which used the concept of entitlement to show that "there *being* not enough food to eat" does not determine starvation, but rather, "people not *having* enough food to eat" is the causal factor. In other words, from the standpoint of a person or family, the issue is not food availability in general, but food access through own production, purchase, gift, barter or other entitlement. Secondly, the concern with "the standpoint of the person or family" actually involved in food production and exchange led other researchers to argue for local participation in development processes in order for change to be appropriate and sustainable (e.g. Rhoades and Booth, 1982; Chambers et al., 1989, 1994; Scoones and Thompson, 2009). The focus on participation built on earlier farming systems research and emphasized the importance of learning with farmers and tapping into local and indigenous technical knowledge. This "Farmer First" paradigm has become further elaborated through the sustainable livelihoods framework, which applies an assets-based and systems approach in which agriculture, health and nutrition are considered in a broader environmental and ecological context (e.g. Farrington et al., 1999). Similar paradigm shifts, from "ecology first" to "people first" perspectives (O'Riordan and Stoll-Kleemann, 2002) have occurred in biodiversity conservation planning and management (Hunter and Heywood, 2011).

Meanwhile, a significant consequence of the rapid expansion of industrial agriculture was the growing reliance on chemical inputs to reduce pest attack and sustain production. Dramatic impacts on human health, ecology and biodiversity were catalogued and described by Rachael Carson in *Silent Spring* (Carson, 1962). The book was to become a major influence in creating greater awareness of environmental issues and how people perceived the impact of human activities on the environment and led to the development of numerous environmental organizations. In 1983, the World Commission on Environment and Development (the Brundtland Commission) was convened by the United Nations to address increasing concern about such impacts on the natural world and human welfare. In establishing the commission, the UN recognized that environmental problems were global in nature and determined that it was in the common interest of all nations to establish policies for sustainable development. Among these environmental problems were growing concerns about the degradation of ecosystems and the loss of biological diversity.

In 1992, the importance of biological diversity conservation and its sustained utilization and development were central to the United Nations Conference on the Environment and Development (UNCED) held in Rio de Janeiro, Brazil, and it was here that the Convention on Biological Diversity (CBD) was opened for signature to enhance the conservation of biological diversity, the sustainable use of its components and the fair and equitable sharing of the benefits arising out of the utilization of genetic resources. The Convention entered into force in December 1993. Subsequently, there was an increasing recognition of both the growing erosion of plant genetic resources and their importance for food and nutrition security, together with the growing interdependence between countries on the use of genetic resources as the building blocks for sustainable agriculture. This led to the adoption of the International Treaty on Plant Genetic Resources for Food and Agriculture (ITPGRFA) in 2001 (Hunter and Heywood, 2011).

In the 1960s and early 1970s the focus of nutrition research was to understand the role of protein in the diet. Nutritionists were preoccupied with levels of protein intake and concerns about protein quality. This led to an emphasis on curative and clinically-based interventions aimed at increasing protein intakes. However, subsequent studies showed that protein intake had in fact been underestimated and that the recommended daily intake had been overestimated (McLaren, 1974). With the exposure of these misconceptions, nutrition research attention then shifted to energy or calorific intake and distributive concerns (UN, 1975). This change in focus was influenced by concerns in the agricultural sector about global food availability. Another nutrition paradigm also opened up during the 1970s; this was related to the central importance of micro-nutrients, and in particular, vitamin A (Latham, 2010). In the late 1980s and 1990s, this interest in micro-nutrients which emerged in the 1970s received a strong boost with additional evidence of the relationship between specific micro-nutrient deficiencies and increased morbidity and mortality. This led to the notion of "Hidden Hunger" (WHO/UNICEF, 1991). There was a strong focus on "do-able" technical fixes through micro-nutrient supplementation and food fortification programmes. During this period there was also increased engagement by the private sector in public nutrition interventions, e.g. increased commercial interests in the production of micro-nutrient supplements (Latham, 2010). Iron fortification and iodization programmes are examples of vertical nutrition interventions which, through collaboration with the private sector, and coupling accessibility of commercial markets with social marketing campaigns, have been successful at going to scale (Bryce et al., 2008).

In parallel with some of these clinical paradigm shifts was a rediscovery of the importance of different sectors for understanding and influencing nutritional health (Garrett and Natalicchio, 2011). The notion of multi-sectoral nutrition planning (MNP) emerged during the early 1970s to help build coordination, mostly between different national-level ministries, including health and agriculture (Joy and Payne, 1975). However, efforts to translate nutrition policies and strategies into operational plans, budgets and effective coordination across sectors encountered both bureaucratic and political difficulties. Each institutional sector with a stake in nutrition issues, e.g. agriculture, health, social welfare, gender, education, water, sanitation and environment, is housed in its own ministry or line organization. These all have their distinct professional approaches and particular organizational cultures. Food and nutrition have more often been separated with mandates under different line ministries. Action by multi-sectoral bodies can also be affected by asymmetric levels of representation or budget authority from each sector for decision making purposes. This compromises the ability to retain staff, and maintain institutional memory, which in turn compounds the challenge to sustain a continuous credible presence as nutrition problems reoccur. Therefore, despite the widely recognized theoretical benefits of system thinking for dealing with the "complex causality of nutrition", public organizations with already weak institutional capacity were overwhelmed by the data demands and coordination needs of multi-sectoral work (Field, 1987; Berg, 1987; Garrett and Natalicchio, 2011). Furthermore, the special units that were responsible for MNP were often institutionally isolated, embroiled in turf wars and under-funded. The 1980s saw a general abandonment of these programmes and a return to "nutrition isolationism".

Meanwhile, another element in the re-convergence of agricultural development and nutrition was occurring over a slightly later time period and at the level of civil society, rather than government. These were "food-based approaches" to nutritional health, which became more commonly discussed and implemented during the late 1970s and 1980s, although in relation to household gardens in particular this is a very ancient strategy for securing household nutritional health (Niñez, 1984; Ruel and Levin, 2002). Food-based approaches, by their nature, require labour and resource intensive efforts to influence behaviour at individual, community and agriculture and health systems levels. They do not have clearly defined biological pathways and are not conducive to vertical delivery strategies that have been successful for some fortification and supplementation interventions (Bhutta et al., 2008).

A more recent trend which also reflects cross-fertilization between sectors is the Right to Food framework (FAO, 2004; De Schutter, 2011a, 2011b), which is a latecomer to the rights-based approaches which came to the forefront in the 1990s. The Right to Food drew in issues of governance, and the need for a legal context to support not just the right to be fed, but the right to feed oneself. Grass-roots movements and networks around food sovereignty, such as La Via Campesina (Oxfam, 2011; Mulvany and Ensor, 2011), emphasized people-focused approaches based on local priorities. The call for strengthened food sovereignty reflects a decline in the self-reliance and dependence on local agricultural diversity and the shift towards increased reliance on external sources for food and/or monetary means to fulfil livelihood requirements.

Since the 1990s, there have also been renewed calls for food- (and life-style) based approaches to address the "double burden" of undernutrition and obesity (Popkin, 1999). The impacts of obesity and linked non-communicable diseases, such as diabetes and cardio-vascular disease, stretch across both developed and developing countries and socio-economic strata to the extent that over- and undernutrition can exist in the same communities. It is increasingly recognized that a diverse and balanced diet will ensure that we can benefit from the other functional elements in foods which have anti-oxidant, anti-cancer and other properties. There is also a return to an appreciation of the social and cultural role that food plays in urban and rural based lives. This has contributed to the growing movement to recognize, understand and value the agricultural biodiversity which has an essential role in sustaining our interlinked local and global food systems.

These shifting disciplinary paradigms have often formed the basis for the vision and mission of the different institutions which deal with nutrition and biodiversity, and in turn have influenced their organizational culture. Ironically, both nutrition and biodiversity are frequently seen as everyone's business but nobody's responsibility. Both nutrition and biodiversity conservation, including agricultural biodiversity, have struggled to find institutional homes, and these have varied according to the currently dominant paradigm or political whim. The uncertain and changing institutional arrangements for housing nutrition and biodiversity, and multi-sectoral coordination bodies, have influenced the capacity for strong technical leadership, continuity of coordination for cross-sectoral and inter-disciplinary partnerships, and contributed to limited financial and political support.

Agriculture, environment and nutrition are each part of changing processes that affect the needs and demands on each other (Hawkes, et al., 2007; Hoddinott, 2011, Pinstrup-Andersen, 2011). While there may have been sufficient convergence of concepts and approaches at some points, dietary diversity is declining, erosion of agricultural biodiversity is increasing and concerns about the sustainability of our agricultural and food systems remain. What are the chances for re-energizing cross-sectoral collaboration to change this scenario and how can the role of agricultural biodiversity be incorporated?

Cross-sectoral directions for the future: Agricultural biodiversity and dietary diversity

This chapter started with an example of an early plea for better cross-sectoral collaboration, yet that call is still echoed today, more than 75 years later. In early 2011, IFPRI's 2020 conference on leveraging agriculture for improving nutrition and health, reiterated calls for greater synergies and partnerships among relevant sectors, and underlined the need for a new paradigm for agricultural development to be driven by nutrition goals (IFPRI, 2011a). One of the achievements of the IFPRI 2020 conference was the participation of high profile keynote speakers to increase visibility for the need for the three sectors to work together. However, there was little detail on the "how" of enabling greater collaboration among these sectors (Fanzo, 2011). Von Braun and colleagues (Von Braun et al., 2011) have explored some of the challenges around bridging the gap between the agricultural and health sectors, and note that these are "researchable issues in themselves".

Learning from partnership research

New findings from research on partnerships can help make current and future cross-sectoral collaboration more effective. A recent review of the partnership literature found that there are few theoretically grounded case studies on partnerships in the context of research for development and there is not in fact a literature, but rather disparate literatures coming from different disciplines with little cross-disciplinary awareness or communication (Horton et al., 2009). This has resulted in the use of different terminologies (partnerships, inter-organizational collaboration, alliances, consortia, networks etc.) and widely different definitions, which can lead to confusion when organizations from different sectors are coming together.

Box 10.1 Definition of partnership in agricultural research for development

"Partnership is a sustained multi-organizational relationship with mutually agreed objectives and an exchange or sharing of resources or knowledge for the purpose of generating research outputs (new knowledge or technology) or fostering innovation (use of new ideas or technology) for practical ends."

Source: Horton et al. (2009)

The exploration of the different literatures led the authors to propose a common definition of partnerships (Box 10.1) which emphasizes key elements identified by many writers, such as: their multi-organizational nature; mutually agreed objectives and sharing of resources or knowledge; and linking research outputs with action. As briefly mentioned above, the multi-disciplinary nature of problems in the realms of nutrition and agricultural biodiversity, influenced earlier efforts to develop holistic and comprehensive approaches to address them. This was often in a context of lack of political ownership, and/or bureaucratic inflexibility. Previous attempts to establish cross-sectoral partnerships for nutrition improvement seem to have often been over-ambitious; to have experienced contradictory objectives among participating agencies and to have lacked the capacity to pool resources (Garrett et al., 2011). Thus, in order to re-energize these partnerships between agriculture and nutrition, there is a need for a robust dialogue to agree on a clearly defined problem which is beyond the scope of a single discipline or sector to solve, and to agree on common objectives around that specific problem.

Building consensus for a common goal will require that the agricultural and biodiversity sectors respond to nutrition priorities. However, it also requires that adopting nutrition goals must bring additional benefits to all stakeholders in the agriculture and biodiversity communities. Many commentators (Pelletier, 2011; Hawkes et al., 2007) have emphasized the need to strengthen the capacity for inter-disciplinary/trans-disciplinary approaches to support effective cross-sectoral collaboration for nutrition and agriculture. This requires the creation of an effective "space" for improved communication across disciplines in order to develop a common conceptual language, and agreement on adapting methods and tools which can work across disciplinary boundaries (Hawkes et al., 2007; IFPRI, 2011a).

It is also seen so often that it is individual champions from the different agriculture and nutrition spheres that have catalysed cross-sectoral collaboration. However, the sustainability of these individual initiatives depends on leadership styles and coordination skills for partnership processes. An appreciation is needed that in addressing the "partnership problematic" it is not only sought to influence the behaviour of others in relation to affecting nutrition outcomes, but there is also a need to change our own behaviour in the partnering process. The first requires a clear understanding of our impact pathway, that is, the boundary partners whose behaviour we are seeking to change, and the type of behaviour change we are seeking, which would lead to actions that would leverage the role of agricultural biodiversity for dietary quality. The second requires a combination of technical leadership skills (across realms of agriculture, environment and nutrition) to provide strategic direction; together with "facilitation leadership" to manage internal partnership processes. This second type of leadership is also related to organizational culture. Building on Maxwell's observations (Maxwell, 2001b), government ministries normally operate under a role culture, with clear hierarchical accountabilities and reporting structures. For inter-disciplinary work, a team-based task culture may be more effective, with leadership playing a more facilitating and enabling role rather than centralizing decision making.

Linking agriculture, nutrition and agricultural biodiversity draws in a larger group of stakeholders, with the risk of making cross-sectoral partnerships unwieldy and difficult to manage. Therefore, the process of the initial scoping and reaching agreement on common objectives and functions of the partnership should directly inform its stakeholder composition, structure (e.g. informal, formal) and governance norms. Collaboration for information sharing and advocacy on the contribution of agricultural biodiversity to improved dietary diversity may result in more flexible and inclusive partnership arrangements, while, on the other hand, collaboration, which demands the delivery of specific research or developmental outputs, will require clear definitions of roles, responsibilities, and agreement on mutual accountabilities. Some partnerships evolve from *ad hoc* informal arrangements to more formal arrangements. A partnership is dynamic and may go through different stages related to scoping and formation, implementation, reflection and transition or exit. Drawing from this to learn from earlier efforts at cross-sectoral partnerships, the deliberate use of a partnership cycle can be a way to assess whether the partnership's original objectives are still relevant; whether these objectives are being met; and whether there is a need to adapt the structure and composition of the partnership.

The study by Horton and colleagues also found that there are strikingly different drivers leading organizations to partner and that these differences have a profound influence on both the partnering processes and results. Drivers can be external, such as donor expectations; institutional, such as an organization's vision and mission; or individual, such as the career benefits that can be gained through involvement with other organizations. It is critical that the actors in a partnership identify the drivers and motivation for their own participation. The inter-disciplinary, and cross-sectoral nature of nutrition problems is not conducive to easy political action (Bryce et al., 2008), and arguably the same might be said for agricultural biodiversity. Experiences from the 1970s show how *ad hoc* political opportunism (as one type of external driver) was insufficient to turn theoretically favoured cross-sectoral collaboration between agriculture and nutrition into sustainable partnerships. Pelletier has argued for the importance of civil society to sustain pressure for accountability improved nutrition outcomes (Pelletier et al., 2011).

Pelletier has also noted that the existence of evidence-based information alone is insufficient for decision making. There is the need to integrate scientific evidence, contextual knowledge, and stakeholder values, interests, and beliefs. External drivers, top-down driven agenda and shifting donor interests will continue to influence cross-sectoral partnerships working for nutrition improvement. However, a systematic exploration of the political landscapes for nutrition and biodiversity can help to identify common areas of interest, potential overlap of political constituencies and opportunities for joint action. An understanding of the political economies for both nutrition and agricultural biodiversity can ensure that external influences are recognized, balanced with evidence-based priorities, and negotiated in a way to be more consistent and integrated with locally specific socio-economic conditions and context.

More recently, positive examples of practical cross-sectoral collaboration are emerging. The chapter now turns to briefly examine some case studies of national, multi-country and global cross-sectoral initiatives which could have a high relevance for the role agricultural biodiversity can play in improving dietary quality.

Synergies between agricultural biodiversity and dietary diversity: Emerging examples

At a country level, Brazil provides a window on what might be possible for effective cross-sectoral partnering to mobilize agricultural biodiversity for improved nutrition and food security. Brazil has designed and implemented several highly innovative multi-sectoral platforms and policy instruments

---

Box 10.2 The Zero Hunger Programme in Brazil

The Zero Hunger Programme was developed by the federal administration in Brazil as a public policy aimed at eradicating hunger and social exclusion. The programme is made up of a set of actions that are being gradually implemented by a cross-sectoral platform made up of the federal administration involving various ministries, other spheres of government (state and municipal administrations), and civil society in the following main areas: (1) implementation of public policies; (2) participatory development of a food and nutrition security policy and (3) self-help action against hunger. The Food and Nutrition Security Policy, which is a multi-sectoral policy, since it involves actions of different governmental sectors such as the health, education, labour, agriculture, and environment sectors among others, involves actions designed to foster the production, trade, quality control, access and use of food products. The National Food Security Council (CONSEA) plays a leading role in implementing this policy and both the PNAE (School Meals National Programme) and the PAA (Food Acquisition Programme) are members of this council.

Source: Grisa et al. (2011)

---

to enhance food security. Most of these fall under the "Fome Zero" or "Zero Hunger" programme launched in 2003 (Box 10.2) which has significantly reduced the number of undernourished people in the country (Grisa et al., 2011).

The PAA, or Food Acquisition Programme, has been one of the most important elements of "Fome Zero" and has had many important benefits including revitalization of local biodiversity and its consumption. The PAA was developed with the aim of ensuring that people facing food or nutritional insecurity have access to a regular supply of high quality food through social programmes such as the PNAE (the School Meals National Programme) and other programmes supplying food to hospitals etc. The PAA is stimulating a counter movement in Brazil by helping farmers to diversify their production using organic or agro-ecological approaches. The PAA purchases a diverse range of fruits, vegetables, processed goods and animal products from family farms and has also contributed to the revalorization and revival of many local products which have little or no commercial value in commodity markets. The programme also promotes the production and distribution of seeds of local varieties thereby supporting the conservation and management of agricultural biodiversity. Research undertaken in different regions of the country clearly demonstrates that farmers linked to the PAA programme are consuming more diverse diets and that schools receiving food from the PAA have significantly changed the composition and quality of meals they provide to students and that there are improvements in dietary diversity for children (Grisa et al., 2011 and case study in this volume). The contribution that the PAA may have made to the dramatic reduction in underweight, wasting and stunting is difficult to separate out from the overall Zero Hunger programme, and the general macro-economic improvements in growth and employment in Brazil. The prevalence of stunting among children less than five years old has reduced from 13.5 per cent in 1996 to 7.1 per cent in 2006–7 (Monteiro et al., 2010). Studies suggest that family purchasing power has increased and that socio-economic inequalities have been reduced (Acosta, 2011). Policy continuity, political leadership and coalition building, legislative coordination, decentralization, active civil society engagement and conditional and targeted funding have all been key factors in ensuring that nutrition issues are prioritized on the political agenda and addressed in a multi-sectoral way (Acosta, 2011; Silva et al., 2010).

However, in the Brazilian case there is also a growing disconnect between the on-going political discourse on undernutrition and the current nutritional epidemiological profile. This shows that the majority of Brazilian mothers and children are overweight and at risk of non-communicable diseases such as diabetes, cardio-vascular disease and some cancers (Bryce et al., 2008).

The United Nations Environment Programme (UNEP)/Food and Agriculture Organization (FAO) implemented Global Environment Facility (GEF) "Mainstreaming biodiversity conservation and sustainable use for improved human nutrition and well-being" project (Box 10.3), is a multi-country project (Brazil, Kenya, Sri Lanka and Turkey) starting in 2012. It will be an important vehicle for the implementation of the Convention on Biological Diversity (CBD) cross-cutting initiative on biodiversity for food and nutrition to integrate and mainstream awareness and understanding of the nutritional value of local agricultural biodiversity through cross-sectoral collaboration. The CBD cross-cutting initiative provides a global reference point within a legally binding convention, and also provides an overarching framework for the implementation of country projects.

At the global level, the Consultative Group on International Agricultural Research (CGIAR) reform process aims to develop improved research-for-development synergies with multiple actors and is prioritizing cross-sectoral collaboration. Within its new strategic results framework, the CGIAR has committed to making agriculture research accountable for improving human health and nutrition. While the new CGIAR Collaborative Research Programme "Agriculture for improved nutrition and health" (CRP4) (IFPRI, 2011b) is the main vehicle for achieving this, other CGIAR Research Programmes will also contribute to this goal (e.g. the commodity CRPs will also develop bio-fortified varieties). The CRP4 is explicitly trying to capitalize on the potential synergies across the agriculture, nutrition and health sectors and has two of four components (Value Chains for Enhanced Nutrition, and Integrated Agriculture, Nutrition and Health Programmes and Policies) where agricultural biodiversity has been accorded significant recognition.

The value chains for nutrition approach is based on the premise that improved coordination among actors involved in the chain will help to identify bottlenecks, negotiate trade-offs between nutrition and economic value and

Box 10.3 Mainstreaming biodiversity conservation and sustainable use for improved human nutrition and well-being (UNEP/FAO-GEF)

This multi-country Global Environment Facility (GEF) funded project will support sustainable biodiversity conservation and use for improved human nutrition and well-being by enabling planners and practitioners from agriculture, health and environment sectors to work together to mainstream agricultural biodiversity into nutrition, food, and livelihood security strategies and programmes at the national and global level. It will be led by Brazil, Kenya, Sri Lanka and Turkey and coordinated by Bioversity International, with implementation support from the United Nations Environment Programme (UNEP) and the Food and Agriculture Organization of the United Nations (FAO). Brazil, Kenya, Sri Lanka and Turkey contain unique agricultural biodiversity that is crucial to the world's food supply. However, in these countries, as in almost every country, the contribution agricultural biodiversity makes to local food security and nutrition, especially in poor rural communities, is undervalued resulting in lost opportunities to reduce hunger and malnutrition. The project will address these issues by undertaking assessments of the nutritional composition of prioritized biodiversity for food and nutrition as well as associated traditional knowledge, the development of national and global information systems and the establishment of new markets for biodiversity foods with high nutritional value. Mainstreaming biodiversity for food and nutrition will be supported by the development of cross-sectoral national policy platforms and other related promotional and scaling-up activities.

Source: www.b4fn.org , accessed 10 January 2013

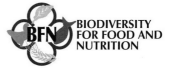

improve the efficiency of the chain (Hawkes and Ruel, 2011). The value chain can act as an organizing principle to bring different stakeholders together and provide an impact pathway linking agricultural production and nutritional change. Thus, it has the potential to harmonize "competing" paradigms of an agricultural production "supply-side" focus and the consumer "demand side". A value chain for nutrition partnership may contribute to addressing the nutrition and partnership problematic raised in earlier sections of this chapter. It provides a conceptual base to bridge the agriculture–nutrition divide; to bring public and private actors together; and the opportunity to scale out and scale up to achieve increased population and geographical coverage.

Box 10.4 Research for improved nutrition through agricultural biodiversity: the value chain approach of the CGIAR's CRP4

The research undertaken in this component will attempt to characterize and understand the role of markets and value chains in improving nutrition and dietary diversification both (1) directly, through an increase in the supply, marketing, access, and consumption/demand of nutritious foods sourced from biodiverse systems, and (2) indirectly, through an increase in income for smallholder famers. Likewise, smallholder farmers can diversify their diets and improve their nutritional status either by producing more biodiverse sourced foods directly or by accessing more nutritious and diverse foods in markets through a rise in their disposable incomes. There will be an emphasis on understanding what role nutritious local and traditional foods (LTFs) and neglected and underutilized species (NUS) play in creating demand for food products sourced from biodiverse landscapes by rural and periurban consumers and in boosting disposable incomes for smallholder farmers.

Source: IFPRI (2011b CRP4 Annex 6, p.83)

African leafy vegetables provide an example of a "value chain for nutrition" approach which has incorporated the promotion of agricultural biodiversity. Strengthening this value chain has involved a wide range of actions such as agronomic and nutrition studies to identify key constraints, seed dissemination, activities related to cultivation and conservation, and demand creation marketing strategies together with a range of actors including farmers, international organisations and local NGOs. These actions took place in a wider socio-economic context of increasing concerns about lifestyle and nutrition practices, and a changing awareness of the contribution that traditional and indigenous foods can make to better dietary diversity and quality (Weinberger and Pichop, 2009; IFPRI, 2011b; Case Study 3).[4] One of the areas of research under CRP4 will be to explore in more depth value chains for nutrition through agricultural biodiversity. The objectives of this are outlined in Box 10.4.

As mentioned earlier, in its overall partnership strategy, CRP4 identifies "value chain actors (and representatives)" as one type of partner. However, the configuration of these actors, their relationship to other types of actor, such as decision makers, development specialists (including health sector workers) or research partners and their utilization of agricultural biodiversity will vary according to the type of value chain. For example, among high-income consumers there is greater nutrition awareness of the contribution that dietary diversity can make to healthy lifestyles and thus increased demand for these products. This is being met through the commercial production and marketing of niche products (with promotion often based on biodiversity and health credentials) in select outlets. In contrast, there is the situation where underutilized species and traditional foods may be available at the local level through women's production and/or collection efforts and female mediated exchange networks and informal markets. In this scenario, there may still be some stigma attached to eating these "wild" or "famine foods", but women remain the custodians of knowledge about collection sites, safe preparation and preservation practices. These examples present different challenges for cross-sectoral collaboration for scaling up benefits to both the producers and the consumers.

The CRP4 proposal recognizes that effective, cross-sectoral partnerships will be central to successful implementation. It identifies four broad categories of partners: enablers (policy and decision-makers); development implementers (government and non-government); value-chain actors (and representatives); and research partners. The CRP4 intends to implement its partnership approach through the development of a partnership strategy at the beginning of the programme, which will include a stakeholder mapping and a landscape analysis of public health, agriculture, and nutrition research and development actors and opportunities.

While the CRP4 proposal does not discuss the earlier challenges in cross-sectoral work, IFPRI, as the lead organization for the CRP, has supported evaluations and case studies of earlier experiences and new efforts involving cross-sectoral partnerships (Benson, 2007; Garrett et al., 2011). The CRP4 offers the chance to build on these assessments to ensure that different disciplinary paradigms do not reinforce certain types of institutional arrangements, which in turn undermine efforts for cross-sectoral collaboration. The CRP4 should also actively institutionalize "new ways of working" such as encouraging inter-disciplinary and trans-disciplinary research-for-development approaches, through both incentive structures and capacity strengthening activities, which are already included as a strong component of the programme. Finally, as CRP4 becomes operational, it will hopefully ensure research space on the cross-sectoral partnering process itself.

In a post-conference statement on the way forward after IFPRI 2020, the authors questioned whether the global and regional institutions that play key roles in the governance of the agriculture, health and nutrition sectors might also need to be reformed for greater effectiveness and integration of efforts, greater openness and transparency. The statement highlighted the need to develop clear guidelines for stakeholder responsibilities (IFPRI, 2011a).

The UN is one of these global institutions, and the United Nations Standing Committee on Nutrition (UNSCN) was set up to act as a point of convergence and initiative in harmonizing nutrition policies and activities in response to nutritional needs of countries. The UNSCN has a mandate to promote cooperation among UN agencies and partner organizations in support of community, national, regional, and international efforts to end malnutrition in all of its forms. The UNSCN consists of UN agencies, "aid recipient" governments, multilaterals, bilateral donor agencies, the academic community, and civil society, all of which have divergent views. Within the UN itself, the mandate for nutrition is spread across several organizations and programmes including FAO, WFP, WHO and UNICEF. This has caused duplication, competition and created a lacuna in terms of effective coordination. One example of an effort to address this situation is Renewed Efforts Against Child Hunger (REACH), an interagency initiative between FAO, WFP, WHO and UNICEF to better align and coordinate nutrition actions at the country level. The initiative was piloted in 2008 in two countries and is currently operational in 13 countries to address malnutrition through a multi-sectoral lens. However, as Müller and Coitinho have argued, the UNSCN has gradually lost its capacity to perform its function to promote cooperation. They consider that part of the problem, and possibly its solution, rests in the UNSCN itself, and they argue that the current reform of the UNSCN will not only strengthen UN coordination in nutrition, but also promote a broader dialogue and partnership with other key stakeholders and constituencies (Müller and Coitinho, 2011). The UNSCN reform proposals have been hotly debated, reflecting in essence the differing paradigms as to how nutrition should be addressed, together with a concern that existing institutional mandates and governance structures should not be tampered with. The reform proposals included the following areas: the extent of true power-sharing among the UNSCN constituencies, and in particular the contentious role of "big food industry" influence in the UNSCN, the role of the UNSCN vis-à-vis harmonization to ensure scientific consensus on current issues or a more activist role in coordination; securing consistent core funding to ensure independence from donor-driven agendas; and the accountability and reporting relationship to the UN Chiefs' Executive Board (CEB). The Chair of the UNSCN has remained within the "4+1" (FAO, WFP, WHO, UNICEF, and World Bank), and it remains to be seen whether the reforms will result in a substantive change in the UNSCN's position and influence in global nutrition governance (UN Standing Committee on Nutrition, 2010; Longhurst, 2010).

However, currently, at the global level, it is the Scaling Up Nutrition (SUN) movement (Box 10.5) which has taken up the initiative to rally political attention and action to address the problem of undernutrition through cross-sectoral action. Many have argued that such a partnership can be the game changer, if mechanisms are put in place to hold partners accountable for delivering on their responsibilities effectively.

Discussion and conclusion

Currently there is renewed global political interest in addressing nutrition issues (e.g. SUN, IFPRI 2020 conference, REACH, the new CGIAR CRP4, and the CBD cross-cutting initiative). As pointed out in the introduction to this chapter, there has also been a growing convergence around the understanding that the current dominant model of agricultural production is not sustainable, and this presents an opportunity to re-evaluate the contribution that food-based approaches can make to improving dietary quality and diversity. While the evidence for food-based approaches (FAO, 1997; Low et al., 2007) and

> **Box 10.5** Global alliances to end malnutrition – the SUN initiative
>
> The Framework for Scaling-Up Nutrition (SUN) is a response to the continuing high levels of undernutrition in the world and the uneven progress towards Millennium Development Goal 1 to halve poverty and hunger by the year 2015. The SUN framework has been developed by specialists from governments, academia, research institutions, civil society, private companies, development agencies, UN organizations and the World Bank. It has been endorsed by more than 100 organizations and was unveiled in Washington in April 2010 at a meeting co-hosted by Canada, Japan, USAID and the World Bank. The SUN Framework's stakeholders intend that it be used within both industrialized, middle income, developing and least-developed countries whose people are affected by undernutrition. The Framework encourages a broad range of local and national level entities to work together in order to realize its different elements, and to do this by working within the context of an overarching national strategy for food, health and nutrition security. One of the elements of the SUN Framework is to promote broader multi-sectoral nutrition-sensitive approaches to development that acts to counter the determinants of undernutrition, including promoting agriculture and food insecurity to improve the availability, access to and consumption of nutritious foods.
>
> Source: http://www.scalingupnutrition.org/, accessed July 2012

the contribution that agricultural biodiversity can make to diets and dietary diversity is growing, there is a need for much further research (Penafiel et al., 2011; Termote et al., 2012). Moreover, there is a need to build an understanding on how to work with partners to scale food and agricultural biodiversity based approaches effectively.

It has been argued that the differing intellectual and ideological paradigms that shape thinking and action in particular disciplines and sectors has strongly influenced earlier efforts at cross-sectoral collaboration between agriculture, health and nutrition. In the renewed efforts to partner for improved nutrition outcomes, these differences will need to be addressed through capacity strengthening for inter-disciplinary approaches and in the institutional arrangements, structures and dynamics of cross-sectoral collaboration.

Finding examples of inter-disciplinary and cross-sectoral partnerships where biodiversity, agriculture and health sectors are collaborating to leverage agricultural biodiversity for dietary diversity has been a challenge. There is also a need for examples of partnership mechanisms which can take into consideration the need to have reinforcing actions across the local–national–global scales. There is a need to continue to document and disseminate examples of these practices.

This would help us to understand what types of stakeholders are involved and their interactions, what factors drive collaboration, and what methods and tools they are using to do this. Working in partnership can improve accountability to the individual partners involved. However, it can also complicate accountability, because of the diverse, and in some cases conflicting, interests and accountability requirements of the different partners. Therefore there is also a need to be able to assess whether investments in cross-sectoral partnership processes and performance are worthwhile and what their contribution is to the partnership, the objectives of the different individual partners and the value added to development goals (Horton et al., 2009).

Finally, we have also seen the political capital for nutrition and agricultural biodiversity vacillate. The fact that neither nutrition nor biodiversity are clearly linked with particular sectors has tended to make them less politically attractive rather than be supportive natural opportunities for cross-sectoral action. This is particularly so when, across the agriculture, environment and health sectors, nutrition problems are low on the list of political and financial priorities (Bryce et al., 2008). There needs to be an understanding of, if and where there might be a convergence of opportunity across the political landscape for both biodiversity and nutrition. Hotspots of agricultural biodiversity often overlap with nutritionally vulnerable populations, as for example in the Andes (De Haan, 2009). There is also growing political interest in strengthening the role that small-holder farmers play in maintaining biodiversity, and linking this more formally to climate adaptation and mitigation programmes, using carbon finance mechanisms (Padulosi et al., 2011). These are examples that could provide opportunities to select adaptive agricultural practices which promote the sustainable use of biodiversity and can also contribute to addressing priority nutrition problems.

Notes

1 A Southern Africa delicacy: *Gonimbrasia belina* is a species of moth found in much of Southern Africa, whose large edible caterpillar, the mopani or mopane worm, is an important source of protein. The availability of canned mopane worms epitomizes the struggle (and victory) to retain biodiversity, habitats, cultural values, and the use of technology to overcome seasonal shortages of the fresh product.

2 Inter-disciplinary collaboration involves the connection and integration of several academic schools of thought, professions, or technologies – along with their specific perspectives – in the pursuit of a common task.

3 Cross-sectoral collaboration is defined as the linking or sharing of information, resources, activities, and capabilities by organizations in two or more sectors to achieve jointly an outcome that could not be achieved by organizations in one sector separately. Available at: http://www.hhh.umn.edu/people/jmbryson/pdf/cross_sector_collaborations.pdf, accessed July 2012.

4 This can be compared with multi-sectoral collaboration where there is no integration among sectors and each sector retains its approach and assumptions without change or development from other sectors within the multi-sectoral collaboration. http://www.cgiarfund.org/cgiarfund/sites/cgiarfund.org/files/Documents/PDF/CRP4_%20Oct06%202011_Revised.pdf, accessed July 2012.

References

Acosta, A.M. (2011) Examining the political, institutional and governance aspects of delivering a national multi-sectoral response to reduce maternal and child malnutrition. *Analysing Nutrition Governance: Brazil Country Report*, Institute of Development Studies, http://www.ids.ac.uk/idsproject/analysing-nutrition-governance, accessed July 2012.

Benson, T. (2007) Cross-sectoral coordination failure: How significant a constraint in national efforts to tackle malnutrition in Africa? *Food and Nutrition Bulletin*, vol 28, no 2 (supplement), United Nations University.

Berg, A. (1987) Nutrition planning is alive and well, thank you, *Food Policy*, vol 12, no 4, November, pp.365–375.

Bernstein, H. (eds) (1973) *Under-development and Development*, Penguin Books, Harmonsworth.

Berry, V. and Petty, C. (1992) *The Nyasaland Survey Papers 1938–1939, Agriculture, Food and Health*, Academy Books, London.

Berti, Peter, R., Krasevec, J. and FitzGerald, S. (2004), A review of the effectiveness of agriculture interventions in improving nutrition outcomes, *Public Health Nutrition*, vol 7, pp.599–609.

Bhutta, Z.A., Tahmeed, A., Black, R.E., Cousens, S., Dewey, K., Giugliani, E., Haider, B.A., Kirkwood, B., Morris, S.S., Sachdev, H.P.S. and Shekar, M., for the Maternal and Child Undernutrition Study Group (2008) What works? Interventions for maternal and child undernutrition and survival, *Lancet*, vol 371, pp.417–440, doi: 10.1016/S0140-6736(07)61693-6.

Biggs, S.D. (1990) A multiple source of innovation model of agricultural research and technology promotion, *World Development*, vol 18, pp.1481–1499.

Blasbalg, T.L., Wispelwey, B. and Deckelbaum, R.J. (2011) Econutrition and utilization of food-based approaches for nutritional health, *Food and Nutrition Bulletin,* vol 32, pp.S4–S13.

Bryce, J., Continho, D., Darnton-Hill, I., Pelletier, D. and Pinstrup-Andersen, P. (2008) Maternal and child undernutrition: effective action at national level, *Lancet*, vol 371, no 9611, pp.510–526.

Carson, R. (2002) *Silent Spring*, Mariner Books, ISBN 0-618-24906-0 [1st published by Houghton Mifflin, 1962].

Chambers, R., Pacey, A. and Thrupp, L.A. (1989) *Farmer First: Farmer Innovation and Agricultural Research*, Intermediate Technology Publications.

Chambers, R., Scoones, I. and Thompson, J. (1994) *Beyond Farmer First: Rural People's Knowledge, Agricultural Research and Extension Practice*, Intermediate Technology Publications.

Collette, L., Hodgkin, T., Kassam, A., Kenmore, P., Lipper, L., Nolte, C., Stamoulis, K. and Steduto, P. (2011) *Save and Grow: A policy makers guide to sustainable intensification of smallholder crop production*, FAO.

DeClerck, F., Fanzo, J., Palm, C. and Remans, R. (2011) Ecological approaches to human nutrition, *Food and Nutrition Bulletin,* vol 32, pp.S41–S50.

De Haan, S. (2009) *Potato Diversity at Height: Multiple dimensions of farmer-driven in situ conservation in the Andes*, PhD thesis, Wageningen University, The Netherlands.

De Schutter, O. (2011a) *Agroecology and the Right to Food*, Report presented at the 16th Session of the United Nations Human Rights Council [A/HRC/16/49], 8 March 2011.

De Schutter, O. (2011b) *The right to an adequate diet: the agriculture–food–health nexus*, Report presented at the 19th Session of the United Nations Human Rights Council, 26 December 2011.

Fanzo, J. (2011) IFPRI's (2020) conference on leveraging agriculture for improving nutrition and health: keeping the momentum and translating ideas into action, doi 10.1007/s12571-011-0122-7.

FAO (1997) *Preventing Micronutrient Malnutrition: A guide to food based approaches, A manual for policy makers and programme planners*, FAO and International Life Sciences Institute, Washington.

FAO (2004) *Voluntary guidelines to support the progressive Realization of the Right to Adequate Food in the Context of National Food Security (the Right to Food Guidelines)*.

Farrington, J., Carney, D., Ashley, C. and Turton, C. (1999) Sustainable Livelihoods in Practice: Early applications of concepts in rural areas, *ODI – Natural Resource Perspectives*, vol. 42, p.13, AQ5.

Field, J.O. (1987) Multi-sectoral planning: a post-mortem, *Food Policy*, vol 12, no 1, February, pp.15–28.

Frison, E., Cherfas, J., and Hodgkin, T. (2011) Agricultural biodiversity is essential for a sustainable improvement in food and nutrition security, *Sustainability*, vol 3, pp.238–253.

Garrett, J. and Natalicchio, M. (eds) (2011) *Working Multi-sectorally in Nutrition, Principles, Practices and Case Studies*, International Food Policy Research Institute, Washington DC, USA

Garrett, J., Bassett, L. and Levinson, F.J. (2011) Multi-sectoral Approaches to Nutrition: Rationale and Historical Perspectives, in J. Garrett and M. Natalicchio (eds) *Working Multi-sectorally in Nutrition, Principles, Practices and Case Studies*, International Food Policy Research Institute, Washington DC.

Grisa, C., Schmitt, C.J., Mattei, L.F., Sérgio Maluf, O.R. and Pereira Leite, S. (2011) Brazil's PAA, Policy driven food systems, *Farming Matters*, 9/2011, 27.3.

Hawkes, C. and Ruel, M.T. (2011) Value chains for nutrition. Conference Brief 4. Leveraging Agriculture for Improving Nutrition and Health. New Delhi, India, 10–12 February 2011, http://2020conference.ifpri.info/publications/briefs/, accessed July 2012.

Hawkes, C., Ruel, M. and Babu, S. (2007) Agriculture and health: Overview, themes and moving forward, *Food and Nutrition Bulletin*, vol 28, no 2 (supplement), United Nations University.

Hoddinott, J. (2011) Agriculture, Health, and Nutrition: Toward conceptualizing the linkages, 2020 Conference Brief 2. Leveraging Agriculture for improving Nutrition and Health. New Delhi, India, 10–12 February 2011, http://2020conference.ifpri.info/publications/briefs/, accessed July 2012.

Horton, D., Prain, G. and Thiele, G. (2009) Perspectives on Partnership: A Literature Review, Working Paper 2009-3, International Potato Centre (CIP), Lima, Peru.

Hunter, D. and Heywood, V. (2011) *Crop Wild Relatives: A Manual of In Situ Conservation*, Earthscan.

FPRI (International Food Policy Research Institute) (2011a) Leveraging Agriculture for Improving Nutrition and Health: The Way Forward, Washington DC, http://2020conference.ifpri.info, accessed July 2012.

IFPRI (International Food Policy Research Institute) (2011b) CGIAR Research Programme 4 Agriculture for improved nutrition and health, Revised proposal submitted October 2011.

Jackson, L., Pascal, U. and Hodgkin, T. (2007) Utilizing and conserving agro-biodiversity in agricultural landscapes; *Agriculture, Ecosystems and Environment 121* (2007) 196–210. Elsevier. (doi:10.1016/j.agee.2006.12.017)

Johns, T., Smith, I.F. and Eyzaguirre, P.B. (2006) Understanding the links between agriculture and health for food, agriculture and the environment, Agrobiodiversity, Nutrition, and Health, IFPRI 2020 Vision, Focus 13, Brief 12.

Joy, L. and Payne, P. (1975) Food and Nutrition Planning, *Nutrition Consultants Reports Series*, no 35 ESN CRS/75/35 FAO, Rome.

Latham, M. (2010) Commentary: The Great Vitamin A Fiacso, World Nutrition, *Journal of the World Public Health Nutrition Association* vol 1, no 1, www.wphna.org, accessed July 2012.

Lipton, M. (1977) *Why poor people stay poor: Urban bias and world development*, Temple Smith and Harvard University Press.

Longhurst, R. (2010) Global Leadership for Nutrition: The UN's Standing Committee on Nutrition (SCN) and its Contributions, IDS Discussion Paper, Volume 2010 Number 390.

Low, J.W., Arimond, M., Osman, N., Cunguara, B., Zano, F. and Tschirley, D. (2007) A food-based approach introducing orange-fleshed sweet potatoes increased vitamin A intake and serum retinol concentrations in young children in rural Mozambique, *Journal of Nutrition,* vol 137, pp.1320–1327.

Maxwell, D. (2001a) The Evolution of Thinking about Food Security, in D. Deveraux and D. Maxwell (eds) *Food Security in Sub-Saharan Africa*, ITDG, London.

Maxwell, D. (2001b) Organisational Issues in Food Security Planning, in D. Deveraux and D. Maxwell (eds) *Food Security in Sub-Saharan Africa,* ITDG, London.

McLaren, D.S. (1974) The Great Protein Fiasco, *Lancet* 304 (7872) pp.93–96.

McNeely, J. and Scherr, S. (2003) *Eco-agriculture: Strategies to Feed the World and Save Wild Biodiversity*, Island Press, Washington DC.

Monteiro, C.A., D'Aquino Benicio, M.H., Conde, W.L., Konno, S., Lovadino, A.L., Barros, A.J.D. and Vitora, C.G. (2010) Narrowing socio-economic inequalities in child stunting: the Brazilian experience, 1974–2007, *Bulletin of the World Health Organization* 88:305-311, doi: 10.2471/BLT.09.069195.

Müller, A. and Coitinho, D.C. (2011) Commentary: Global nutrition: What should change? in David L. Pelletier (ed.) Mainstreaming Nutrition in National Policy Agendas: Successes, Challenges, and Emergent Opportunities, *Food and Nutrition Bulletin,* vol 32, no 2 (supplement).

Mulvany, P. and Ensor, J. (2011) Changing a dysfunctional food system: Towards ecological food provision in the framework of food sovereignty, *Food Chain* (2011), vol 1, no 1, pp.34–51.

Niñez, V.K. (1984) *Household gardens: theoretical considerations on an old survival strategy*, International Potato Center, Lima.

O'Riordan, T. and Stoll-Kleemann, S. (2002) *Biodiversity, Sustainability and Human Communities: Protecting Beyond the Protected*, Cambridge University Press, UK.

Oxfam (2011) *Growing a Better Future, Food justice in a resource-constrained world*, Oxfam International, www.oxfam.org/grow, accessed July 2012.

Padulosi, S., Heywood, V., Hunter, D. and Jarvis, A. (2011) Underutilized crops and climate change – current status and outlook, in S. Yadav, B. Redden, J.L. Hatfield and H. Lotze-Campen (eds) *Crop Adaptation to Climate Change*, Wiley-Blackwell, Ames, IA, pp.507–521.

Penafiel, A.D.D., Lachat, C., Espinel, R., Van Damme, P., Kolsteren, P. (2011) A systematic review on the contributions of edible plant and animal biodiversity to human diets, *Eco-health*, vol 8, no 3, pp.381–399.

Pelletier, D.L., Frongillo, E.A., Gervaise, S., Hoey, L., Menon, P., Ngo, T., Stoltzfus, R.J., Ahmed, A.M.S. and Ahmed, T. (2011) Nutrition agenda setting, policy formulation and implementation: lessons from the Mainstreaming Nutrition Initiative, *Health Policy and Planning 2011*, pp.1–13, doi:10.1093/healpol/czr011.

Pinstrup-Andersen, P. (2011) The food system and its interaction with human health and nutrition, IFPRI 2020 conference brief 13.

Popkin, B.M. (1999) Urbanization, lifestyle changes and the nutrition transition, *World Dev*, vol 27, pp.1905–1916.

Pretty, J. (1995) *Regenerating Agriculture*, Earthscan, London.

Quinn, V.J. (1994) Nutrition and National Development, An evaluation of nutrition planning in Malawi from 1936 to 1990, Thesis, Department of Human Nutrition, Wageningen Agricultural University, Wageningen, The Netherlands.

Rhoades, R.E. and Booth, R.H. (1982) Farmer back to farmer: a model for generating acceptable agricultural technology, *Agricultural Administration*, vol 11, pp.127–137.

Richards, A. (1939) *Land, Labour, and Diet in Northern Rhodesia: an economic study of the Bemba tribe*, Oxford University Press, Oxford.

Rist, G. (1997) *The history of development: from western origins to global faith*, Zed Books, London.

Rostow, W.W. (1960) *The Stages of Economic Growth: A Non-Communist Manifesto* Cambridge University Press.

Ruel, M.T. and Levin, C.E. (2002) Food-Based Approaches for Alleviating Micronutrient Malnutrition: An Overview, in Palit K. Kataki and Suresh Chandra Babu (eds) *Food Systems for improved human nutrition: linking agriculture, nutrition and productivity*, The Haworth Press, New York.

Scherr, S. and McNeely, J. (2007) Farming with Nature: The Science and Practice of Eco-agriculture.

Scoones, I., and Thompson, J. (2009) *Farmer First Revisited: Innovation for Agricultural Research and Development*, Intermediate Technology Publications.

Sen, A. (1981) *Poverty and Famines: An Essay on Entitlement and Deprivation*, Clarendon Press, Oxford.

Silva da, J. G, Grossi del, E. and Franca de, C.G. (2010) *The Fome Zero (Zero Hunger) Program: The Brazilian experience*, Ministry of Agrarian Development. Brasília, NEAD Special Series 13, FAO, ISBN 978-85-60548-82-8.

Termote, C., Bwama Meyi, M., Dhed'a Djailo, B., Huybregts, L., Lachat, C., Kolsteren, P. and Van Damme, P. (2012) A Biodiverse Rich Environment Does Not Contribute to a Better Diet: A Case Study from DR Congo, *PLoS ONE*, vol 7, no 1, e30533. doi:10.1371/journal.pone.0030533.

UN (1975) *Report of the World Food Conference, New York*, 5–16 November 1974, Rome.

UN Standing Committee on Nutrition (2010) Is it necessary to re-invent it? [Editorial] *World Nutrition*, June (2010) **1**, 2: 46–52, www.wphna.org, accessed July 2012.

Von Braun, J., Ruel, M. and Gillespie, S. (2011) Bridging the gap between agriculture and health sectors, IFPRI 2020 conference brief 14.

Weinberger and Pichop (2009) Marketing of African Indigenous Vegetables along Urban and Peri-Urban Supply chains in Sub-Saharan Africa, in *African Indigenous Vegetables in Urban Agriculture*, Earthscan.

WHO (2005) Ecosystems and Human Wellbeing – Health Synthesis, A report of the Millenium Ecosystem Assessment, Geneva.

WHO/UNICEF (1991) Proceedings: ending hidden hunger (A policy conference on micronutrient malnutrition), Montreal, Canada.

Part III

Case studies

Agricultural biodiversity and
food-based approaches to
improving nutrition

Case study 1

Traditional foods of the Pacific: Go Local, a case study in Pohnpei, Federated States of Micronesia

Lois Englberger and Eminher Johnson

Context and statement of the problem

Overall background

In recent years, throughout the Pacific Islands there has been an alarming shift towards consumption of low quality imported processed foods accompanied by a neglect of traditional food systems. This has led to serious health problems, food security risk and losses of agricultural biodiversity, traditional knowledge, customs and culture. Global and regional problems of climate change, population pressure, food and fuel price increases and unstable economic conditions exacerbate the Pacific's problems related to food imports and highlight the need to protect traditional food systems and agricultural biodiversity (Pacific Food Summit, 2010; Hezel, 2010; Coyne, 2000).

This case study focuses on Pohnpei, one of the four states of the Federated States of Micronesia (FSM), a nation of 607 islands (volcanic and atoll)[1] spread over a million square miles of water in the western Pacific Ocean. FSM's total population is ~107,000, including Pohnpei, the seat of the national capital, ~34,500; Chuuk 53,600; Yap 11,200 and Kosrae 7,700 (FSM, 2002) and includes many cultural identities. The nation was established in 1986, supported by a Compact of Free Association with the United States. Subsistence farming and fishing are the primary economic activities (CIA, 2011).

Pohnpei State, total land area 355 sq km (Englberger et al., 2009b), consists of the main island Pohnpei and five outer atoll island groups. The main island has a rugged mountainous terrain, year-round heavy rainfall, warm temperatures and rich tropical vegetation.

Dietary and life-style changes and related health problems

Pohnpei has remarkable plant diversity with 133 breadfruit varieties, 55 bananas, 171 yams, 24 giant swamp taros, nine tapiocas and many pandanus varieties documented (Adam et al., 2003; Raynor, 1991). The traditional diet was based on these crops, coconut, fish and seafood, and fresh fruits and sugar cane and pandanus as snacks. However, along with increasing modernization in the

1970s, there has been a neglect of traditional foods and a shift towards the consumption of unhealthy imported processed foods (Englberger et al., 2003d). The introduction of easily prepared, costly, imported processed western foods decreased the need of growing traditional healthy food.

White rice, in particular, has become a staple food, along with white flour. The consumption of sweet, salty and refined foods, as well as imported fats and fatty meats has also dramatically increased. Lifestyles have changed: physical activity has decreased, along with an increase in office jobs, shopping for food, and use of motorized vehicles, boats, and mechanized equipment. These dietary and lifestyle changes have led to serious problems of overweight and obesity, diabetes, heart disease, cancer, vitamin A deficiency (VAD) and anaemia (WHO, 2008; Englberger et al., 2003d, 2009b). Over 70 per cent of Pohnpei adults between 25 and 64 years of age are overweight (with 42.6 per cent obese) and 32.1 per cent have diabetes (WHO, 2008), causing increased health costs.

While few Pohnpeians reach the World Health Organization (WHO) criteria for severe vitamin A deficiency (WHO, 2009a),[2] over half of Pohnpei children between 24 and 48 months old in a population-based survey were identified as VAD, with low serum retinol levels ($< 20 \mu g/dl$) (Yamamura et al., 2004) and increased risk of contracting eye infections and other health conditions.

Why agricultural biodiversity was used as a solution

In 1998 efforts were initiated to identify local foods that could be promoted to alleviate problems associated with VAD deficiency. Local experts mentioned the rare Karat and other yellow-fleshed bananas. Analyses showed that Karat, a variety traditionally given to infants, is rich in beta-carotene, the most important of the provitamin A carotenoids, with amounts much higher than in common white-fleshed bananas (Englberger, 2001). Karat soon received international acclaim for its rich nutrient content (Coghlan, 2004; Kuhnlein, 2004), creating additional interest at home. Further studies showed that there are many varieties of yellow-fleshed banana, giant swamp taro, breadfruit and pandanus that are rich in beta-carotene and other carotenoids, nutrients and fibre (Table C1.1) (Newilah et al., 2008; Englberger et al., 2003a, b, c, 2006, 2008, 2009a; Kritchevsky, 1999; McLaren and Frigg, 2001; Coyne et al., 2005; WCRF/AICR, 2007).

Although familiar with many of these traditional crop varieties, Pohnpeians (and other Micronesians) were largely unaware of their inherent health benefits. As one Pohnpei farmer said, "If we farmers had known about the importance of the yellow-fleshed varieties, we would have planted more."

The study mainly focuses on terrestrial species, but marine agricultural biodiversity was also taken into account as it documented and promoted fish, seafood consumption, and the traditional animal protein of the islands. Consequently, both these types of agricultural biodiversity[3] were used as a solution to the problem of imported foods through the overall "Go Local" promotion of locally-available foods, from land and sea.

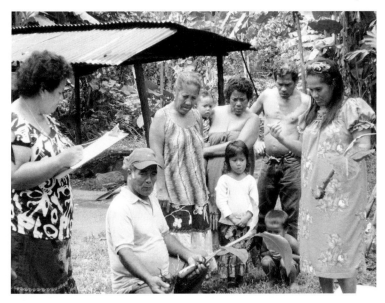

Figure C1.1 Traditional knowledge and skills are preserved in the community by collecting, sharing, and distributing different local varieties of banana. Photo credit: Chizuru Seki

Delivery mechanism to mobilize agricultural biodiversity

Our campaign used an inter-agency, ethnographic, participatory, and community-based approach in understanding the problems and addressing the solutions. This approach also increased stakeholder involvement. An important early activity was forming the Island Food Community of Pohnpei (IFCP) as a non-governmental organization to coordinate activities (IFCP, 2004).

Two slogans were all-important: the first, "Go Yellow", focused on the yellow-fleshed varieties, including Karat (Englberger, 2006; IFCP and Micronesian Seminar, 2006); the second, "Let's Go Local" was broader, promoting production and consumption of all local food. To strengthen the campaign, the "CHEEF" acronym was created to refer to the benefits of local food: culture, health, environment, economic and food security (Englberger et al., 2010c).

Many methods were used to mobilize agricultural biodiversity including: workshops; container garden demonstration plots; school visits; planting material distribution; planting, cooking and weight loss competitions; posters; youth clubs; breastfeeding clubs; billboards; mass media (newspaper, radio, television, video, emails, and the website www.islandfood.org); leaflets, newsletters and booklets; songs; recipes; national postal stamps of Karat, other yellow-fleshed bananas and other foods; postcards, telephone cards, t-shirts, pens and pencils; gene bank; and charcoal ovens (Englberger et al., 2009b, 2010b, c, d; Ormerod, 2006; Hanson, 2010).

In 2005, the IFCP joined a global project on traditional food systems and health, using specific guidelines (Kuhnlein et al., 2006) and led by the Centre

Table C1.1 Carotenoid content of selected Pohnpei, FSM traditional staple food cultivars compared to rice (*μg*/100 g edible portion)

Cultivar	Species	Flesh color[a]	β-carotene	α-carotene	β-crypto xanthin	β-carotene equivalents[b]	RE[c]	RAE[d]	Total Carotenoids[e]
Banana									
Utin Iap	*Musa spp*	Orange: 15	8508	na	na	8508	1418	709	na
Karat	*Musa spp*	Yellow/orange: 8	2230	455	30	2473	412	206	4320
Giant swamp taro									
Mwahng Tekatek Weitahta	*Cyrtosperma merkusii*	Yellow: 1	4486	na	na	4486	748	374	na
Mwahngin Wel	*Cyrtosperma merkusii*	Yellow: 4	2930	2040	120	4010	668	334	5630
Breadfruit									
Mei Kole	*Artocarpus mariannensis*	Yellow	868	142	na	939	132	78	na
Pandanus									
Luarmwe	*Pandanus tectorius*	Yellow	310	50	20	345	58	29	5200
Imported food									
Rice, white or brown	*Oryza sativa*	White	na	na	na	0	0	0	0

na – not analyzed

Notes: Analyses were conducted at different laboratories, see published papers. All used state-of-the art techniques, including high performance liquid chromatography (HPLC). Samples were as eaten: raw ripe (banana, pandanus); cooked ripe (breadfruit) and cooked as mature (taro). All samples were composite samples: 3-6 fruits or corms per sample, collected from Pohnpei State, Federated States of Micronesia. Data are from: Englberger et al. 2009a (pandanus), Englberger et al. 2008 (giant swamp taro), Englberger et al. 2006 (banana), Englberger et al. 2003a (breadfruit). Imported food: rice: Dignan et al. 2004. Imported rice has now become a common staple food in Pohnpei.

a Raw flesh color was described visually and estimated using the DSM Yolk Color Fan, numbers ranging from 1 to 15 for increasing coloration of yellow and orange.

b β-carotene equivalents: content of β-carotene plus half of α-carotene and β-cryptoxanthin.

c Retinol Equivalents (conversion factor 6:1 from β-carotene equivalents to RE). The estimated Recommended Dietary Intake (RDI) for a non-pregnant, non-lactating female is 500 μg RE/day and for a child 1-3 years old is 400 μg/day (FAO/WHO 2002).

d Retinol Activity Equivalents (conversion factor 12:1 from β-carotene equivalents to RAE)

e This includes estimates of identified and unidentified carotenoids levels.

for Indigenous Peoples' Nutrition and Environment (CINE). A target Pohnpei community in Mand,[4] Madolenihmw, was selected and a three-month documentation of the traditional food system and health problems was carried out, followed by a two-year intervention (Englberger et al., 2009b, 2010a). Much was learned in this project, which has contributed to our on-going work.

In developing the methods, the focus was on maximizing resources, capturing interest and increasing involvement. For example, posters hung up in public places could be seen for an extended period and media messages reached many people.

Evidence of impact of the intervention

There is substantial evidence of the intervention's impact. Karat was not sold at local markets prior to the discovery in 1998 of its rich nutrient content. Since 1999, Karat has appeared in the markets and its availability is steadily increasing. In 2006, Karat was sold in eight of 14 local markets (Parvanta et al., 2006). Currently, Karat is being sold and is available in all the local food markets and other food marts that also carry imported food.

Another Pohnpei case study as part of the CINE global health study showed that in the target community there were significant increases in banana and giant swamp taro consumption and dietary diversity, and an improved attitude towards local foods (Kaufer et al., 2010; Englberger et al., 2010a). It is notable that in 2009, two years after the intervention, a further assessment showed that the giant swamp taro consumption increase was sustained and imported foods consumption significantly decreased from the first assessment in 2005 (Bittenbender, 2010).

An increase in cooked local food take-outs is now seen (Naik, 2008), and local vendors report that their sales have been helped by the campaign. The daily available selection of cooked local foods includes: pounded banana, banana cream, pilolo, mashed giant swamp taro, fresh sashimi both reef and ocean fish, fried or sautéed reef fish/tuna, coconut cream clamps, tapioca, soft taro, yam in different recipes, coconuts, local cinnamon tea, etc. These locally cooked foods are mostly being sold on roadside in town and also in urban communities.

It is at present too early to report the extent to which these increases have impacted the consumption and utilization of local food.

Efforts for scaling up

Since the initial project in Mand Community started in 2005, the project has been taken to five further Pohnpei communities, including a Pohnpei atoll, and to communities in the other three FSM states (Johnson, 2010; Suda et al., 2010; Tara, 2010). There are now many more requests for the IFCP to speak about their work and approach to schools, communities and other groups.

Additionally interest in the "Go Local" approach has spread to other Pacific Island countries where "Go Local" workshops have been held (SPC LRD, 2008) and projects have been planned (WHO, 2009a). The approach has been presented

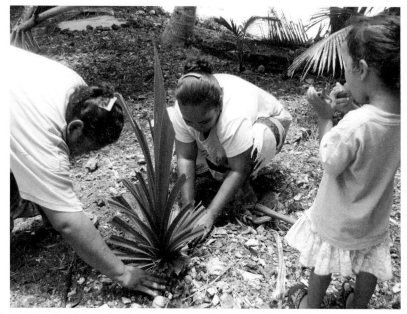

Figure C1.2 Pandanus planting to prevent soil erosion. Photo credit: Chizuru Seki

at many regional and international meetings (Pacific Food Summit, 2010) and the Food and Agriculture Organization (FAO) asked IFCP to prepare guidelines on how to implement a "Go Local" project so that the FSM experience could be taken to other Pacific Island countries (Englberger, 2011). In addition, our work identifying carotenoid-rich banana varieties has created interest in similar research elsewhere (Fungo et al., 2010; Amorim et al., 2009; Davey et al., 2009).

There are considerable barriers for scaling up: limited funding and resources, geographic dispersion, and different cultures and languages within the FSM and other Pacific Island cultures, but the movement is definitely spreading.

The FSM National Government approved two projects to be carried out in 2012 under the Resources and Development (R&D) Department: the Coconut Rehabilitation and FSM Food Security projects. During their meeting, which took place in 2011, the projects adopted the Island Food Let's "Go Local" approach inviting R&D experts to work on these projects along with other relevant partners.

Stakeholder involvement to ensure success

The IFCP was built upon an inter-agency approach with wide stakeholder involvement, involving governmental, non-governmental and private sector agencies along with community participation (IFCP, 2004). Intervention activities have involved wide participation from the agriculture, education and health sectors, as well as other groups. Such activities include farmers' workshops, classroom presentations, inter-agency meetings, information boxes and poster displays at local shops. Stakeholders are involved through an on-going awareness campaign to increase local food production and consumption at home, in the community, state, national and international functions, e.g. FAO's "Go Local" tool kit as guidelines to help in scaling up the non-communicable diseases (NCD) prevention strategies. They are also asked to become IFCP members, providing membership fees and strengthening ties and commitments.

Impact on relevant policies

Prior to the launching of the "Go Local" campaign, there was never any promotion on utilizing local food. After these local foods were analyzed and proved to be healthy, it boosted an initiative to raise this awareness that led to finding a slogan that can best describe the goal of this campaign.

The "Go Local" awareness has been heard and made a great impact on community, state and national policies. In 2010, Mand Community adopted a policy that bans serving soft drinks at community functions, followed by similar policies by the Pingelap People's Organization, and the Kolonia Kosrae Congregational Church.

In 2005, the Pohnpei State Governor proclaimed Karat as the Pohnpei State Banana (David, 2005) and in 2010, the FSM President proclaimed that the utilization of local foods is encouraged at all government events and festivities (Mori, 2010).

Key lessons learned

Repetition, colour, fun, many types of activities, using mass media but also face-to-face communication, and the community- and inter-agency approach with wide stakeholder involvement are all used. Research on the nutrient composition of foods and varietal differences is important in creating interest in local food crops and to expand data available on traditional knowledge and characterization of the food crops and varieties. As always, research is needed for project evaluation, for example, status on local food intake and planting of rare varieties. Social marketing tools, such as our IFCP Go Local t-shirts, pens and pencils, attract great interest and provide entry points for discussions.

A key lesson is that passion and dedication are needed, and that the message needs to reach the hearts of the people in order to start to change attitudes and behaviour by having champions in positions of influence.

Finally, it is important to continue to share the overall message, to "Go Local" for all of the "CHEEF" benefits of local food. This way agricultural biodiversity can be effectively used to improve health and nutrition.

Acknowledgements

Warm thanks are extended to all community, government and non-government agency partners and funding agencies and to Harriet V. Kuhnlein for reviewing the manuscript.

The photos (Figures C1.1 and C1.2) are from two ongoing projects in Pohnpei: "Pandanus planting for climate change adaptation" and "Food security and income generation for women". This tree crop produces nutrient-rich fruits; it can be planted close to the coastline to prevent erosion and leaves are used to handcraft mats, jewellery, baskets and purses.

Notes

1 An atoll is a ring-shaped low-lying coral island or group of islands, often consisting of only a narrow strip of land with seawater on both sides, circling a lagoon. Atoll island climates are considered among the harshest in the world due to the poor rainfall and poor soils.
2 Vitamin A deficiency increases vulnerability to infection and poor eye health and vision (McLaren and Frigg, 2001).
3 Agricultural biodiversity has been defined as "the variety and variability of animals, plants and micro-organisms that are used directly or indirectly for food and agriculture, including crops, livestock, forestry and fisheries" (FAO, 2004).
4 Mand Community is a rural community reached by a 40-minute drive on a paved road from the commercial centre of the main island Pohnpei.

References

Adam, I.E., Balick, M.J. and Lee, R.A. (2003) 'Useful plants of Pohnpei: A literature survey and database', New York, Institute of Economic Botany, New York Botanical Garden.

Amorim, E.P., Vilarinhos, A.D., Cohen, K.O., Amorim, V.B.O., dos Santos-Serejo, J.A., e Silva, S.O., Pestana, K.N., dos Santos, V.J., Paes, N.S., Monte, D.C., and dos Reis, R.V. (2009) 'Genetic diversity of carotenoid-rich bananas evaluated by Diversity Arrays Technology (DArT)', *Genetics and Molecular Biology*, vol 32, no 1, pp.96–103.

Bittenbender, A. (2010) 'Evaluation of the Mand Nutrition and Local Food Promotion Project: Pohnpei, Federated States of Micronesia', Internship Report Submitted to the Faculty of the Mel and Enid Zuckerman College of Public Health in Partial Fulfillment of the Requirements for the Degree of Masters of Public Health, University of Arizona.

Central Intelligence Agency (2011) *CIA Factbook*, www.cia.gov/library/publications/the-world-factbook/geos/fm.html, accessed January 20, 2011.

Coghlan, A. (2004) 'Orange banana to boost kids' eyes', *New Scientist*, www.newscientist.com/article/dn6120-orange-banana-to-boost-kids-eyes.html, accessed January 20, 2011.

Coyne, T. (2000) 'Lifestyle diseases in Pacific communities', Noumea, New Caledonia, Secretariat of the Pacific Community.

Coyne, T., Ibiebele, T.I., Baade, P.D., Dobson, A., McClintock, C., Dunn, S., Leonard, D. and Shaw, J. (2005) 'Diabetes mellitus and serum carotenoids: findings of a population-based study in Queensland, Australia', *American Journal of Clinical Nutrition*, vol 82, pp.685–693.

Davey, M.W., Van den Bergh, I., Markham, R., Swennen, R., Keulemans, J. (2009) 'Genetic variability in Musa fruit provitamin A carotenoids, lutein and mineral micronutrient contents', *Food Chemistry*, vol 115, pp.806–813.

David, J.P. (2005) Proclamation of World Food Day 2005: Karat as the Pohnpei State Banana. Office of the Governor, Pohnpei State Government, Kolonia, Pohnpei.

Dignan, C., Burlingame, B., Kumar, S., and Aalbersberg, W. (2004) *The Pacific Islands Food Composition Tables*, 2nd edn, Food and Agriculture Organization of the United Nations, Rome.

Englberger, L. (2001) 'Varieties of bananas and taro in Micronesia are found high in provitamin A carotenoids', *Proceedings of the First South East Asia and Pacific Regional Meeting on Carotenoids*, 2–5 August 2000, Bangkok, Thailand, Institute of Nutrition, Mahidol University in collaboration with the International Carotenoid Society, supported by the FAO Regional Office for Asia and the Pacific, pp.27–33.

Englberger, L. (2006) 'Going Yellow video promotes healthy food in Micronesia', *Sight and Life Newsletter* 1/2006, pp.31–33.

Englberger, L. (2011) *Let's Go Local. Guidelines for Promoting Pacific Island Food*, FAO, Rome, Italy. http://www.fao.org/docrep/015/an763e/an763e.pdf

Englberger, L., Aalbersberg, W., Ravi, P., Bonnin, E., Marks, G.C., Fitzgerald, M.H., and Elymore, J. (2003a) 'Further analyses on Micronesian banana, taro, breadfruit and other foods for provitamin A carotenoids and minerals', *Journal of Food Composition and Analysis*, vol 16, no 2, pp.219–236.

Englberger, L., Aalbersberg, W., Fitzgerald, M.H., Marks, G.C., and Chand, K. (2003b) 'Provitamin A carotenoid content of different cultivars of edible pandanus fruit tectorius', *Journal of Food Composition and Analysis*, vol 16, no 2, pp.237–247.

Englberger, L., Schierle, J., Marks, G.C., and Fitzgerald, M.H. (2003c) 'Micronesian banana, taro, and other foods: newly recognized sources of provitamin A and other carotenoids', *Journal of Food Composition and Analysis*, vol 16, no 1, pp.3–19.

Englberger, L., Marks, G.C., and Fitzgerald, M.H. (2003d) 'Insights on food and nutrition in the Federated States of Micronesia: a review of the literature', *Public Health Nutrition*, vol 6, no 1, pp.3–15.

Englberger, L., Schierle, J., Aalbersberg, W., Hofmann, P., Humphries, J., Huang, A., Lorens, A., Levendusky, A., Daniells, J., Marks, G.C., and Fitzgerald, M.H. (2006) 'Carotenoid and vitamin content of Karat and other Micronesian banana cultivars', *International Journal of Food Science and Nutrition*, vol 57, pp.399–418.

Englberger, L., Schierle, J., Kraemer, K., Aalbersberg, W., Dolodolotawake, U., Humphries, J., Graham, R., Reid, A.P., Lorens, A., Albert, K., Levendusky, A., Johnson, F., Paul, Y., and Sengebau, F. (2008) 'Carotenoid and mineral content of Micronesian giant swamp taro (Cyrtosperma) cultivars', *Journal of Food Composition and Analysis*, vol 21, pp.93–106.

Englberger, L., Schierle, J., Hoffman, P., Lorens, A., Albert, K., Levendusky, A., Paul, Y., Lickaneth, E., Elymore, A., Maddison, M., deBrum, I., Nemra, J., Alfred, J., Vander Velde, N., and Kraemer, K. (2009a) 'Carotenoid and vitamin content of Micronesian atoll foods: pandanus (*Pandanus tectorius*) and garlic pear (*Crataeva speciosa*) fruit', *Journal of Food Composition and Analysis*, vol 22, no 1, pp.1–8.

Englberger, L., Lorens, A., Levendusky, A., Pedrus, P., Albert, K., Hagilmai, W., Paul, Y., Nelber, D., Moses, P., Shaeffer, S., and Gallen, M. (2009b) 'Chapter 6: Documentation of the Traditional Food System of Pohnpei', pp.109–138. in: H.V. Kuhnlein, B. Erasmus and D. Spigelski (eds) *Indigenous Peoples' Food Systems: the Many Dimensions of Culture, Diversity and Environment for Nutrition and Health*, FAO, Rome.

Englberger, L., Kuhnlein, H.V., Lorens, A., Pedrus, P., Albert, K., Currie, J., Pretrick, M., Jim, R., and Kaufer, L. (2010a) 'Pohnpei, FSM case study in a global health project documents its local food resources and successfully promotes local food for health', *Pacific Health Dialog*, vol 16, no1, pp.121–128.

Englberger, L., Lorens, A., Pretrick, M., Spegal, R., and Falcam, I. (2010b) ' "Go Local" Island Food Network: Using email networking to promote island foods for their health, biodiversity, and other "CHEEF" benefits', *Pacific Health Dialog*, vol 16, no 1, pp.41–47.

Englberger, L., Joakim, A., Larsen, K., Lorens, A., and Yamada, L. (2010c) 'Go local in Micronesia: Promoting the "CHEEF" benefits of local foods', *Sight and Life Magazine* 1/2010, pp.40–44.

Englberger, L., Lorens, A., Pretrick, M., Raynor, B., Currie, J., Corsi, A., Kaufer, L., Naik, R.I., Spegal, R., and Kuhnlein, H.V. (2010d) Chapter 13: Approaches and Lessons Learned for Promoting Dietary Improvement in Pohnpei, Micronesia, in: B. Thompson and L. Amoroso (eds) *Combating Micronutrient Deficiencies: Food-based Approaches*, Food and Agriculture Organization of the United Nations.

FAO (2004) 'What is Agrobiodiversity Factsheet' developed from the Training Manual Building on Gender, Agrobiodiversity and Local Knowledge, Food and Agriculture Organization.

FSM Department of Economic Affairs (2002) *2000 Population and housing census report: National census report, Palikir*, Pohnpei, FSM National Government.

Fungo, R., Kikafunda, J.K., and Pillay, M. (2010) 'Beta-carotene, iron and zinc content in Papua New Guinea and East African Highland Bananas', *African Journal of Food, Agriculture and Nutrition Development*, vol 10, no 6, www.ajfand.net/Issue36/PDFs/Fungo5060.pdf, accessed February 1, 2010.

Hanson, M. (2010) 'New FSM Postal Stamps Promote Local Foods', *Kaselehlie Press*, vol 10, no 21, p.15.

Hezel, F.X. (2010) 'Disease in Micronesia: A historical survey', *Pacific Health Dialog*, vol 16, no 1, pp.11–25.

IFCP (2004) Articles of Incorporation of the Island Food Community of Pohnpei (IFCP), Pohnpei, Federated States of Micronesia.

IFCP and Micronesian Seminar (2006), Going Yellow (video), Kolonia, Pohnpei, FSM.

Johnson, E. (2010) 'Yap community of Ruu holds Go Local workshop', *Kaselehlie Press*, vol 10, no 15, p.15.

Johnson, E. (2011) 'Let's Go Local Spurs up Action at the Calvary Christian Academy', *Kaselehilia Press*, vol 11, no 9.

Kaufer, L., Englberger, L., Cue, R., Lorens, A., Albert, K., Pedrus, P., and Kuhnlein, H.V. (2010) 'Evaluation of a traditional food for health intervention in Pohnpei, Federated States of Micronesia', *Pacific Health Dialog*, vol 16, no 1, pp.61–73.

Kritchevsky, S.B. (1999) 'Beta-carotene, carotenoids and the prevention of coronary heart disease', *Journal of Nutrition*, vol 129, pp.5–8.

Kuhnlein, H.V. (2004) 'Karat, pulque and gac: three shining stars in the traditional food galaxy', *Nutrition Reviews*, vol 62, pp.439–442.

Kuhnlein, H.V., Smitasiri, S., Yesudas, S., Bhattacharjee, L., Li Dan, Ahmed, S. and collaborators (2006) *Documenting Traditional Food Systems for Indigenous Peoples: International Studies*. Guidelines for Procedures. Centre for Indigenous Peoples' Nutrition and Environment, McGill University, Canada http://www.mcgill.ca/cine/research/global/ (accessed 29 October 2012)

McLaren, D.S., and Frigg, M. (2001) *Sight and Life Manual on Vitamin A Deficiency Disorders (VADD)*, 2nd edn, Basel, Task Force Sight and Life.

Mori, M. (2010) Proclamation to encourage awareness on food security issue in the Federated States of Micronesia. Office of the President, Pohnpei, Federated States of Micronesia.

Naik, R.I. (2008) An Assessment of Local Food Production in Pohnpei, Federated States of Micronesia. B.S. Thesis, University of California, Santa Barbara.

Newilah, G.N., Lusty, C., Van den Bergh, I., Akyeampong, E., Davey, M., and Tomekpe, K. (2008) 'Evaluating bananas and plantains grown in Cameroon as a potential source of carotenoids', *Food*, vol 2, no 2, pp.135–138.

Ormerod, A. (2006) 'The case of the yellow bananas', *Eden Project Friends*, vol 23, pp.6–7.

Pacific Food Summit (2010) Framework for Action on Food Security in the Pacific, A framework agreed by participants at the Pacific Food Summit, April 21–23, 2010, www.foodsecurepacific.org, accessed February 2011.

Parvanta, A., Englberger, L., Lorens, A., and Yamada, L. (2006) *Report on a Banana Volume Market Study and Health/Awareness Campaign*, Island Food Community of Pohnpei, Kolonia, Pohnpei.

Raynor, B. (1991) 'Agroforestry Systems in Pohnpei – Practices and Strategies for Development: RAS/86/036 Field Document 4', FAO/UNDP South Pacific Forestry Development Programme.

SPC LRD News (2008) 'Go Local: Working to improve the nutritional security of Solomon Islands and PNG local communities', Secretariat of the Pacific Community (SPC) Land Resources Division (LRD), *News*, vol 4, no 3, p.22.

Suda, E., Ragus, L., and Englberger, L. (2010) 'Go Local Project is Initiated in Chuuk as a Collaborative Effort', *Kaselehlie Press*, vol 10, no 14, p.15.

Tara, M. (2010) 'Kosrae holds Go Local agroforestry and health workshop', *Kaselehlie Press*, March 31, vol 10, no 9, p.15.

World Cancer Research Fund (WCRF)/American Institute for Cancer Research (AICR) (2007) *Food, Nutrition, Physical Activity and the Prevention of Cancer: A Global Perspective*, AICR, Washington DC.

WHO (2008) 'Federated States of Micronesia (Pohnpei) NCD risk factors STEPS report', Suva, WHO Western Pacific Region.

WHO (2009a) 'Global prevalence of vitamin A deficiency in populations at risk 1995–2005. WHO Global Database on Vitamin A Deficiency', Geneva, World Health Organization, whqlibdoc.who.int/publications/2009/9789241598019_eng.pdf, accessed January 31, 2011.

WHO (2009b) 'Nutrition, Diet and Lifestyle: Scaling up action in the Pacific', Summary report of regional meeting, Tanoa International Hotel, Nadi, Fiji, 23–27 February 2009.

Yamamura, C., Sullivan, K.M., van der Haar, F., Auerbach, S.B. and Iohp, K.K. (2004) 'Risk factors for vitamin A deficiency among preschool aged children in Pohnpei, Federated States of Micronesia', *Journal of Tropical Pediatrics*, vol 50, no 1, pp.16–19.

Case study 2

The role of integrated home gardens and local, neglected and underutilized plant species in food security in Nepal and meeting the Millennium Development Goal 1 (MDG)

Roshan Pudasaini, Sajal Sthapit, Rojee Suwal and Bhuwon Sthapit

Introduction

Agriculture is the main source of livelihood in Nepal for nearly 76 per cent of the people (CBS, 2001), and is largely subsistence-oriented. With large variations in agro-ecological conditions and socio-cultural circumstances, a great diversity of farming systems exists. Farmers are predominantly smallholders owning on average less than one hectare of cultivated land. The land is usually of low productivity and has to support large families. Consequently, many households face food shortage in most years (Food Security Monitoring Task Force, 2010).

Low food intake, together with infections and diseases are the immediate causes of malnutrition (UNICEF, 1990). However, eating adequate calories does not ensure that sufficient micronutrients are consumed in order to keep the body healthy.

A survey on food consumption in Nepal carried out in 1970 shows that 83 per cent of the total calories consumed was from cereals, mainly rice, wheat and maize. The intake of pulses, vegetables, fruits and animal products was very low (Krishna, 2004:47). The consumption of such nutritious food is limited because of high and rising commodity prices (SEWA, 2009).

Nutritious food is difficult to find in the poorer rural areas where most people are dependent on staple foods with little diversity (Krishna, 2004; Johns and Sthapit, 2004; Talukder et al., 2004). It is especially a challenge in the far western and mid-western mountains of Nepal, where the hunger index is categorized as extremely alarming (Food Monitoring Task Force, 2010). Hunger in these areas is mostly caused by undernourishment (WFP, 2009). Geographic remoteness, education levels and poor economic conditions are the main obstacles that limit access to nutritious food among these families (Talukder et al., 2004). Furthermore, there are gender-based inequalities in the access to food. Distribution of food in the household is often uneven and women usually eat last in 70 per cent of the households. Protein energy malnutrition (PEM), iodine deficiency disorders (IDD), vitamin A deficiency (VAD), and iron deficiency anaemia (IDA) are the common forms of malnutrition experienced by women. Nearly three-quarters of all women are anaemic, and prevalence is especially high among pregnant women. Nepal is one of few countries where the life expectancy rate of women is lower than that of men especially in poor rural areas. As young and able men are forced to migrate in search of opportunities outside their villages, women are left to do more agricultural work in rural areas (Food Security Monitoring Task Force, 2010). These factors of inequalities in health and nutrition are also valid for other excluded groups based on caste and class (FIAN, 2011).

Poor nutrition status of women impacts on the health and well-being of their children, too. Not surprisingly, children also exhibit high malnutrition rates in Western Nepal. Almost 50 per cent of children under five years of age are stunted and nearly 40 per cent are underweight (Food Security Monitoring Task Force, 2010). Undernutrition at this stage of life can have long-term implications continuing through adulthood. Poor nutrition in pre-school days can significantly reduce cognitive capacity and consequently human, social and economic potential in later lives of these children (Ruel and Hoddinott, 2008).

Role of home gardens

Home gardening is a traditional land use practice carried out around a homestead consisting of several species of plants that are grown and maintained by the family members with the primary objective of fulfilling the family's consumption needs (Abdoellah et al., 2002; Eyzaguirre and Linares, 2004; Shrestha et al., 2004; Gautam et al., 2004). Home gardening is one of the key components of the Nepalese farming system with over 70 per cent of households maintaining home gardens at varying scales, ranging from 2 to 11 per cent of the family's landholding (Gautam et al., 2004; Sunwar et al., 2006; Gautam et al., 2008). The size of individual home gardens in Nepal is so small that the impact of production is deemed insufficient in commercial terms to receive priority from government and donors.

Despite their size, if production is diversified with more species and managed well, home gardens can increase dietary diversity (Trinh et al., 2003) and help address household malnutrition. By promoting increased consumption of the available diversity, nutrition of farming families can be improved (Johns and Sthapit, 2004; Shrestha et al., 2002, 2004a; Sthapit et al., 2004a). As home gardens are predominantly managed by women, they can also play an important role in ensuring proper diets of women and children, especially in rural areas (Suwal et al., 2008). Hence, the real value of home gardens is in ensuring proper health of women and children first and foremost, who can then have more fulfilling lives to contribute as productive citizens.

In addition to the family's food needs, home gardens also augment household income, especially for women, from the sale of surplus produce. Even with small cash incomes, women in villages can exercise greater economic agency in controlling small family expense. Women also tend to spend money differently

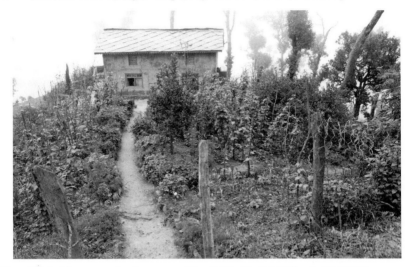

Figure C2.1 A home garden in western Nepal. Credit: Sajal Sthapit, LI-BIRD

than men by giving prioiry to food, healthcare and education for their children (Meinzen-Dick et al., 2011).

Home gardens also make the homestead aesthetically pleasing and help maintain species of ethnic, cultural and religious importance (Soemarowoto, 1987; Abdoellah et al., 2002; Trinh et al., 2003; Sthapit et al., 2008). In Nepal, the home gardens involve the management of multipurpose trees, shrubs, annual and perennial vegetables and fruits, spices, herbs and medicinal plants, birds and animals on the same land units in a spatial or temporal sequence (Shrestha et al., 2002; Gautam et al., 2004; Suwal et al., 2005). Traditionally people supplement food from wild and uncultivated crops besides cultivated species in gardens and arable farming systems (Daniggelis, 2003). Many neglected and underutilized species, from a research perspective, are appreciated by local populations and food culture for their taste and nutritional value (Sthapit et al., 2008; Johns and Sthapit, 2004). The home garden therefore provides a bridge between the social and the biological, linking cultivated spaces and natural ecosystems, combining and conserving species diversity and cultural diversity.

The project on home gardens was initiated to understand the scientific basis of management of agricultural biodiversity in home garden ecosystems; Phase I (2002–2004). Phase II (2006–2008) concentrated on the enhancement of family nutrition and income of resource poor and disadvantaged groups of farmers and Phase III (2009–2013) aimed to mainstream home gardens in an inclusive development programme of the country (Table C2.1). Figure C2.3 shows the distribution of case study sites in Nepal during Phases II and III.

Some level of awareness activities on the relationships between nutrition, health, dietary diversity and biodiversity are important for the communities. Organizing existing women's groups for collective action on these activities can be effective.

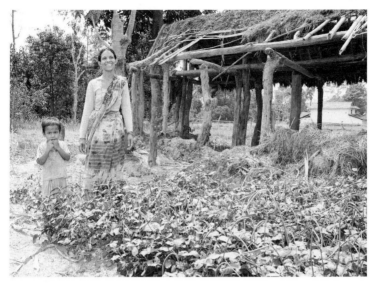

Figure C2.2 A farmer and her daughter in their home garden in Rupandehi, Nepal. Credit: Sajal Sthapit, LI-BIRD

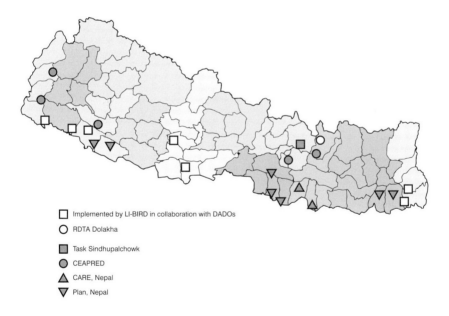

Figure C2.3 Map of the project sites of home gardens in Nepal implemented through partnership of a range of government and NGO partners

Table C2.1 Main objectives, partners involved and survey sites included in Phases I, II and III of the Home garden project in Nepal

Title	Major Objective	Foci	Name partners involved	Number of sites and target Households (HH)
Phase I Enhancing contribution of home gardens to on-farm management of plant genetic resources and improve livelihood of Nepalese farmers (2002–2004)	Understand and document the dynamics (historical perspective, structure, composition, utilization and underlying indigenous knowledge systems) of home gardens	Understanding the dynamics (structure, size, composition and use) of home garden Measuring the potential of home gardens to contribute in livelihood enhancement of resource poor Developing technologies, approaches and methods for a sustainable on-farm management of plant genetic resources for improving food security, nutrition and income of resource poor farmers	Bioversity International implemented by Local Initiatives of Biodiversity, Research and Development (LI-BIRD) in partnership with Nepal Agricultural Research Council (NARC),Department of Agriculture (DoA) and Helen Keller International (HKI)	Jhapa (Gauriganj-5 community; 355 HH) Ilam (Panchkanya 4–6 community: 366 HH) Rupandehi (Dudrakshya1, 8 community; 634 HH) Gulmi (Durbardevisthan 2, 3 and 5 communities; 800 HH)
Phase II Enhancing Family Nutrition and Income for improved livelihoods of Resource Poor and Disadvantaged Groups through Integrated Home Gardens in Nepal (2006–2008)	Improvement of nutrition and income of poor and disadvantaged families through promotion of integrated home gardens	Experiences and good practices of integrated home garden from first phase scaled up to a wider geographic region Enhanced capacity of disadvantaged groups to increase access to livelihood assets, decision making and benefits from collective action Improving access of poor to quality diets	Local Initiatives of Biodiversity, Research and Development (LI-BIRD) directly implanted in partnership with Nepal Agricultural Research Council (NARC), Department of Agriculture (DoA), SDC funded projects (TUKI, CEPREAD) and Bioversity International and HKI technical backstopping.	Experiences and good practices of integrated home garden approach of the first phase (2002–2005) of the project were scaled out in 12 districts extended from eastern to far-western regions of Nepal through different partners. Ilam (5 communities; 801 HH) Jhapa (3 communities; 465 HH) Gulmi (5 communities; 660 HH) Rupendehi (3 communities; 426 HH) Bardiya (2 communities; 344 HH) Kailali (1 community; 120 HH) Kanchanpur (1 community; 146 HH) Dolkha (5 communities; 421 HH) Sindhulpalchowk (4 communities; 357 HH)

Phase III Linking Home garden in inclusive development programme for contributing to securing livelihoods of resource poor and disadvantaged groups of Nepal (2009-2013)	Supportive institution and policy environment development for mainstreaming of home garden promotion concept	Mainstreaming home garden into national agriculture development programme Encouraging local government and local service providers to support and adopt home garden into their livelihood enhancement programmes	Local Initiatives of Biodiversity, Research and Development (LI-BIRD) directly implanted in partnership with Nepal Agricultural Research Council (NARC), Department of Agriculture (DoA), SDC funded projects (TUKI, CEPREAD) and Bioversity International and HKI technical backstopping.	Ilam (7 communities; 1031 HH) Jhapa (6 communities; 1174 HH) Gulmi (8 communities; 978 HH) Rupendehi (5 communities; 608 HH) Bardiya (4 communities; 555 HH) Kailali (3 communities; 324 HH) Kanchanpur (3 communities; 280 HH) Dolkha (3 communities; 700 HH) Sindhulpalchowk (6 communities; 557 HH) Ramechhap (2 communities; 245 HH) Okhaldhunga (2 communities; 219 HH) Kabhrepalanchok; 2 communities 100 HH Surkhet; 1 community 50 HH Baitadi; 2 communities 100 HH) Dadeldhura; 3 communities 150 HH)

Increasing diversity using home garden diversity kits

Diversity kits include small quantities of seeds or saplings of different kinds made available to farmers to complement the available resources (seeds and saplings of vegetables, fruits, fodder and other home garden species) (Sthapit et al., 2006). Analysis of the nutritional gap, demand of farmers, agro-ecology and farmers' capacity are the basis for determining the composition of diversity kits for home gardens. The composition of diversity is a mixture of local and underutilized crops species both perennial and annual that are not easily available from commercial seed companies.

Specific foods are required for use in traditional ceremonies and rituals in Nepal. As a result, social customs require Nepalese farmers to maintain a wide variety of fruits and plants in their home gardens for use at festivals. Celebration and commercialization of local festivals also create local demand for unique species grown in home gardens. For example, during Maghesankranti (January/February), the demand for and hence the price of root crops such as yams, sweet potatoes and taros climb steeply. Likewise, a wide range of citrus fruits, especially pommello and pseudo lemon are necessary for the celebration of the Diwali and Chhath festivals. Promoting diversity kits that include crops of cultural importance is often ignored, but can play a big role in maintaining home garden diversity.

Technology transfer for low-cost home garden management

One of the basic tenets for successful home gardening for the rural smallholders is to make it as cost effective as possible. Therefore external inputs (fertilizers, seeds and other chemical and physical materials) are not promoted. Instead, focus is placed on locally available seeds, compost, farmyard manure and local production technologies to ensure secure access to production inputs as well as safe and healthy food for family well-being.

Kitchen waste, water management, multi-layer cropping, combination of perennial and annual crops, local bio-pesticide, vermi compost and sack farming in flood-prone areas are some proven techniques used in low-cost home garden management. A year-round refresher training at the local resource centre, cross-site exchange visits and travelling seminars are a few mechanisms employed for transferring skills and promoting local innovations.

Establishing resource home gardens as knowledge sharing and exchange centres

Although home gardens are very common, only a small proportion are managed efficiently to get the maximum output for their size. Those gardens which are producing diverse food products throughout the year and are well managed can be utilized as demonstration sites. The owners of such home gardens are identified and developed as resource home gardeners to provide management and material inputs to other home gardeners. The owners of such home gardens are role models in the area for other farmers to aspire to.

They can train other fellow farmers and also act as local sources for seeds/ saplings and knowledge.

A home garden alone cannot address all the livelihood requirements of a family. Due to its diversity and with the guidance of a proper nutritional calendar, home gardens contribute to the quality of food consumption (safe, nutritious and preferred), especially in terms of fulfilling the micronutrient requirements of the family. However, due to their small size, fulfilling the required quantity of food security might be beyond the scope of many home gardens (Gautam et al., 2008). Therefore, other programmes and projects that are related to the livelihood of those particular farmers should be implemented collaboratively to increase impact. Major demand of staple food and income generation in higher degree should be addressed by such particular projects and home garden production will complement them by providing diversified food and nutrition, and supplementary income. Home gardens would be the ideal entry point for developing the confidence of poor and marginal farming communities.

Food-based approach to better nutrition

The success of home gardens has been measured as an increase in diversity. However, from a nutritional perspective, it is important to look at whether the diversity is increasing in functional categories (DeClerck et al., 2011). The home garden project in Nepal examined how increases in biodiversity correlates with increased functional and nutritional diversity.

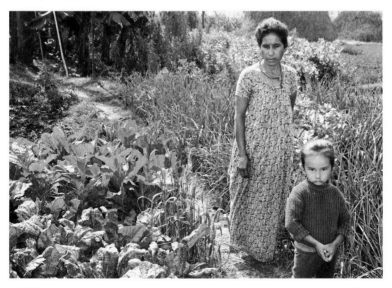

Figure C2.4 A resource home gardener and her son in their home garden in Rupandehi, Nepal. Credit: Sajal Sthapit, LI-BIRD

Mean home garden (household) species richness increased in 10 out of 11 sites between 2006 and 2011 (Table C2.2).

Food culture and cooking traditions play important roles in the availability of nutrients in food (Englberger et al., 2010; Rijal, 2010). Bioavailability of nutrients also depends on how the food is prepared, what other foods it is consumed with and the health status of the person eating it. The approach used in this study did not address the different levels of bioavailability of the nutrients and this limitation is acknowledged.

Table C2.2 Mean household (HH) species richness of edible and all species found in home gardens in 2006 and 2011

Site	Altitude (metres above sea level)	Mean HH edible species richness (range)		Mean HH species richness (range)	
		2006	2011	2006	2011
Eastern Hills					
Ilam district					
Chulachu VDC	173	20 (1–36)	27 (13–50)	27 (3–50)	34 (15–72)
Gorkhe VDC	1717	17 (3–31)	24 (14–43)	24 (3–42)	35 (21–66)
Sumbek VDC	1413	17 (8–29)	25 (1–37)	18 (9–30)	35 (6–60)
Eastern Terai					
Jhapa district					
Chakchaki VDC	95	9 (2–21)	14 (2–33)	13 (3–11)	19 (2–58)
Duwagadhi	116	18 (5–39)	25 (8–59)	21 (5–49)	36 (12–97)
Western Hills					
Gulmi district					
Amarpur VDC	1180	6 (2–11)	21 (9–48)	no records	27 (10–63)
Hardineta VDC	1132	6 (1–13)	17 (7–46)	no records	24 (7–64)
Western Terai					
Kailali district					
Godawari VDC	679	13 (2–24)	13 (4–40)	no records	14 (4–54)
Rupandehi district					
Khadawa Bangain VDC	120	10 (5–20)	20 (1–45)	no records	24 (4–60)
Siktahan VDC	115	4 (1–8)	23 (13–37)	no records	30 (15–55)
Bardia district					
Taratal VDC	167	3 (1–7)	18 (8–31)	No records	22 (8–38)

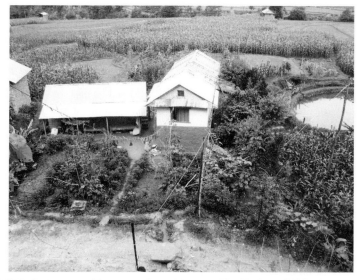

Figure C2.5 An integrated home garden with vegetables fruits and fisheries extended to crops. Credit: Mahesh Shrestha, LI-BIRD

However, by promoting a greater range of diversity, with foods that are prepared and consumed in a variety of ways, better nutrition can be achieved (Frison et al., 2011; Fanzo and Pronyk, 2011). Increasing awareness of the importance of nutritious diets and providing access to safe fruit and vegetables will be needed to attain the long-term outcome of diet diversification: to have a healthy, balanced diet fulfilling the recommended per capita consumption rate of 400 g of fruit and vegetables per day (Keatinge et al., 2010).

Species available before (2006) and after (2011) the implementation of the home garden project were categorized depending on nutrients provided (such as proteins, iron, folate, vitamin A, etc.). For each nutrient category, the number of species providing the nutrient were counted to determine the increase in number of choices for each nutrient.

Along with an increase in household species richness (Table C2.2), the number of species contributing sources of nutrients were found to also increase for all nutrients and all seasons considered.

Hence, it was found that in this project "Enhancing family nutrition and income for improved livelihoods of resource poor and disadvantaged groups through integrated home gardens in Nepal" (see Table C2.1), increasing species richness of home gardens also increased the sources of nutrients available to households.

Scaling up

The Nepal Agricultural Research Council (NARC) has identified the home garden as a research area for targeting poor and marginal farmers (NARC strategic planning meeting, 2005). This is an important change because historically home gardens were ignored by research in Nepal. There is a great need to involve stakeholders from health sectors to use home gardens as a food-based approach to nutrition that can complement dietary supplements. Therefore, a partnership between the agro-biodiversity, agriculture and food, health and environment sectors needs to be cultivated at the national and local levels.

One of the great achievements of the second phase of the home garden project is the acceptance by the government's planning commission to apply the concept all over the country. The Ministry of Agriculture and Co-operatives approved the norms for home garden establishment and management and has also issued a circular to District Agriculture Development Offices (DADOs) for the protection, management and utilization of biodiversity for supporting livelihoods of local people. The traditional Kitchen Garden programme that promoted hybrid vegetable seeds from exotic sources has now been revamped to an integrated home garden scheme that encourages the use of indigenous crops and varieties of vegetable, fruits, small ruminants and trees. The initiation of the government could be further capitalized on and used as an opportunity by providing technical support in future.

The government sector found the home garden project an attractive intervention to reach the agriculture programme for socially excluded and disadvantaged groups of society and also a way to meet objectives and MDGs. Most strategies to address malnutrition in Nepal are rooted within the health sector. While critical, these programmes generally address disease-related effects and emphasize the immediate determinants of undernutrition. Addressing undernutrition through the production of diverse foods within the agricultural sector, such as home gardening for family well-being, has been an eye-opener for policy makers.

Lessons learned

Access to a wide range of local crop diversity through community actions such as biodiversity fairs, diversity kits and establishing community-based home garden resource centres are important lessons learned. The lessons learned from the project fall within two key areas.

First, situation analysis within the four main areas (assessment, access, use and benefit) can, and most probably will, lead to a number of different community actions. Second, the decision to implement a particular community action, and therefore its success, will depend on farmers and the farming community having the knowledge and leadership capacity to evaluate the benefits that this action will have for them. This in turn emphasizes the importance of strengthening and empowering local institutions so as to enable farmers to take a greater role in the management of agricultural biodiversity in home gardens.

Much can be learned from the projects profiled in this case study that might assist countries that are currently off-track in meeting the hunger component of the MDG1 target. The main objective of Phase II was to improve the nutrition and income of the families from disadvantaged groups (DAG) in remote and conflict-affected areas through the promotion of integrated home gardens. The project focused on families of DAG with a particular focus on women in an effort to promote the mainstreaming of social equity, governance and gender at grassroots levels. The past three years of the project have focused much on land-poor farmers, mostly women, to enable them to utilize their land resources effectively and to empower them economically and socially through organization, voice and influence to enhance social capital of smallholder women farmers. The term "social capital" captures the idea that social bonds and norms are critical for sustainability. Where social capital is high in formalized women groups, people have the confidence to invest in collective activities, knowing that others will do so too. Modest investments in capacity building and targeted training, and engaging different sectors in setting priorities, would have a significant pay-off. With technical support from LI-BIRD, the Department of Agriculture and other donor-funded projects scale up good practices of the home gardening programme in 17 districts through respective DADOs under their third thematic area of "Livelihood improvement of disadvantaged families". Vulnerable groups usually lack enough land to grow staple crops, but many of them have access to small plots which they can cultivate intensively. Home gardening can be a means for reaching excluded people, but it cannot address all their problems. More structural means, such as rights-based approaches, are necessary to complement more direct interventions such as support for home gardening. Policy support guided by outcome based upon large number beneficiaries per unit of investment might require rethinking.

Acknowledgements

The financial support of SDC Nepal and the technical assistance of Bioversity is gratefully acknowledged. The authors would also like to thank Resham Gautam, Pratap Shrestha and Leyla Kutlu for their technical contribution during the project implementation.

References

Abdoellah, O.S., Parikesit, Gunawan, B. and Hadikusumah, H.Y. (2002) 'Home gardens in the Upper Citarum Watershed, West Java: a challenge for *in situ* conservation of plant genetic resources', in J.W. Watson and P.B. Eyzaguirre (eds) *Home gardens and in situ conservation of plant genetic resources in farming systems,* pp.140–148, International Plant Genetic Resources Institute, Rome.

CBS (2001) *Statistical Year Book of Nepal,* Centre Bureau of Statistics, Kathmandu, Nepal.

Daniggelis, E. (2003) 'Women and wild foods: Nutrition and household security among Rai and Sherpa forager farmers in Eastern Nepal,' in P.L. Howard (ed.) *Women and Plants: Gender Relations in Biodiversity Management and Conservation,* pp. 83–95, London and New York: Zed Books.

DeClerck, F.A.J., Fanzo, J., Palm, C., and Remans, R. (2011) 'Ecological approaches to human nutrition,' *Food and Nut. Bull,* vol 32, no 1, pp.S41–S50.

Englberger, L., Joakim, A., Larsen, K., Lorens, A., and Yamada, L. (2010) 'Go Local in Micronesia: Promoting the "CHEEF" benefits of local foods,' *Sight and Life Magazine* 1/2010, pp.40–44.

Eyzaguirre, P. and Linares, O.F. (2004) *Home gardens and agrobiodiversity*, pp.296, Smithsonian Books, Washington.

Fanzo, J.C. and Pronyk, P.M. (2011) 'A review of global progress toward the Millennium Development Goal 1 Hunger Target,' *Food and Nutrition Bulletin*, vol 32(2), pp.144–158.

FIAN (2011) 'Parallel Report the Right to Adequate Food of Women in Nepal,' Combined fourth and fifth periodic report of States Parties, Submitted to CEDAW's 49th Session.

Food Security Monitoring Task Force (2010) *The Food Security Atlas of Nepal*, National Planning Commission, Government of Nepal.

Frison, E.A., Cherfas, J. and Hodgkin, H. (2011) 'Agricultural biodiversity is essential for a sustainable improvement in food and nutrition security', *Sustainability* 2011, vol 3, pp.238–253; doi:10.3390/su3010238.

Gautam, R., Suwal, R. and Basnet, S.B. (2005) 'Enhancing contribution of home gardens to on-farm management of plant genetic resources and to the improvement of the livelihoods of Nepalese farmers: findings of baseline survey of four project sites (Jhapa, Ilam, Rupandehi and Gulmi),' Local Initiatives for Biodiversity, Research and Development, Pokhara.

Gautam R., Suwal R. and Basnet S.B. (2004) *Status of home gardens of Nepal: Findings of a baseline survey conducted in four sites of Home Garden Project*. LI-BIRD.

Gautam, R., Sthapit, B., Subedi, A., Poudel, D., Shrestha, P. and Eyzaguirre, P. (2008) 'Home gardens management of key species in Nepal: A way to maximize the use of useful diversity for the well being of poor farmers,' *Plant Genetic Resources Characterization and Utilization NIAB 2008,* pp.1–12, doi.10.1017/S1479262108110930.

Gautam, R., Suwal, R., and Sthapit, B.R. (2009) 'Securing family nutrition through promotion of home gardens: underutilized production systems in Nepal,' in H. Jaenicke, J. Ganry, I. Höschle-Zeledon, and R. Kahane (eds) *Acta Horticulture,* vol 806, *Underutilized Plants for Food, Nutrition, Income and Sustainable Development,* Proceedings of International Symposium, Arusha, Tanzania, 3–7 March 2008, International Society for Horticultural Science. Leuven, Belgium. p.739.

Johns, T. and Sthapit, B.R. (2004) 'Biocultural diversity in the sustainability of developing country food systems,' *Food and Nutrition Bulletin,* vol 25, no 2, pp.143–155.

Keatinge, J.D.H., Waliyar, F., Jamnadas, R.H., Moustafa, A., Andrade, M., and Drechsel, P. (2010) 'Relearning Old Lessons for the Future of Food—By Bread Alone No Longer: Diversifying Diets with Fruit and Vegetables,' *Crop Science,* vol 50, pp.S51–S62; doi: 10.2135/cropsci2009.09.0528.

Krishna, G.C. (2004) 'Home gardening as a household nutrient garden', in R. Gautam, B. Sthapit, and P. Shrestha (eds) *Home Gardens in Nepal: Proceedings of a national workshop,'* 6–7 August, LI-BIRD, Biodiversity International, SDC, Pokhara, Nepal.

Meinzen-Dick, R., Behrman, J., Menon, R., and Quisumbing, A. (2011) 'Gender: A key dimension linking agricultural programs to improved nutrition and health,' 2020 Conference Brief 9, IFPRI.

NARC (2005) 'NARC strategic planning meeting report', Khumaltar, Nepal.

Rijal, D. (2010) 'Role of food tradition in conserving crop landraces on-farm,' *Journal of Agriculture and Environment,* vol 11, Jun.

Ruel, M. and Hoddinott, J. (2008) 'Investing in early childhood nutrition,' IFPRI Policy Brief 8.

SEWA (2009) 'Impact of price rise on poor households,' SEWA, http://www.sewa.org/pdf/ IMPACT OF PRICE RISE ON POOR HOUSE HOLDS – Survey by SEWA. pdf, accessed July 2012.

Shrestha, P., Gautam, R., Rana, R.B., and Sthapit, B.R. (2002) 'Home gardens in Nepal: Status and scope for research and development,' in J.W. Watson and P.B. Eyzaguirre (eds) *Home gardens and in situ conservation of plant genetic resources in farming systems,* Proceeding of the second international home gardens workshops, Witzenhausen, 17–19 July 2001, pp.105–124, Federal Republic of Germany: International Plant Genetic Resources Institute, Rome.

Shrestha, P., Gautam, R., Rana, R.B. and Sthapit, B.R. (2004) 'Managing diversity in various ecosystems: Home gardens in Nepal', in P.B. Eyzaguirre and O.F. Linares, (eds) *Home Gardens and Agrobiodiversity*, Smithsonian Books, Washington.

Soemarowoto, O. (1987) 'Homegardens: A traditional agro-forestry system with a promising future,' in H.A. Steppler and P.K.R. Nair (eds) *Agro-forestry: A decade of development*, pp.157–170, ICRAF, Nairobi, Kenya.

Sthapit, B., Resham, G. and Eyzaguirre, P. (2004a) 'The value of home gardens to small farmers' in: Home Gardens in Nepal: Proceedings of a national workshop, 6–7 August 2004, in R. Gautam, B. Sthapit, and P. Shrestha (eds) LI-BIRD, Bioversity International, SDC, Pokhara, Nepal.

Sthapit, B., Rana, R.B., Hue, N.N. and Rijal, D.K. (2004b) 'The diversity of taro and sponge gourds in home gardens of Nepal and Vietnam,' in P.B. Eyzaguirre and O.F Linares (eds) *Home Gardens and Agrobiodiversity*, pp.234–255, Smithsonian Books, Washington.

Sthapit, B., Rana, R.B., Subedi, A., Gyawali, S., Bajracharya, J., Chaudhary, P., Joshi, B.K., Sthapit, S., Joshi, K.D., and Upadhyay, M.P. (2006) 'Participatory four cell analysis (FCA) for local crop diversity,' in B.R. Sthapit, P.K. Shrestha, and M.P. Upadhyay, (eds) *Good practices: On-farm management of agricultural biodiversity in Nepal*, NARC, LI-BIRD, IPGRI and IDRC.

Sthapit, B.R., Rana, R., Eyzaguirre, P., and Jarvis, D. (2008) 'The value of genetic diversity to resource-poor farmers in Nepal and Vietnam,' *International Journal of Agricultural Sustainability*, vol 6, no 2, pp.148–166, doi: 10.3763/ijas.2007.0291.

Sunwar, S., Thornstrom, C., Subedi, A., and Bystrom, M. (2006) 'Home gardens in western Nepal: opportunities and challenges for on-farm management of agrobiodiversity', *Biodiversity and Conservation* 15: 4211–38.

Suwal, R., Gautam, R., Sunwar, S., Basnet, S.B. and Subedi, A. (2005) 'Enhancing the contribution of home gardens to on-farm management of plant genetic resources and to improvement of the livelihoods of Nepalese farmers', Site Selection Report, Local Initiatives for Biodiversity, Research and Development, Pokhara, Nepal.

Suwal, R., Regmi, B.R., Shrestha, A., and Sthapit, B.R. (2008) 'Home gardens are within the reach of marginalized people (24 September 2008)', *LEISA* 24.3 September, p.34.

Talukder, A., Sapkota, G., Srestha, S., Pee, S., de and Bloem, M.W. (2004) 'Homestead production program in Central and Far Western Nepal increases food and nutrition security: An overview of program achievements,' in Home Gardens in Nepal: Proceedings of a national workshop', 6–7 August 2004, in R. Gautam, B. Sthapit, P. Shrestha (eds), LI-BIRD, Biodiversity International, SDC, Pokhara, Nepal.

Trinh, L.N., Watson, J.W., Hue, N.N., De, N.N., Minh, N.V., Chu, P., Sthapit, B.R. and Eyzaguirre, P.B. (2003) 'Agro-biodiversity conservation and development in Vietnamese home gardens', *Agriculture, Ecosystems and Environment* 2033, pp.1–28.

UNICEF (1990) *Strategy for improved nutrition of children and women in developing countries*, Policy Review Paper E/ICEF/1990/1.6, UNICEF, New York; JC 27/UNICEF-WHO/89.4 New York.

WFP Nepal (2009) 'A sub-regional hunger index for Nepal', *Nepal Food Security Monitoring System,* World Food Programme.

Case study 3

Diversity of indigenous fruit trees and their contribution to nutrition and livelihoods in sub-Saharan Africa: examples from Kenya and Cameroon

Katja Kehlenbeck, Ebenezar Asaah and Ramni Jamnadass

Introduction

In sub-Saharan Africa (SSA), growing both domesticated and wild fruit species on farms diversifies the crop production options of small-scale farmers and can bring significant health, ecological and economic revenues (Keatinge et al., 2010; Weinberger and Lumpkin, 2005). Dozens of indigenous fruit tree species (IFTs), although relatively unknown in global markets, are locally of large importance for food/nutrition security and income generation. Akinnifesi et al. (2008) showed the high potential of many wild fruit species from different African regions for undergoing domestication followed by successful on-farm production. Fruit markets in SSA are estimated to grow substantially due to economic and human population growth and increasing urbanisation rates, e.g. by 5.7 per cent per year in Kenya (calculation of ICRAF based on Ruel et al., 2005). Women are often strongly involved in and benefit from fruit processing and trade, particularly with regard to indigenous fruits (Schreckenberg et al., 2006). With appropriate promotion, the contribution of fruits to the livelihoods and health of African farmers and consumers could be substantially increased.

Currently, fruit consumption in SSA – with a daily average of only 36 g per person in Eastern and about 90 g in Western Africa (WHO, 2002) – is far below the recommended daily amount of 200 g per person (WHO, 2003). In sub-Saharan Africa about 30 per cent of inhabitants, most of them women and children, suffer from malnutrition (UNSCN, 2010). Fruits offer not only easily available energy, but also micronutrients such as vitamins and minerals necessary to sustain and support human healthy growth and activity (see examples below). There are, however, a variety of factors that constrain fruit consumption and production in Africa such as:

- Lack of consumer awareness on the health benefits of regular fruit consumption;
- Change of consumer preferences and loss of the traditional nutrition systems based on local agricultural biodiversity, which leads to erosion of both the plant genetic resources and the related traditional knowledge;

- Degradation of natural vegetation used for collecting indigenous fruits in the past;
- Lack of sufficient tree domestication techniques and their dissemination, especially of vegetative tree propagation methods;
- Lack of fruit processing facilities, which leads to high post-harvest losses;
- Poorly organised fruit marketing pathways along the value chain.

Indigenous fruit trees (IFTs) traditionally provide rural communities in SSA's drylands, where cultivation of exotic fruit species often is not possible, with nutritious fruits for self-consumption and sale. Wild fruits are mostly gathered from natural stands only, but IFTs are usually not cultivated on farms (Simitu et al., 2009). Climate change will most probably shift the natural geographic ranges, and reduce density and productivity of some wild fruit species (Dawson et al., 2011). Domestication of selected high value IFT species and their on-farm cultivation in agroforestry systems are prerequisites for enhanced production, processing and marketing of valuable indigenous fruits (Pye-Smith, 2010). In addition, cultivation of IFT species on farms will contribute to climate change mitigation and adaptation of farming systems. Trees such as fruit trees provide many other valuable environmental services (Garrity, 2004). Increased cultivation of IFTs will contribute to diversification of farming systems, improve connectivity of remaining natural habitats for biodiversity conservation and decrease the pressure on natural IFT stands, thus further contributing to conservation of genetic resources of these trees. In the following, the value of fruits for nutrition and income generation is described in more detail.

Fruits for health and food security

Deficiency of iron and vitamin A is prevalent in most parts of SSA. Low intake of vitamin A – around 50 million African children are at risk of deficiency – is considered to be Africa's third greatest public health problem after HIV/AIDS and malaria.[1] Vitamin C from fruits, on the other hand, is essential for absorbing iron, an important mineral that is present in significant quantities in green leafy vegetables. Indigenous fruits contribute to the vitamin and mineral supply of local communities, e.g. baobab (*Adansonia digitata*) for vitamin C, marula (*Sclerocarya birrea*) for vitamin A and white crossberries (*Grewia tenax*) for iron (Table C3.1). A child could cover 100 per cent of its vitamin C requirement by eating only about 10 g of baobab pulp a day. Concerning iron, consumption of 40–100 g white crossberries covers almost 100 per cent of the daily iron requirement of a child less than eight years old. In addition to micronutrients, fruits such as tamarind (*Tamarindus indica*) and baobab contribute much to energy supply due to their sugar content (Table C3.1). However, data on nutrient contents of many indigenous fruits are either unavailable or unreliable. The high variability of nutrient contents given in the literature (Table C3.1) may be caused by using different methods for analysis, but also by the fact that a very high variability

Table C3.1 Nutrient contents of selected indigenous and exotic fruits per 100g edible portion (high values are highlighted in bold).

Species	Energy (Kcal)	Protein (g)	Vit C (mg)	Vit A (RE) (mg)	Iron (mg)	Calcium (mg)
Indigenous fruits						
Adansonia digitata	340	3.1	150–**500**	0.03–0.06	1.7	360
Grewia tenax	N.A.	3.6	N.A.	N.A.	7.4–**20.8**	**610**
Sclerocarya birrea	225	0.5	68–**200**	**0.035**	0.1	6
Tamarindus indica	270	**4.8**	3–9	0.01–0.06	0.7	260
Ziziphus mauritiana	21	1.2	70–165	0.07	1.0	40
Exotic fruits						
Guava (*Psidium guajava*)	68	2.6	**228.3**	0.031	0.3	18
Mango (*Mangifera indica*)	65	0.5	27.7	0.038	0.1	10
Orange (*Citrus sinensis*)	47	0.9	53.0	0.008	0.1	40
Pawpaw (*Carica papaya*)	39	0.6	62.0	**0.135**	0.1	24

Sources: Indigenous fruits: Freedman (1998) Famine foods. http://www.hort.purdue.edu/newcrop/faminefoods/ff_home.html (accessed 13 August 2012); Fruits for the Future Series, ICUC; Fineli (http://www.fineli.fi/, accessed 20 July 2012), etc.; Exotic fruits: Lukmanji & Hertzmark (2008) Tanzania Food Composition Tables.

naturally occurs among different populations of the same species as long as the species is undomesticated.

Tree crops such as fruit trees are contributing not only to nutrition security, but also to food security. Due to their extensive and deep rooting systems, fruit trees are less sensitive to droughts as compared with annual staple crops and give a harvest even when the staple crops fail. Not only during droughts, but especially during the pre-harvest periods of annual staples characterised by food shortages ('hunger gap'), fruits from some IFT species may be ready for harvest to serve as emergency food or to be sold, thus contributing to food and nutrition security (see case study 1 from Kenya and Figure C3.1 from Malawi and Zambia). By combining site-specific portfolios of different exotic and indigenous fruit species for cultivation, a year-round supply of fruits can be achieved.

Fruits for income generation and integrated rural development

Fruit tree cultivation offers great potential for income generation if farmers are (i) linked to markets to reduce input costs and improve prices for their produce, (ii) trained in best on-farm management of existing fruit trees; and (iii) in cultivating improved, high value varieties and species, which best fit present and future market demands (see above). When farmers have access to improved grafted planting material, they can expect a relatively quick return from their

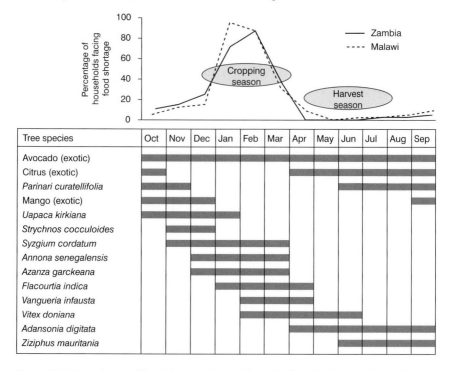

Figure C3.1 Prevalence of food shortage in rural households of Malawi and Zambia and the harvest periods of different exotic and indigenous fruit species of the same region. During the cropping ('hunger') season, fruits of one exotic and four indigenous species are continuously available, fruits of three more species are partly available (data collected by World Biodiversity Centre (ICRAF) staff in the region)

new trees as grafted trees will start fruiting two to three years after planting. Small-scale processing groups, particularly of women, benefit from improved fruit cultivation and help to reduce post-harvest losses. Still, there is a high unexploited potential for enhanced employment, business development and income generation through processing of both exotic and wild or domesticated indigenous fruits. For example, a feasibility study of small-scale juice concentrate processing enterprises calculated a potential net profit of about 28 per cent of the gross production value in Malawi (Jordaan et al., 2008). Domestication of IFTs includes: identification and characterisation of the available genetic diversity of a species; capture, selection and management of the genetic resources; propagation of superior materials and sustainable cultivation of the species in managed agro-ecosystems (Simons and Leakey, 2004). Vegetative propagation methods such as rooting of stem cuttings, grafting and marcotting warrant early fruiting and ensure that the desired traits of superior mother trees are passed to the offspring. Successful projects on domestication of IFTs, for example in Cameroon (see below), show that fruit cultivation and processing have significant impacts on rural development and transforming people's lives.

Case 1 Kenya: High on-farm IFT species diversity, but low consumption of fruits in the drylands

In Kenya, about 400 indigenous fruit tree species occur (Chikamai et al., 2004), which are said to contribute much to livelihoods of rural communities, particularly during the frequent periods of food shortage. However, detailed studies on diversity of IFTs and their consumption in Kenya are scarce. A case study was thus performed by Simitu et al. (2009) in the drylands of Mwingi District, Eastern Kenya, where 104 households were randomly selected to collect data on IFT abundance on farms and fruit consumption data of adults (26 male and 26 female respondents) as well as of children (26 boys and 26 girls < 18 years). All fruit tree species occurring on the farm of the respondent were identified and the individual trees counted. A combination of a semi-structured questionnaire and visual aids were used to collect detailed and reliable data on fruit consumption over a period of one year. A food-frequency questionnaire (FFQ) developed after Agudo (2004) with the names of all available fruit species was used to determine which species were consumed in the periods of the year, when the species could be harvested and how often the respondents consumed the respective fruit during that time. Typical household measures and photos of standard portions were used to help respondents estimate the usual amount of fruits consumed per meal and to calculate mean consumption per day for each of the species.

A total of 57 IFT species were mentioned as being consumed by the respondents; 36 of these species were found on the 104 surveyed farms, 21 species were exclusively collected from the wild. Thirty-three of the species found on farms were maintained from natural regeneration (e.g. trees protected during field clearing, new seedlings spared during weeding), of which 17 species were never planted and 16 species were both protected from natural regeneration and actively planted by respondents. The remaining three species out of the 36 on-farm species were exclusively planted. The most frequent species were *Balanites aegyptiaca* (desert date) occurring on 58 per cent of the surveyed farms, *Adansonia digitata* (baobab; 50 per cent) and *Berchemia discolor* (50 per cent). However, a large proportion of species were each found only on one or two of the surveyed farms. With regard to individual tree numbers, only 1.3 per cent of the counted 4,048 trees on the surveyed farms were actively planted by the respondents, e.g. some tamarind (*Tamarindus indica*) trees. Two crossberry species (*Grewia villosa* and *G. tembensis*) were the most abundant species, representing 20 and 16 per cent of the recorded tree individuals, respectively. Thirteen species were very rare, represented by less than 10 individuals each.

Mean daily consumption of indigenous fruits was 19 g per person, being a little higher for children (about 23 g) than adults. Adults view many indigenous fruits as food for children and consume only fruits from certain, higher valued species such as baobab, tamarind, *Berchemia discolor* or *Lannea alata*. When exotic fruits (which were available only on market days) were included in the calculations, the mean daily consumption increased from 19 g to 28 g of fruits

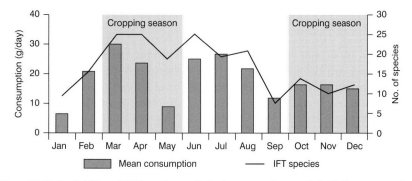

Figure C3.2 Availability of IFT species ready for harvest and mean daily fruit consumption per person during the course of the year in Mwingi district, Eastern Kenya

per person. This is still far below the recommended daily intake of 200 g per person (WHO, 2003). During the course of the year, fruit consumption varied among seasons (Figure C3.2), but 10–25 IFT species were ready for harvest even during the 'hunger gaps' of the two cropping seasons (March to May and October to December). Lean fruit seasons with mean daily consumptions of less than 10 g per day were in January and May, peak consumption seasons with more than 20 g per day in February to April and June to August. Mean daily consumption in a month was positively influenced by number of IFT species ready for harvest in the respective month ($R^2 = 0.543$, $p = 0.006$) (P. Simitu, 2008, pers. comm.). For example, in September, only eight IFT species had mature fruits for harvesting and daily fruit consumption was only 12.8 g per person in the same month, whereas in March 25 species were ready for harvest and the daily consumption was almost 30 g (Figure C3.2).

The study in Kenya showed the urgent need for awareness creation among rural communities about the value of fruit consumption for improved nutrition and health. Many IFT species were available, but they were not used efficiently. Domestication of priority species will help to increase the number of planted IFTs on farms and to improve the perception of IFTs in the rural communities from 'food for children' towards 'valuable fruits for health and wealth'. The first steps of a participatory species priority setting in Kenya resulted in the preliminary selection of *Tamarindus indica, Adansonia digitata, Sclerocarya birrea, Ziziphus mauritania* and *Balanites aegyptiaca* (Chikamai et al., 2004) as well as *Vitex payos* (Muok et al., 2000), *Berchemia discolor* and *Carissa edulis* (Teklehaimanot, 2005). However, species priority settings should also consider regional preferences, nutritional value of fruits, market and value addition potentials, seasonality of fruiting and adaptability of species to climate change and should involve not only farmers, but also fruit traders, processors and exporters, agricultural extension officers, and scientists from several disciplines such as agricultural economics, agronomy, natural resources conservation, ecology, ethno-botany, health and nutrition (Franzel et al., 1996).

Lessons learned and way forward

So far, both government extension services and NGOs in Kenya neglect the value of indigenous fruits for improved livelihoods of rural communities and, instead, focus on the promotion of exotic fruits, such as mango and passion fruit. Integrating the health sector and involving the educational segment in future programmes as well as analysing and developing value chains for indigenous fruits may help to mainstream IFT cultivation, processing, marketing and consumption in Kenya and beyond.

Case 2 Cameroon: Successful participatory fruit tree domestication improved livelihoods of rural communities

Farmers in humid West and Central Africa depend mainly on cacao and coffee cultivation for income generation, but have suffered from low and fluctuating prices for these commodities since the 1980s. Against this background, there was an urgent need to diversify farmers' livelihood options through the development of sustainable poverty reduction strategies, including agroforestry and tree domestication. In agroforestry systems, a combination of annual crops and useful tree and shrub species fulfils diverse production and service functions (Garrity, 2004). Many of these functions were once provided by natural forests, which are declining in Cameroon and elsewhere. The related decline in availability of important forest products such as food, medicine, fodder, timber and fuel wood with its negative impact on traditional diets, health systems and income generating opportunities for the local communities can at least be partly offset by promoting diverse agroforestry systems.

In 1995, the World Agroforestry Centre (ICRAF) conducted a farmers' species preference survey in the humid tropics of West and Central Africa. The priority species identified for domestication and improvement by research were mainly indigenous fruit, nut and medicinal species with a high value for nutrition and income generation such as *Irvingia gabonensis, Dacryodes edulis, Ricinodendron heudelotii, Chrysophyllum albidum, Garcinia kola* and different *Cola* species (Franzel et al., 1996). Contrary to the situation in Kenya (case 1), indigenous fruits are highly valued by farmers and consumers in Cameroon and have a ready market. The combined harvesting seasons of the mentioned species offered a year-round supply with produce for home consumption and sale (Figure C3.3). Fruits and nuts of some of these species are highly nutritious and contribute much to energy, protein and mineral supply of consumers (Table C3.2).

In Cameroon, participatory priority species selection showed a high demand for fruit and nut species such as bush mango (*Irvingia gabonensis*) and African plum (*Dacryodes edulis*). Until the start of the tree domestication programme in 1995, these species were mainly found in forests, from where the fruits were collected for home consumption, processing and sale. However, the number of these valuable trees was decreasing due to deforestation and over-exploitation, among other reasons (Tchoundjeu et al., 2006). After the critical strategic decision

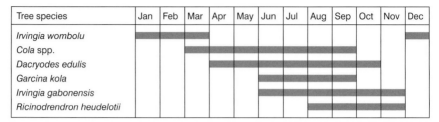

Tree species	Jan	Feb	Mar	Apr	May	Jun	Jul	Aug	Sep	Oct	Nov	Dec
Irvingia wombolu												
Cola spp.												
Dacryodes edulis												
Garcina kola												
Irvingia gabonensis												
Ricinodrendron heudelotii												

Figure C3.3 Harvest periods of selected priority indigenous fruit and nut species of West and Central Africa

Table C3.2 Nutrient contents of selected indigenous fruit and nut species of Central Africa per 100g edible portion.

Species	Energy (Kcal)	Protein (g)	Vit C (mg)	Vit A (RE) (mg)	Iron (mg)	Calcium (mg)
Dacryodes edulis (fruit flesh)	263	4.6	19	N.A.	0.8	43
Irvingia gabonensis (fruit flesh)	61	0.9	74	N.A.	1.8	20
Irvingia gabonensis (kernels)	697	8.5	N.A.	N.A.	3.4	120
Ricinodendron heudelotii (kernels)	530	21.0	0	0	0.4	611

Sources: Leung W.T.W., Busson F., Jardin, C. (1968) Food composition table for use in Africa. FAO, Rome, Italy; Platt B.S. (1962) Tables of representative values of foods commonly used in tropical countries. Special Report Series 302, Medical Research Council, London, UK.

to implement participatory tree domestication rather than the conventional research station approach, the first step of the domestication programme in Cameroon in 1999 was to develop propagation methods for the priority species based on appropriate low-tech methods that did not require running water or electricity and that was adapted to farmers' capacity and competences in remote rural communities (Leakey et al., 1990). In parallel, pilot farmers in selected rural communities – assisted by teams made up of scientists and extension staff from both government and non-governmental organisations – selected superior mother trees with the desired traits (e.g. many large and sweet fruits, early first fruiting) based on simple techniques for the characterisation of tree-to-tree variation developed by the team (Atangana et al., 2002; Tchoundjeu et al., 2006).

In the second step, innovative farmers managing pilot nurseries were trained in participatory tree domestication techniques and their nurseries were upgraded to 'Rural Resource Centres' (RRCs) (Asaah et al., 2011). RRCs manage community-owned nurseries for the production and distribution of high quality tree planting materials, but have additional functions as hubs for the development of propagation techniques and for training of nursery managers, farmers and small-scale processors (Figure C3.4). Also, RRCs serve as collection points and marketing centres for tree products. Each RRC is equipped with a

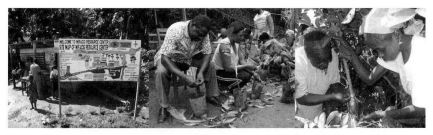

Figure C3.4 Appearance and activities of Rural Resource Centres (RRCs) in Cameroon. Left: entrance to an RRC; middle: farmers are trained in grafting techniques; right: women marcotting a fruit tree (photographs by Charlie Pye-Smith (left and centre) and Julius Atia (right))

Box C3.1 The fruits of success

If you had visited Christophe Missé in the 1990s, on his small farm some 40 kilometres north of the Cameroonian capital, Yaoundé, you would have heard a story of hardship and poverty. "My cocoa crop yielded an income for just three months a year," he recalls, "and even with the extra cash I earned as a part-time teacher, we struggled to make ends meet." Then, in 1999, Missé attended a training session held by the World Agroforestry Centre in Nkolfep, West Region. It was, he says, an experience that changed his life. He learnt about the techniques used to develop superior varieties of indigenous fruit trees. "As soon as I'd completed the training, I realised that it would help me to transform my farm," he says. He set up a nursery with his neighbours and is now selling over 7,000 trees a year. He has also planted hundreds of indigenous fruit trees on his farm such as bush mango and African plum, which now grow besides his main cash crop, cocoa. The African plums are particularly impressive, with some of his most fruitful trees earning 10,000 CFA francs (US$22) a year, five times as much as his individual cocoa bushes. Apart from enhancing the nutrition and food security of his family, Missé has substantially improved his livelihood with the additional income generated from fruit cultivation. "With the money I've made I've built a new house," he says proudly, "and I can now pay for two of my children to go to private school."

Source: Extract from Pye-Smith, 2010

nursery, meeting and training facilities, motherblocks and demonstration plots, and fruit drying/storage facilities, if appropriate. RRCs are also holding a register for newly-developed farmers' fruit tree varieties, in order that local domesticators can assert their rights over selected cultivars. Interested innovative farmers from the villages nearby are trained at the RRCs to become nursery managers and to start 'satellite nurseries' on their farms (Tchoundjeu et al., 2006; Asaah et al.,

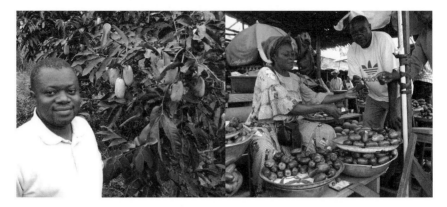

Figure C3.5 Christophe Missé (left) has significantly improved his income by growing superior varieties of indigenous fruit trees, such as African plums on his farm in Cameroon, which are in high demand at the local markets (right) (photographs by Charlie Pye-Smith)

2011; see example in Box C3.1). The trainees are then equipped with a starter kit of high quality germplasm and will construct simple nursery structures with local material at their farms. By this decentralised approach, even farmers in remote locations have access to high quality planting material of fruit trees from the satellite nurseries. Asaah et al. (2011) reported that the programme currently works in seven RRCs with more than 200 farmer groups or associations. ICRAF researchers developed training packages and play a coordinating and mentoring role in managing the RRCs and the local government extension officers. The RRCs are under the day-to-day technical supervision and general management of 17 'relay organisations', which include local NGOs, community-based organisations or well-established farmer groups, sometimes complemented by the involvement of local government extension officers. The relay organisations were trained in different aspects to ensure quality delivery of innovative advisory services to farmers and of community capacity-building activities.

According to Asaah et al. (2011) and Tchoundjeu et al. (2010), the following outcomes of the project were reported:

- In 2008, seven RRCs provided advisory services to about 100 satellite nurseries (8–35 satellite nurseries per RRC) and produced 122,500 indigenous fruit and nut trees that have been planted on the farms (Figure C3.5).
- Annual incomes were about US$21,000 for one RRC (running for 10 years) and an average of US$7,350 for each of 35 farmer-managed satellite nurseries of the same RRC in 2009.
- Around 50 per cent of local adopters integrated 10 fruit trees on average in their farms and reported to have increased their fruit consumption, 30 per cent also mentioned increased income (see Box C3.1 for an

example). The stated increase in fruit consumption is supposed to be due to the enhanced accessibility of a diverse set of different fruit species planted on the farms that fruit almost year-round (Figure C3.3), but no quantitative data are yet available.

- Tree nurseries that had received technical support (e.g. training on propagation techniques, group dynamics, management and marketing techniques) from ICRAF's participatory tree domestication initiative supplied a wider range of fruit trees and propagated in more appropriate ways and with higher purchaser satisfaction than those nurseries that had not received assistance. After about five years of support, RRCs are usually able to generate sufficient income to sustain their activities independently.
- The RRC approach for integrating participatory tree domestication with a broader set of rural services (e.g. training in nursery management and sustainable farming, watershed protection, beekeeping and marketing, providing microfinance, linking farmers to markets) is recognised as one of the best examples of multifunctional agricultural development for the reduction of poverty through conservation of biodiversity, and was accordingly awarded an Equator Prize in 2010.[2]

Lessons learned and way forward

This domestication project and the RRC approach developed within the project proved successful in regard to sustainably improving livelihoods of rural communities. Similar projects were already applied in Nigeria and the Democratic Republic of Congo (Tchoundjeu et al., 2006). RRCs were found to be economically independent after about five years of technical support while producing significant incomes from production of high quality agroforestry seedlings and from providing services such as training of farmers, micro-processors and nursery managers. The same RRC model will now be tested for up-scaling in Kenya, Tanzania, Rwanda and Mali and for its suitability for tree domestication in drylands.

Notes

1 www.worldmapper.org, accessed July 2012.
2 http://www.equatorinitiative.org/index.php?option=com_content&view=article&id=597%3Aribaagroforestryresourcecentre&catid=175&Itemid=339, accessed July 2012.

References

Agudo, A. (2004) Measuring intake of fruit and vegetables, Background paper for the Joint FAO/WHO Workshop on Fruit and Vegetables for Health, 1–3 September 2004, Kobe, Japan, available at: http://www.who.int/dietphysicalactivity/publications/f&v_intake_measurement.pdf, accessed July 2012.

Akinnifesi, F.K., Leakey, R.R.B., Ajayi, O.C., Sileshi, G., Tchoundjeu, Z., Matakala, P., Kwesiga, F.R. (2008) *Indigenous fruit trees in the tropics: domestication, utilization and commercialization*, CAB International, Wallingford, UK, in association with the World Agro-forestry Centre, Nairobi, Kenya.

Asaah, E.K., Tchoundjeu, Z., Leakey, R.R.B., Takousting, B., Njong, J., Edang, I. (2011) Trees, agro-forestry and multifunctional agriculture in Cameroon, *International Journal of Agricultural Sustainability*, vol 9, pp.110–119.

Atangana, A.R., Ukafor, V., Anegbeh, P.O., Asaah, E., Tchoundjeu, Z., Usoro, C., Fondoun, J.M., Ndoumbe, M., Leakey, R.R.B. (2002) Domestication of *Irvingia gabonensis*: 2, The selection of multiple traits for potential cultivars from Cameroon and Nigeria, *Agroforestry Systems* 55, pp.221–229.

Chikamai, B., Eyog-Matig, O., Mbogga, M. (2004) Review and appraisal on the status of indigenous fruits in Eastern Africa, A report prepared for IPGRI-SAFORGEN in the framework of AFREA/FORNESSA, IPGRI (International Plant Genetic Resources Institute) SSA, Nairobi, Kenya.

Dawson, I.K., Vinceti, B., Weber, J.C., Neufeldt, H., Russell, J, Lengkeek, A.G., Kalinganire, A., Kindt, R., Lillesø, J.P.B., Roshetko, J., Jamnadass, R. (2011) Climate change and tree genetic resource management: maintaining and enhancing the productivity and value of smallholder tropical agro-forestry landscapes, A review. *Agroforestry Systems*, vol 81, pp.67–78.

Franzel, S., Jaenicke, H., Janssen, W. (1996) Choosing the right trees: setting priorities for multipurpose tree improvement, ISNAR Research Report 8, The Hague, The Netherlands.

Garrity, D.P. (2004) Agroforestry and the achievement of the Millennium Development Goals, *Agroforestry Systems*, vol 61, pp.5–17.

Jordaan, D.P.S., Akinnifesi, F.K., Ham, C., Ajayi, O.C. (2008) The feasibility of small-scale indigenous fruit processing enterprises in Southern Africa, in F.K. Akinnifesi, R.R.B. Leakey, O.C. Ajayi, G. Sileshi, Z. Tchoundjeu, P. Matakala, F.R. Kwesiga (eds) *Indigenous fruit trees in the tropics: domestication, utilization and commercialization*, CAB International, Wallingford, UK, in association with the World Agroforestry Centre, Nairobi, Kenya, pp.273–287.

Keatinge, J.D.H., Waliyar, F., Jamnadass, R.H., Moustafa, A., Andrade, M., Drechsel, P., Hughes, J.A., Kadirvel, P., Luther, K. (2010) Relearning old lessons for the future of food – by bread alone no longer: diversifying diets with fruit and vegetables, *Crop Science*, vol 50, pp.S51–S62.

Leakey, R.R.B., Mesén, J.F., Tchoundjeu, Z., Longman, K.A., Dick, J.M., Newton, A., Matin, A., Grace, J., Munro, R.C., Muthoka, P.N. (1990) Low-technology techniques for the vegetative propagation of tropical trees, *Commonwealth Forestry Review*, vol 69, pp.247–257.

Lukmanji, Z., Hertzmark, E., Mlingi, N., Assey, V., Ndossi, G., Fawzi, W. (2008) Tanzania food composition Tables. MUHAS-TFNC, HSPH, Dar es Salaam Tanzania https://apps.sph.harvard.edu/publisher/upload/nutritionsource/files/tanzania-food-composition-tables.pdf, accessed July 2012.

Muok, B.O., Owuor, B., Dawson, I., Were, J. (2000) The potential of indigenous fruit trees: Results of a survey in Kitui District, Kenya, *Agroforestry Today*, vol 12, pp.13–16.

Pye-Smith, C. (2010) The fruits of success: a programme to domesticate West and Central Africa's wild fruit trees is raising incomes, improving health and stimulating the rural economy, *Trees for Change*, no 4, The World Agroforestry Centre, Nairobi, Kenya.

Ruel, M.T., Minot, N., Smith, L. (2005) *Patterns and determinants of fruit and vegetable consumption in sub-Saharan Africa: a multi-country comparison*, IFPRI (International Food Policy Research Institute), Washington DC.

Schreckenberg, K., Awono, A., Degrande, A., Mbosso, C., Ndoye, O., Tchoundjeu, Z. (2006) Domesticating indigenous fruit trees as a contribution to poverty reduction, *Forests, Trees and Livelihoods*, vol 16, pp.35–51.

Simitu, P., Jamnadass, R., Kindt, R., Kungu, J., Kimiywe, J. (2009) Consumption of dryland indigenous fruits to improve livelihoods in Kenya, The case of Mwingi District, *Acta Horticulturae*, vol 806, pp.93–98.

Simons, A.J., Leakey, R.R.B. (2004) Tree domestication in tropical agroforestry, *Agroforestry Systems*, vol 61, pp.167–181.

Tchoundjeu, Z., Asaah, E.K., Anegbeh, P., Degrande, D., Mbile, P., Facheux, C., Tsobeng, A., Atangana, R.A., Ngo-Mpeck, M.L., Simons, A.J. (2006) Putting participatory domestication into practice in West and Central Africa, *Forests, Trees and Livelihoods*, vol 16, pp.53–69.

Tchoundjeu, Z., Degrande, A., Leakey, R.R.B., Simons, A.J., Nimino, G., Kemajou, E., Asaah, E., Facheux, C., Mbile, P., Mbosso, C., Sado, T., Tsobeng, A. (2010) Impact of participatory tree domestication on farmer livelihoods in west and central Africa, *Forests, Trees and Livelihoods*, vol 19, pp.217–234.

Teklehaimanot, Z. (2005) Indigenous fruit trees of Eastern Africa, The Leverhulme Trust: a Study Abroad Fellowship report, University of Wales, Bangor, UK .

UNSCN (2010) *6th Report on the world nutrition situation: Progress in nutrition*, United Nations System – Standing Committee on Nutrition, Geneva, Switzerland, http://www.unscn.org/files/Publications/RWNS6/report/SCN_report.pdf, accessed July 2012.

Weinberger, K., Lumpkin, T. A (2005) Horticulture for poverty alleviation – the unfunded revolution, Working Paper No. 15, AVRDC (The World Vegetable Center), Shanhua, Taiwan.

WHO (World Health Organization) (2002) *The World Health Report 2002: Reducing Risks, Promoting Healthy Life*, http://www.who.int/whr/2002/en/, accessed July 2012.

WHO (World Health Organization) (2003) *Diet, nutrition and the prevention of chronic diseases: report of a joint WHO/FAO expert consultation, Geneva, 28 January – 1 February 2002*, Technical Report Series 916, WHO/FAO, http://whqlibdoc.who.int/trs/who_trs_916.pdf, accessed July 2012.

Case study 4

Fish diversity and fish consumption in Bangladesh

Shakuntala Haraksingh Thilsted

Introduction

Bangladesh prides itself on being very rich in fish diversity. Its numerous and diverse inland waterbodies – beels (floodplain depressions and lakes), ponds, rivers, canals, ditches – and paddy fields, are home to over 267 freshwater fish species (Rahman, 1989). In terms of production, it is reported that only China and India outrank Bangladesh in freshwater fisheries. In addition, coastal and marine fisheries also have a large biodiversity. In the mangrove waters in Sundarbans, over 400 fish species, as well as other aquatic animals such as shrimp, prawn and crab are reported (Islam and Haque, 2004). In rivers and estuaries, the fish catch is dominated by one migratory species, hilsa (*Tenualosa ilisha*; "Macher raja ilish – hilsa, the king of fish"), which makes up 11 per cent of the annual total fish production (Department of Fisheries, 2010). Millions of people, especially the rural poor, are dependent to varying degrees on these fisheries for their livelihoods, income and food. These rich fishery resources, which are intrinsically intertwined with rice production, are exemplified in the old proverb "Machee bhatee bangali", literally translated as "Fish and rice make a Bengali". Together with the staple, boiled rice eaten by many at least twice per day and vegetables, fish is an essential and irreplaceable animal-source food in the Bangladeshi diet.

Changes in the rice–fish production system in Bangladesh

With over half of the country comprised of floodplains, in the past, agriculture and capture fisheries complemented one another in a natural cycle of wet and dry season and monsoon rains. During the dry season (approx. May–December), most of the land was cultivated and fish were restricted to beels, rivers and canals. In the monsoon and post-monsoon periods (June–November), the floodplains were inundated and cultivation of deepwater rice was practised. This vast area provided an ideal habitat for the many freshwater fish species and people had access to fish (Payne and Temple, 1996).

In the early 1970s, Bangladesh was unable to produce enough rice to feed its population of 75 million. In the following three decades, rice production tripled,

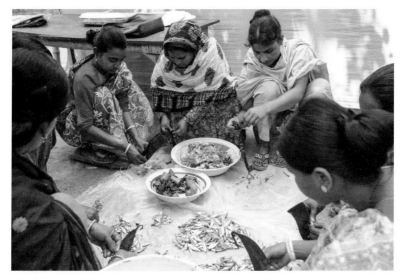

Figure C4.1 Bangladeshi women preparing a fish curry. Photograph by Finn Thilsted

and today, with a population of 160 million, the country is considered almost self-sufficient in rice. This has changed the overall agricultural production and management of land and water drastically, favouring rice production: high-yielding rice varieties were introduced, more areas were brought under rice production, irrigation was expanded greatly, areas were drained and protected by flood control embankments, and fertilizer and pesticide use increased. Increased agricultural production intensity brought about reduction in soil fertility, decrease in groundwater level and siltation. These changes have been at the expense of inland fisheries; the area of inland waterbodies and the duration of inundation have fallen, with degradation and loss of fish habitat, as well as obstruction in fish movement to floodplains (Craig et al., 2004).

In the past 25 years, freshwater aquaculture has grown, and many households with a pond practise varying intensities of pond polyculture. Mostly, a mixture of carps was stocked, with silver favocarp (*Hypophthalmichthys molitrix*) being the most popular species. In recent years, the monoculture of the introduced species, Nile tilapia (*Oreochromis niloticus*) and pangas (*Pangasianodon hypophthalmus*) in ponds and closed waterbodies has been growing rapidly. Also, large areas near the coast have been converted to shrimp farms. Marine and coastal catches have grown to a certain extent due to the use of mechanized trawlers and new gears; however, in recent years, decline in catches has been reported, due to overfishing (Mazid, 2002).

Trends in fish intake

Official national data for fish production and catch are an inadequate proxy for intake, as it is well-recognized that these data fail to capture fish bought in small,

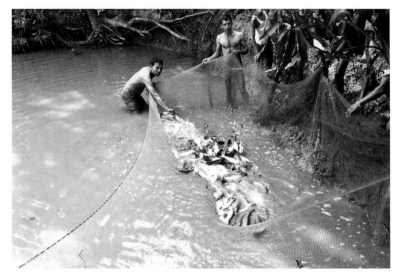

Figure C4.2 Pond polyculture in Bangladesh. Photograph by Finn Thilsted

rural markets, as well as fish caught by household members for consumption. Data from consumption surveys carried out in rural Bangladesh are used. In national rural consumption surveys conducted in 1962–1964 and 1981–1982, the average fish intake was 28 g fish/capita/d and 23 g fish/capita/d, respectively (Thompson et al., 2002). Data from household (rural and urban) income and expenditure report fish intakes of 38 g fish/capita/d and 40 g fish/capita/d, in 2000 and 2005, respectively (Bangladesh Bureau of Statistics, 2005).

Several rural surveys have shown the effect of location, seasonality, year and household socio-economic status on fish consumption. In a survey conducted in 1997–1998, in Kishoreganj, an area in northern Bangladesh with rich fisheries resources, the average fish intake in the peak fish production season (October), 82 g raw, edible parts/person/d, was more than double that in the lean season (July). Fish intake data were collected by size of fish: small indigenous fish species (SIS, growing to a maximum length of 25 cm) and large fish; the intake of SIS was two-thirds of total fish intake (Roos, 2001). Surveys in Mymensingh, in 1996–1997, in three different seasons, among households practising pond polyculture of carps showed that in the low-income tertile households, the average intake of SIS was 76 g raw fish/capita/d, more than twice that of large fish. The high-income tertile consumed 44 per cent more fish in total than the low-income tertile, with a smaller proportion of SIS, 60 per cent of total fish intake, than large fish (Bouis et al., 1998). In a survey conducted in two rural upazilas in northern Bangladesh, in one upazila, in October 2007–May 2008, and in the other, in January–June 2007, the usual mean fish intake in women ($n = 455$) was estimated at 12 g fish/woman/d (5th–95th percentile: 2.1–34.2) (Yakes et al., 2011). It is important that fish intake data are collected at species level, and both interviewees and interviewers pay special attention to the intake of small fish, consumed fresh, as well as dried and fermented (M.A.R. Hossain, personal communication, 20 October 2010).

The frequency of fish consumption in Bangladesh is high, ranking second (after rice) or third (after rice and vegetables). In a survey on biodiversity of fisheries and nutrition in four rural areas, in 520 households in total, during three seasons in 1992 (a drought year, the lowest flood levels in the preceding 20 years), 7 days' household food frequency consumption was conducted (Minkin et al., 1997). Fish was consumed by 85 per cent of households at least once per week; and the average number of days per week of fish consumption was 3.5. In the Nutrition Surveillance Project implemented by Helen Keller International (HKI), the frequency of consumption in seven days preceding an interview of four nutrient-rich foods – eggs, fish, green leafy vegetables and lentils – was collected for over 51,000 rural children, aged 12–59 months, twice a month, in 2000. The fish was the most frequently eaten of these four foods (HKI, 2002). A similar food frequency consumption pattern was recorded in mothers of children less than five years of age, in rural Bangladesh in 2005. Fish was the second most frequently consumed food, after rice; followed by milk, lentils, green leafy vegetables, eggs, red/orange/yellow vegetables and fruits, chicken and meat, in descending order of frequency of consumption (J. Waid, personal communication, 28 February 2011).

The diversity of fish species consumption in Bangladesh is very high. In the above-mentioned study in Kishoreganj, 44 common names for fish and two common names for shrimp were recorded (Roos, 2001). One SIS, puti (*Puntius* spp), consumed both fresh and fermented, covering 10 species accounted for 26 per cent of the total fish intake; and five species, puti, silver carp, taki (*Channa punctata*), baim/chikra (*Macrognathus aculeatus, M. pancalus, Mastacembalus armatus*) and mola (*Amblypharyngodon mola*); in descending order of proportion of total weight of fish consumption made up 57 per cent of total fish intake (Roos et al., 2003). In the above-mentioned study in four rural areas, a total of 75 fish species were consumed; small fish accounted for 43 per cent of the total fish intake (kg/household/y); catfish and carp, 13 per cent; hilsa, 9 per cent; and snakehead, 7 per cent (Minkin et al., 1997).

Even though the quantity of fish consumed may be low and probably continues to decrease among the rural poor, the high frequency of fish consumption and diversity of fish species consumed perhaps reflect the positive perceptions of fish, in particular SIS, for good nutrition, health and well-being (Thilsted and Roos, 1999; Deb and Haque, 2011).

The nutritional contribution of fish consumption

Fish, especially SIS, are a rich animal-source food of multiple, essential, highly bioavailable nutrients; animal protein, and some, for example hilsa, have a high content of fat and beneficial polyunsaturated fatty acids. As shown in Table C4.1, some common SIS – mola, chanda (*Chanda nama, Parambassis ranga, Pseudambassis baculis*), dhela (*Ostreobrama cotio cotio*) and darkina (*Esomus*

Table C4.1 Vitamin A, calcium, iron, and zinc contents in selected, common fish species in Bangladesh

		Contents per 100 g raw, cleaned parts (mean ± SD (n)[a]				
Common name[b]	Scientific name	Vitamin A RAE[c]	Calcium g	Calcium[d] g	Iron mg	Zinc mg
Small indigenous fish species						
Baim/Chikra	Macrognathus aculeatus	90 ± 15 (3)	0.4 ± 0.1 (5)	0.2 ± 0.0 (5)	2.4 ± 0.4 (5)	1.2 ± 0.2 (5)
	Macrognathus pancalus	30 90 (1)	—[e]	—	—	—
	Mastacembalus armatus	(1)	—	—	—	—
Chanda	Parambassis ranga	1679 ± 1000 (3)	1.0 ± 0.3 (5)	0.9 ± 0.3 (5)	1.8 ± 0.7 (5)	2.3 ± 0.6 (5)
	Parambassis baculis	340 ± 105 (3)	—	—	—	—
	Chanda nama	170 (1)	—	—	—	—
Darkina	Esomus danricus	890 ± 380 (3)	0.9 ± 0.4 (3)	0.8 ± 0.3 (3)	12.0 ± 9.1 (3)	4.0 ± 1.0 (3)
Dhela	Rohtee cotio	937 (1)	1.3	—	—	—
Kachki	Corica soborna	90 ± 20 (7)	0.5 ± 0.0 (2)	0.4 ± 0.0 (2)	2.8 ± 1.2 (2)	3.1 ± 0.5 (2)
Mola	Amblypharyngodon mola	2680 ± 390 (7)	0.9 ± 0.1 (3)	0.8 ± 0.0 (3)	5.7 ± 3.7 (3)	3.2 ± 0.5 (3)
Puti	Puntius sophore	60 ± 20 (3)	1.2 ± 0.2 (4)	0.8 ± 0.1 (4)	3.0 ± 0.9 (4)	3.1 ± 0.5 (4)
	Puntius chola	70 (1)	—	—	—	—
	Puntius ticto	20 (1)	—	—	—	—
Taki	Channa punctatus	140 ± 45 (3)	0.8 ± 0.2 (3)	0.3 ± 0.1 (3)	1.8 ± 0.4 (3)	1.5 ± 0.2 (3)

Commonly cultured large fish species: carp

Mrigal	*Cirrhinus cirrhosus*	< 30 (1)	1.0 ± 0.1 (3)	0.0 ± 0.0 (3)	2.5 ± 1.3 (3)	—
Silver carp	*Hypophthalmichthys molitrix*	< 30 (3)	0.9 ± 0.4 (3)	0.0 ± 0.0 (3)	4.4 ± 1.8 (3)	—

Notes
a n: number of samples. For small indigenous fish species, a sample consisted of 10–300 fish and for large fish, 1–2 fish.
b Fish species are listed in alphabetical order in each sub-group.
c RAE: retinol activity equivalent
d In raw, edible parts, after correcting for calcium in the plate waste (mainly bones)
e —: not measured
Sources: Thilsted et al., 1997; Roos et al., 2007a

danricus) – have high contents of vitamin A. As most SIS are eaten whole, with bones, they are also a very rich source of highly bioavailable calcium. Darkina has a high iron and zinc content (Roos et al., 2007a). In the above-mentioned study in Kishoreganj, SIS contributed 40 per cent and 31 per cent of the total recommended intakes of vitamin A and calcium, respectively, at household level, in the peak fish production season (Roos et al., 2006). In addition, fish enhances the bioavailability of iron and zinc from the other foods in a meal (Aung-Than-Batu et al., 1976). The edible parts of large cultured fish such as silver carp, tilapia and pangas do not contain vitamin A, iron or zinc, and as the bones of large fish are discarded as plate waste, they do not contribute to calcium intake (Roos et al., 2007b).

Measures to promote and protect fish biodiversity and fish consumption

Reduction in biodiversity of indigenous freshwater fish species in Bangladesh is a major concern, with 15 per cent of species reported to have disappeared, 20 per cent critically endangered, and the rate of disappearance increasing in recent years (IUCN Bangladesh, 2000). Over the last six decades, 23 fish species have been introduced in Bangladesh, mainly for cultivation in closed pond systems. It is reported that the escape of these species to rivers and floodplains during the monsoon and floods is a threat to the biodiversity of SIS, as some are highly carnivorous and predatory (Hossain and Wahab, 2010). Many other factors contribute to decreasing fish biodiversity and production, including rapid population growth, water pollution by industry, natural disasters, sea intrusion, salinity, overexploitation of fisheries, use of harmful gears and dewatering of waterbodies.

Conservation and management of common fishery resources and fish migration routes are crucial for promotion and protection of biodiversity, as well as fish consumption. Community-based and community-managed fisheries approaches, ensuring fishers access rights and tackling the diverse interests of various stakeholders, offer opportunities for improving fish diversity and increasing fish intake, in particular of SIS. These approaches are important for the rural poor – 60 per cent being functionally landless, lacking access to land and water for agricultural production, and dependent, to some extent, on common resources for their livelihoods and food.

Work initiated in 1994 in Sigharagi Beel, north-central Bangladesh, on the re-establishment of fish migratory routes, through rehabilitating a channel to floodplains by desiltation resulted in restoration of fish habitats. A five-fold increase in total fish production, a doubling of the proportion of fish (mainly SIS) caught and consumed by the landless and small farmers, and an increase in the number of fish species (mainly SIS) from 46 to 64, pre- to post-restoration were recorded (Center for Natural Resource Studies, 1996).

The Management of Aquatic Ecosystems through Community Husbandry (MACH) projects (1998–2003) included interventions to restore three major

Box C4.1 Shefali and her family no longer depend on Hail Haor (wetlands ecosystem) for their livelihood and income

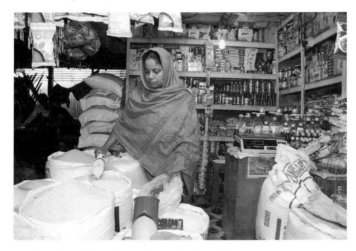

Figure C4.3 Shefali in her shop, selling rice to a villager

"The Hail Haor (a large shallow lake in north-east Banagladesh) resources were disappearing day by day due to overexploitation by the people. Our livelihood was under great threat and our daily income was decreasing. We had little money and many days we did not have enough food to eat". These were the words of Shefali Khatun (about 35 years of age), a woman from Hajipur village, Maulvi Bazar district, describing the dependence of her family – and many others – on the Hail Haor, before the MACH project. "I was a housewife and mother of a son; my husband, Korom Ali, was a fisherman and he also caught birds in the Haor. Our livelihood was fully dependent on the Hail Haor", Shefali said, in an interview in 2004.

"I heard about the MACH project and got interested to protect the Haor. I became a member of the Machranga Mohila Samity, a Resource User Group (RUG) for women. My husband and I received skill development training. Afterwards, I took a small loan of BDT 5,000 and began buying and selling rice. As my business grew, I took more loans and bought some cows. As my savings grew, I opened a small shop. My husband helps me with my work, especially in buying goods for my shop from the market."

Shefali has paid back all her loans. She has supported her husband in starting a small business, buying and selling dried small fish. He no longer catches fish or birds in the Haor. "Today, my family lives well; I have purchased a small piece of land and leased a fish pond for two years. My son goes to school and is in fifth grade. We are all happy."

Box C4.2 Shanti has expanded her fish pond after one year of fish farming

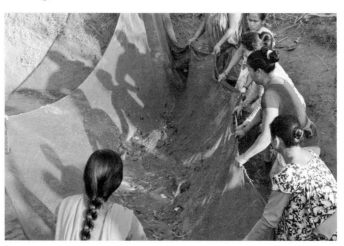

Figure C4.4 Shanti and her neighbours harvesting fish from her pond

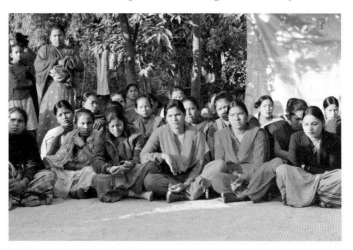

Figure C4.5 Shanti and other Nepalese women farmers attend a field trip in Bangladesh

Shanti Mahato lives with her husband, two young sons and her parents-in-law in Khairini village, Chitwan, Nepal. She received project support to dig a pond (100 m²) in 2010 and stock carps and small fish. Together with other women in her village, she received training in pond polyculture. In a period of 9 months, Shanti and her family consumed about 20 kg of fish and sold 25 kg for NPR 4,200. She reported that her family enjoys eating fish, especially small fish as they are tasty. Together with about 20 women farmers, Shanti visited Bangladesh on a one-week trip in 2011. She was pleasantly surprised to see that pond polyculture was very popular in Bangladesh and the farmers knew a lot about fish production. She found the growing of many different vegetables on the dykes of the ponds very interesting and began this practice when she returned home. However, as her pond is small, not many vegetables could be planted on the dykes. She also expanded her pond to 130 m². Shanti is an active member of a women's farmer group and spends time going to nearby villages to teach women farmers about fish production in ponds. She likes fish farming and plans to convert a rice field to a big fish pond.

wetland habitats, ensure sustainable productivity and improve the livelihoods of the poor who depend on these wetlands, through community based co-management. Activities included forming community organizations and links to local government, excavation of beels and canals to expand dry season water holding, establishment of fish sanctuaries and a closed fishing season, release of indigenous fish species, and tree planting. In Hail Haor, north-east Bangladesh, data were collected for the baseline year (April 1999 – March 2000) and intervention years (April 2000 – March 2003). The number of fish species increased from 71 (baseline year) to 85 (average of three intervention years); average fish consumption increased from 45 g/capita/d (baseline year) to 61 g/capita/d (third intervention year); small fish species, consumed fresh, dried and fermented, accounted for 85 per cent of average total consumption; and the proportions of fish consumed which were caught or bought from rural markets were 30 per cent and 70 per cent, respectively (Anonymous, 2003).

Conclusions

Biodiversity of fish species is important for nutrition and livelihoods of the rural poor in Bangladesh. There are promising fisheries technologies which have been developed and are being practised for improving fish biodiversity and nutrition. More stakeholders are becoming aware of the importance of small fish species, both freshwater and marine, for improving human nutrition, and the implications for national development. The Bangladesh Country Investment Plan (CIP), a roadmap towards investment in agriculture, food security and nutrition (2011–2016), the CGIAR Research Programs, and other initiatives such as Feed the Future and Scaling Up Nutrition (SUN): 1,000 Days provide good opportunities for developing and implementing interventions which can improve fish biodiversity and increase fish consumption in Bangladesh.

Box C4.3 Practices to increase production of small fish species

Carp production, together with management of indigenous fish species, including enforcement of fishing regulatory measures were carried out in a large beel (40 ha), in north-west Bangladesh. This approach resulted in a total fish production of over 25 tonnes in 6 months, of which 45 per cent were non-stocked fish, mainly SIS (Rahman et al., 2008). Depending on geographical location and season, different culture practices with fish and rice can increase fish diversity, as well as the nutritional quality of the combined rice and fish production. Allowing fish in ponds access to rice fields with water, as well as concurrent or rotational rice–fish culture technologies are being practised (Dewan et al., 2003; Kunda et al., 2009).

Recognizing the above-described nutritional contribution of SIS, polyculture of carps and SIS, especially mola, in small ponds was introduced in the late 1990s. No significant difference in total fish production was seen between ponds stocked with carps and mola, and those with carps alone. However, the nutritional quality of the total fish production improved considerably in the ponds with mola. In this production system, the eradication of indigenous species, the majority being SIS by repeated netting, dewatering, and the use of a piscicide, rotenone, prior to stocking of carp fingerlings – based on the rationale that competition exists between native and stocked fish – was stopped. In addition to the production of carps, production of the vitamin A rich-mola of only 10 kg/pond/y in the estimated 4 million small, seasonal ponds in Bangladesh can meet the annual recommended vitamin A intake of 6 million children (Roos et al., 2007b). This production technology of carp–mola pond polyculture has gained wide acceptance by the government and development partners in Bangladesh, and is also being practised in Sundarbans, West Bengal and Terai, Nepal.

References

Anonymous (2003) MACH Completion report: Management of Aquatic Ecosystems through Community Husbandry, Fish catch & consumption survey report, Vol 3, http://pdf.usaid.gov/pdf_docs/PDACK308.pdf, accessed August 2012.

Aung-Than-Batu, Thein-Than, Thane-Toe (1976) "Iron absorption from Southeast Asian rice-based meals" *American Journal of Clinical Nutrition*, vol 29, pp.219–225.

Bangladesh Bureau of Statistics (BBS) (2005) *Report of the Household Income and Expenditure Survey 2005*, BBS, Dhaka.

Bouis, H., De la Briére, B., Halman, K., Hassan, N., Hels, O., Quabili, W., Quisumbing, A., Thilsted, S.H., Zihad, Z.H., Zohir, S. (1998) "Commercial vegetable and polyculture fish production in Bangladesh: their impacts on income, household resource allocation and nutrition" Final project report to DANIDA and USAID, International Food Policy Research Institute (IFPRI), Washington DC.

Center for Natural Resource Studies (CNRS) (1996) "Community-based fisheries management and habitat restoration project" Annual report July 1995 – June 1996, CNRS, Dhaka.

Craig, J.F., Halls, A.S., Bean, C.W. (2004) "The Bangladesh floodplain fisheries" *Fisheries Research*, vol 66, no 2–3, pp.271–286.

Deb, A.K. and Haque, C.E. (2011) "Every mother is a mini-doctor: ethnomedicinal use of fish, shellfish and some other aquatic animals in Bangladesh" *Journal of Ethnopharmacology*, vol 134, no 2, pp.259–267.

Department of Fisheries (2010) *Fisheries Statistical Year Book of Bangladesh*, Fisheries Resource Survey System, Dhaka.

Dewan, S., Chowdhury, M.T.H., Mondal, S., Das, B.C. (2003) "Monoculture of *Amblypharyngodon mola* and *Osteobrama cotio cotio* in rice fields and their polyculture with *Barbodes gonionotus* and *Cyprinus carpio*", in Md. A. Wahab, S.H. Thilsted, Md. E. Hoq (eds) *Small Indigenous Species of Fish in Bangladesh: Culture Potentials for Improved Nutrition and Livelihood*, Bangladesh Agricultural University, Mymensingh.

Helen Keller International (HKI) (2002) "Eggs are rarely eaten in rural Bangladesh: why and how to improve their availability" *Nutritional Surveillance Project Bulletin*, no 11, HKI, Dhaka.

Hossain, M.A.R. and Wahab, M.A., (2010) "The diversity of cypriniforms throughout Bangladesh: present status and conservation challenges", in G.H. Tepper (ed.) *Species Diversity and Extinction*, Nova Science Publishers, New York.

Islam, Md. S. and Haque, M. (2004) "The mangrove-based coastal and near shore fisheries of Bangladesh: ecology, exploitation and management" *Reviews in Fish Biology and Fisheries*, vol 14, pp.153–180.

IUCN Bangladesh (2000) *Red list of threatened animals of Bangladesh*, IUCN–The World Conservation Union, IUCN Bangladesh.

Kunda, M., Azim, M.E., Wahab, M.A., Dewan, S., Majid, M.A., Thilsted, S.H. (2009) "Effects of including catla and tilapia in a freshwater prawn-mola polyculture in a rotational rice-fish culture systems" *Aquaculture Research*, vol 40, no 9, pp.1089–1098.

Mazid, M.A. (2002) "Development for fisheries in Bangladesh: plan and strategies for income generation and poverty alleviation" N. Mazid, Dhaka.

Minkin, S.F., Rahman, M.M., Halder, S. (1997) "Fish biodiversity, human nutrition and environmental restoration in Bangladesh", in C. Tsai and M.Y. Ali (eds) *Openwater Fisheries of Bangladesh*, The University Press Limited, Dhaka.

Payne, A.I. and Temple, S.A. (1996) "River and floodplains fisheries in the Ganges Basin: final report", London Overseas Development Administration Fisheries Science Management Programme.

Rahman, A.K.A. (1989) *Freshwater fishes of Bangladesh*, Zoological Society of Bangladesh, Dhaka.

Rahman, M.F., Barman, B.K., Ahmed, M.K., Dewan, S. (2008) "Technical issues on management of seasonal floodplains under community-based fish culture in Bangladesh" 2nd International Forum on Water and Food, Addis Ababa, Ethiopia, 10–14 November 2008, Proceedings of the CGIAR Challenge Programme on Water and Food, II, pp.258–261.

Roos, N. (2001) "Fish consumption and aquaculture in rural Bangladesh: nutritional contribution and production potential of culturing small indigenous fish species (SIS) in pond polyculture with commonly cultured carps" PhD thesis. Royal Veterinary and Agricultural University, Frederiksberg.

Roos, N., Islam, M., Thilsted, S.H. (2003) "Small fish is an important dietary source of vitamin A and calcium in rural Bangladesh" *International Journal of Food Sciences and Nutrition*, vol 54, pp.329–339.

Roos, N., Wahab, M.A., Chamnan, C., Thilsted, S.H. (2006) "Fish and health", in C. Hawkes and M.T. Ruel, (eds) *2020 Understanding the Links between Agriculture and Health*, Focus 13, Brief 10, International Food Policy Research Institute (IFPRI), Washington DC.

Roos, N., Wahab, M.A., Chamnan, C., Thilsted, S.H. (2007a) "The role of fish in food-based strategies to combat vitamin A and mineral deficiencies in developing countries" *Journal of Nutrition*, vol 137, pp.1106–1109.

Roos, N., Wahab, M.A., Hossain, M.A.R., Thilsted, S.H. (2007b) "Linking human nutrition and fisheries: incorporating micronutrient dense, small indigenous fish species in carp polyculture production in Bangladesh" *Food and Nutrition Bulletin*, vol 28, no 2 Supplement, pp.S280–S293.

Thilsted, S.H. and Roos, N. (1999) "Policy issues on fisheries and food and nutrition", in M. Ahmed, C. Delgado, S. Sverdrup-Jensen, R.A.V. Santos (eds) *Fisheries Policy Research in Developing Countries. Issues, Policies and Needs* ICLARM Conference Proceedings, vol 60, pp.61–69.

Thilsted, S.H., Roos, N., Hassan, N. (1997) "The role of small indigenous fish species in food and nutrition security in Bangladesh" *Naga, ICLARM Quarterly*, vol 20, nos 3 and 4 Supplement, pp.82–84.

Thompson, P., Roos, N., Sultana, P., Thilsted, S.H. (2002) "Changing significance of inland fisheries for livelihoods and nutrition in Bangladesh", in P.K. Kataki and S.C. Babu (eds) *Food Systems for Improved Human Nutrition: Linking Agriculture, Nutrition and Productivity*, Haworth Press, New York.

Yakes, E.A., Arsenault, J.E., Islam, M.M., Hossain, M.B., Ahmed, T., German, J.B., Gillies, L.A., Rahman, A.S., Drake, C., Jamil, K.M., Lewis, B.L., Brown, K.H. (2011) "Intakes and breast-milk concentrations of essential fatty acids are low among Bangladeshi women with 24–48-month-old children", *British Journal of Nutrition*, vol 105, no 11, pp.1660–1670.

Case study 5

The introduction of orange-fleshed sweet potato in Mozambican diets: a marginal change to make a major difference

Jan Low, Mary Arimond, Ricardo Labarta, Maria Andrade and Sam Namanda

Statement of the problem

Vitamin A is an essential micronutrient for human health. Vitamin A deficiency (VAD) can limit growth, weaken immunity, cause xeropthalmia leading to blindness, and increase mortality (Sommer and West, 1996). VAD is widespread among young children in sub-Saharan Africa (SSA), and in Mozambique the problem is severe with an estimated prevalence of 71 per cent in children 6–59 months of age (Nutrition Division in Department of Community Health, 2003). Food-based approaches to combating VAD aim to increase access to and intake of vitamin A-rich foods. They complement supplementation and food fortification approaches, particularly for reaching rural households with limited incomes for purchasing fortified products, but solid evidence for their effectiveness is limited (Ruel and Levin, 2000).

Why use orange-fleshed sweet potato (OFSP) as the key entry point?

There are two types of vitamin A available in foods: preformed retinol (vitamin A itself) typically found in animal foods such as eggs, liver, and milk; and pro-vitamin A carotenoids found in plant foods such as dark green leafy vegetables and yellow and orange vegetables and fruits (McLaren and Frigg, 2001). Poor households typically cannot afford to consume the highly bioavailable animal foods on a regular basis. β-carotene is the major pro-vitamin A carotenoid among plant sources and the bioavailability of that beta-carotene which is converted into vitamin A (retinol) varies considerably. Among plant sources, OFSP have good to excellent amounts of beta-carotene, which is highly bioavailable (Jaarsveld et al., 2005; Haskell et al., 2004). Just 100–125 g of boiled or steamed OFSP meet the daily recommended intake levels of vitamin A for children under five years of age (Low et al., 2009). Moreover, unlike many vegetables, the sweet potato has significant amounts of energy as well as vitamin A. Hence, OFSP is considered a biofortified staple food crop that can tackle the problem of inadequate caloric intake as well as VAD.

Sweet potato (*Ipomoea batatas (L.)*) exhibits a wide range of varietal diversity that results in it being grown from sea level to 2,300 m above sea level in SSA. Over 5,000 accessions are found in the germplasm bank maintained at the International Potato Center in Lima, Peru. Flesh colors cover the gamut of white, cream, yellow, orange, and purple. In SSA, the dominant landraces grown are white-fleshed, lacking in beta-carotene. The promotion of OFSP in SSA centers around asking households to make a marginal change in their sweet potato growing and consuming practices—eating orange instead of or in addition to white.

Delivery mechanism

The Towards Sustained Nutrition Improvement (TSNI) action research project was initiated in September 2002. Recognizing that the causes of VAD and undernutrition among young children are diverse, from the outset an integrated approach was adopted with three distinct pathways:

1 *Agriculture: Introduction of a new source of vitamin A and energy biofortified OFSP*
   Intervention farmers receive (principally through groups) planting material of high-yielding OFSP varieties, combined with lessons on how to improve crop management and storage practices to maximize the availability of OFSP in the diet throughout the year (Figure C5.1).

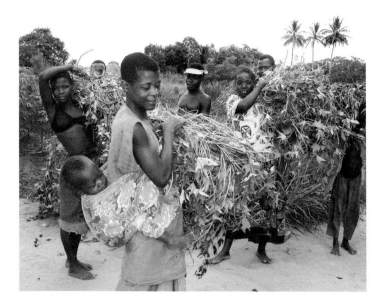

Figure C5.1 The project specifically targeted women with small children to receive OFSP vines. Credit: J.Low

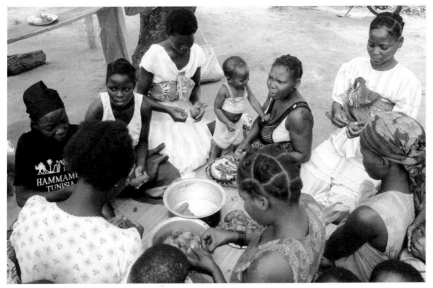

Figure C5.2 Women preparing sweet potato as part of porridge preparation during a group nutrition session. Credit: J.Low

2   *Nutrition: Demand creation and empowerment through knowledge*

At the village level, principal caregivers, both women and men, are encouraged and enabled to improve infant and young child feeding practices, hygiene practices, and diversify the household diet. A nutrition extensionist conducts monthly group sessions for a year (Figure C5.2). Demand creation efforts focus on building awareness among the broader community to create: 1) demand for the new OFSP cultivars and their derivatives, 2) demand for other vitamin A-rich foods, and 3) a supportive environment to accelerate behavior change at the household level. For the TSNI, these included six province-wide radio programs, three community theater performances (Figure C5.3), painted stalls and signs in local markets, t-shirts, caps and long cloths worn by women as skirts decorated with the slogan "O doce que dá saúde" (the sweet that gives health).

3   *Marketing: Market development for OFSP roots and processed products*

This component aims to link farmers to traders and to inform consumers about where they can purchase OFSP (Figure C5.4). Farmers with identified market outlets are more likely to expand the area under production. Thus, generated demand combined with market development stimulates production, enhances producer income and spreads the health benefits of OFSP to a wider population, all of which contribute to farmers' willingness to retain OFSP and expand production. Demand for OFSP is enhanced if profitable processed products using OFSP as a major ingredient are developed.

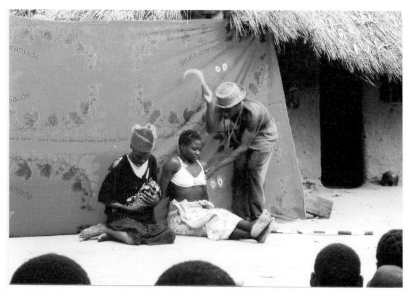

Figure C5.3 Community theater seeks to create a supportive environment for mothers to adopt improved caregiving practices. Credit: J.Low

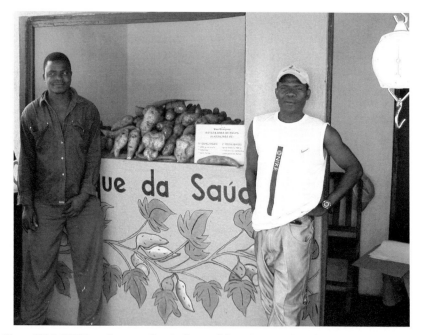

Figure C5.4 OFSP traders standing in front of their decorated roadside sales stall. Credit: J. Low

The intervention lasted 18 months in two of the poorest districts in rural Zambézia, Mozambique. World Vision, an international NGO, posted pairs of extensionists, one for agriculture and marketing, the other for nutrition at the community level, each pair serving 14 farmers groups. In total there were 498 mother–child pairs captured in the study that were compared with 243 mother–child pairs from "control" areas where no intervention was made.

Evidence of impact

The effectiveness of the intervention was evaluated after two agricultural cycles and findings published (Low et al., 2007). In the second year, 90 per cent of intervention households produced OFSP. Vitamin A intakes among intervention children ($n = 498$) were much higher than those of control children ($n = 243$) (median 426 vs. 56 μg retinol activity equivalents, $P < 0.001$). OFSP contributed 35 per cent of the total vitamin A intake of all children in the intervention area and 90 per cent among those who had consumed it the previous day. Serum retinol data were obtained as a proxy for vitamin A status. Controlling for infection/inflammation and other confounders, a 15 per cent decline in the prevalence of VAD was attributable to the integrated intervention. OFSP was well accepted and liked by both adults and children.

Scaling-up effort

The TSNI case study used an intensive package of activities that enabled us to demonstrate the potential for success in a community setting. The cost per beneficiary, however, was high (US$79 per direct plus indirect beneficiaries) (Labarta and Low, 2007) and hence the follow-up action research project, known as the Reaching End Users (REU) project (led by HarvestPlus), sought to lower the cost by introducing the use of village promoters and using existing church or farmers groups instead of engaging in new group formation. The integrated approach was retained, although the marketing component was restricted to areas with better market access. By working through promoters, extension personnel could reach a larger number of beneficiaries per extensionist and substantially reduce costs. Positive results were found, confirming that vitamin A intakes can be doubled in key target groups for a reasonable cost using the integrated approach with promoters (Hotz et al., 2011; HarvestPlus, 2010). In addition to the REU study, OFSP dissemination has been taking place on a broader scale in Mozambique but without the resources to measure the household-level consumption impact. Seminars and workshops have been held to disseminate findings and promote adoption. The monitoring of OFSP adoption is captured as part of the national agriculture survey, which is conducted periodically. As of 2008, 138,000 households were growing OFSP (Departamento de Estatística (Direcção de Economia), 2008).

Relevant stakeholders

From the outset of the OFSP effort, there was strong buy-in from the nutrition division of the Ministry of Health, because nutritionists doubted the financial sustainability of twice-yearly vitamin A supplement distribution and felt strongly that the underlying causes of vitamin A deficiency (inadequate intakes and disease) should be addressed. A nurse from the Ministry of Health was seconded to the project to lead the blood sampling and assist in the implementation of the nutrition component. The NGO, World Vision, collaborated with public sector agriculture extension in the establishment of maintenance of key vine multiplication sites. Another NGO, Helen Keller International, was contracted to develop the behavior change strategy and produce the radio programs. The Institute of Agronomic Research for Mozambique (INIA) was a full partner, providing the initial cuttings of the eight OFSP varieties used in the project. INIA, now reorganized and known as IIAM (Institute for Agrarian Research in Mozambique), is backstopped by a resident sweet potato breeder from the International Potato Center.

Policy impact

A stakeholder's workshop was held at the onset of the OFSP promotion effort and a six-page policy brief was disseminated on the potential for OFSP in Mozambique (Low et al., 2000). The use of food-based approaches and OFSP is recognized as an excellent source of vitamin A in the government's current nutrition strategy. The sweet potato is recognized in agriculture policy documents for its role as a crop to mitigate drought and to recover from floods. The Food and Nutritional Security Strategy II 2008–2015 (ESAN) has incorporated the basic human right to adequate food and recognizes the need to increase local production of adequate food to cover nutritional needs in terms of quantity (energy) and quality (which ensures all essential nutrients) (Bulletin of the Republic, 2007). Mozambique has a Technical Secretariat for Food Security and Nutrition (SETSAN) that coordinates, promotes, monitors and evaluates the activities carried out by line organizations of the Government and others involved in food and nutrition security. A SETSAN representative is a member of the Sweetpotato Support Platform (SSP) for Southern Africa, created in 2010 for sharing experiences and backstopping varietal development and seed systems. The SSP for Southern Africa is based in Maputo due to Mozambique's decade-long experience in developing and promoting OFSP.

The Mozambican experience, combined with findings from other studies in Uganda and Kenya, has provided vital evidence that is being used by members of the Vitamin A for Africa (VITAA) platform and others to attract funding for the development and use of locally adapted OFSP varieties and their promotions. Currently, 15 countries are actively engaged in OFSP-related activities (Kenya, Ethiopia, Uganda, Tanzania, Rwanda, Malawi, Zambia, Mozambique, Madagascar, DR Congo, Angola, South Africa, Burkina Faso, Ghana, Nigeria) and are exchanging information through the Sweet potato for Profit and Health Initiative (launched in October 2009) and the Sweet potato Knowledge Portal (www.sweetpotatoknowledge.org, accessed July 2012). The extent of activities within a given country varies, driven by available human and financial resources.

Key lessons learned

There have been four major lessons growing out of the OFSP promotion experience to date in Mozambique. First, all age groups enjoy consuming OFSP and it can make significant impacts on vitamin A intakes and status when it is available. The orange color proved to be an advantage, not a disadvantage, for an agriculture intervention with a clear nutritional message. Second, adults and children can differ in their varietal preferences. Adults in general prefer more floury textures (higher dry matter content) than young children do. This is relevant because introduced OFSP germplasm from the Americas tends to have lower dry matter content than existing African varieties, including the limited number of OFSP African varieties that have been collected and used in promotion programs in SSA. Third, the most important constraint to expanded and sustained sweet potato production is the timely availability of quality planting material at the beginning of the rains. We tested various distribution methods and found that for drought-prone areas establishing trained farmer multipliers with water access to serve their local communities is preferable to periodic mass distribution efforts. In addition, a new method (the Triple S method) of storing small but healthy roots in a bucket of sand during the dry season and re-sprouting in protected seed beds prior to the rains is a promising solution for rural farmers with limited dry season water access. Fourth, for sustained adoption, it is necessary to invest in actual breeding efforts in Africa to have materials that are sufficiently adapted to local conditions. It has been discovered that the most preferred variety found in the TSNI project for its taste, yield, and excellent shape for marketing, Resisto, did not have vines sufficiently vigorous as the local varieties to withstand the dry season or alternatively, re-sprout in adequate amounts at the beginning of the rains. This led to the seeking and obtaining of funds to launch an accelerated breeding effort to produce more drought-tolerant OFSP for Mozambique. In early 2011, 15 new improved OFSP varieties were released and will form the foundation for a major dissemination effort to reach 120,000 households beginning in December 2011.

References

Bulletin of the Republic (2007) Resolution Nr. 56/2007 Food and Nutrition Security Strategy, Maputo: Government of Mozambique.

Departamento de Estatistica (Direcção de Economia) (2008) *Trabalho do Inquérito Agrícola 2008* [*National Agricultural Survey for Mozambique 2008*], Maputo: Ministério da Agricultura.

Harvestplus (2010) *Disseminating Orange-Fleshed Sweet Potato: Findings From a HarvestPlus project in Mozambique and Uganda*, Washington DC: HarvestPlus.

Haskell, M.J., Jamil, K.M., Hassan, F., Peerson, J.M., Hossain, M.I., Fuchs, G.J. and Brown, K.H. (2004) "Daily consumption of Indian spinach (*Basella alba*) or sweet potatoes has a positive effect on total body vitamin A stores in Bangadeshi men" *American Journal of Clinical Nutrition*, vol 80, pp.705–714.

Hotz, C., Loechl, C., Braum, A.D., Eozenou, P., Gillagan, D., Moursi, M., Munhaua, B., Van Jaarsveld, P., Carriquiry, A. and Meenakshi, J.V. (2011) "A large-scale intervention to introduce orange sweet potato in rural Mozambique increases vitamin A intakes among children and women" *British Journal of Nutrition*, pp.1–14, doi: 10.1017/S0007114511005174.

Jaarsveld, P.V., Faber, M., Tanumihardjo, S.A., Nestel, P., Lombard, C.J. and Benade, A.J. (2005) "Beta-carotene-rich orange-fleshed sweet potato improves the vitamin A status of primary school children assessed with the modified-relative-dose-response test" *American Journal of Clinical Nutrition*, vol 81, pp.1080–1087.

Labarta, R. and Low, J.W. (2007) "Can integrated agriculture-nutrition extension programs deliver cost-effectively? Evidence from the dissemination of vitamin A rich orange-fleshed sweet potato in Mozambique", Working Paper, International Potato Center.

Low, J., Uaiene, R., Andrade, M.I. and Howard, J. (2000) Orange-flesh Sweet Potato: Promising Partnerships for Assuring the Integration of Nutritional Concerns into Agricultural Research and Extension in Mozambique [Online]. Maputo: Ministry of Agriculture and Rural Development (Mozambique), Directorate of Economics, Flash No. 20E, http://ageconsearch.umn.edu/bitstream/55215/2/flash20e.pdf, accessed August 2012.

Low, J.W., Arimond, M., Osman, N., Cunguara, B., Zano, F. and Tschirley, D. (2007) "A food-based approach introducing orange-fleshed sweet potatoes increased vitamin A intake and serum retinol concentrations in young children in rural Mozambique" *J Nutr*, vol 137, pp.1320–1327.

Low, J.W., Lynam, J., Lemaga, B., Crissman, C., Barker, I., Thiele, G., Namanda, S., Wheatley, C. and Andrade, M. (2009) "Sweetpotato in Sub-Saharan Africa", In: G. Loebenstein and G. Thottappilly (eds) *The Sweet potato*, Dordrecht: Springer Science + Business Media BV.

McLaren, D.S. and Frigg, M. (2001) *Sight and Life guidebook on vitamin A in health and disease*, Basel, Switzerland, Task Force Sight and Life.

Nutrition Division in Department of Community Health (2003) National survey about vitamin A deficiency, anaemia prevalence, and malaria in children 6–59 months of age and their respective mothers, Maputo: Ministry of Health (Mozambique).

Ruel, M.T. and Levin, C.E. (2000) "Assessing the potential for food-based strategies to reduce vitamin A and iron deficiencies: a review of recent evidence", FCND Discussion Paper No. 92. Washington DC: Food Consumption and Nutrition Division, International Food Policy Institute.

Sommer, A. and West, K.P. (1996) *Vitamin A deficiency: health, survival, and vision*, Oxford University Press, UK.

Case study 6

Diversifying diets: using indigenous vegetables to improve profitability, nutrition and health in Africa

C. Ojiewo, A. Tenkouano, J. d'A. Hughes and J.D.H. Keatinge

Introduction

The picture of malnutrition in Africa is quite depressing: 20–25 per cent of the population's nutrient intake falls below minimum dietary requirements, 25–30 per cent of children under five years of age are underweight, 33–45 per cent suffer from vitamin A deficiency (VAD), while a further 30–50 per cent are stunted. There is more than 25 per cent goitre prevalence among 6–11 year olds, 13–20 per cent have low birth weights, and infant mortality rates stand at an unacceptable 5.5–13.5 per cent (Kean et al., 1999). Even more alarming is an 18 per cent rise in the number of malnourished children projected by 2020 (IFPRI, 2001).

Imbalanced diets lead to nutrient deficiencies. Efforts to combat micronutrient deficiencies through biofortification of staple crops or by diet supplementation with vitamins or minerals are relatively expensive and can target only a few nutritional factors. Indigenous vegetables are rich in provitamin A and vitamin C, several mineral micronutrients, other micronutrients and nutraceuticals (Yang and Keding, 2009). Diversifying diets with indigenous vegetables is a sustainable way to supply a range of nutrients to the body and combat malnutrition and associated health problems, particularly for poor households. The relative increased costs of crop diversification would be one-off and minor in relation to the ongoing costs of supplementation through drug treatment or through artificial food additives.

Genetic diversity and health-related benefits of indigenous vegetables in Africa

There are about 400 well-defined plant species encompassing 53 botanical families that are primarily used as vegetables in Africa (PROTA, 2004). More than 90 per cent of these species are either indigenous or ancient introductions to Africa and only 8 per cent are recent introductions regarded as standard global vegetables (PROTA, 2009).

Most indigenous vegetables are collected from the wild, or occur as volunteer plants in crop fields; more recently domestication and cultivation has been on a steady rise (Chweya and Eyzaguirre, 1999; Oniang'o et al., 2006). Amaranth, spider plant, African nightshade (*Solanum scabrum*), African eggplant, vegetable cowpea (*Vigna unguiculata*), and jute mallow (*Corchorus olitorius*) are considered as the most important crop species across communities and borders (PROTA, 2004). The genebank collection of the World Vegetable Center (AVRDC) in Arusha, Tanzania, holds 2,659 indigenous vegetable accessions of 48 species (Table C6.1), the largest in Africa to date. This genebank acts as the primary source of breeding material for the development of new varieties by AVRDC and its partners in the public and private sectors. It is an essential resource for the participatory, farmer-focused variety selection process that AVRDC and its partners have adopted.

High levels of minerals, especially calcium, iron and phosphorus, vitamins A and C and proteins are found in indigenous vegetables (Nesamvuni et al., 2001). These are of particular health value to vulnerable groups such as pregnant and nursing mothers (Table C6.2). Spider plant, roselle and hair lettuce are excellent sources of iron (Weinberger and Msuya, 2004) while African nightshade, jute mallow, and moringa (*Moringa oleifera*) are substantive sources of provitamin A (Muchiri, 2004). Within poor households, approximately 50 per cent of all vitamin A requirements and 30 per cent of iron requirements are provided by the consumption of indigenous vegetables (Weinberger and Msuya, 2004). Spider plant has been reported to retain up to 90 per cent of its vitamin C when boiled (Sreeramulu et al., 1983).

Many indigenous vegetables also contain a variety of nutraceuticals such as allylic sulfides, beta-carotene, flavonoids, genistein, isothiocyanates, limonoids, lycopene, phenolic acids, and phytoestrogens, many of which are antioxidants that prevent or ameliorate disease symptoms. Strong associations between these nutraceuticals and immunity enhancement and prevention of chronic diseases have been reported (German and Dillard, 1998). Indigenous vegetables have been reported to show antioxidant, antiviral, antibacterial, anti-inflammatory and anti-mutagenic activities (Yang and Keding, 2009).

Nutritionally well-balanced diets improve the control of HIV infection and mitigate the health impact of AIDS (FAO, 2002). Chronic malnutrition, especially micronutrient deficiency, has a progressive and synergistic relationship with HIV/AIDS (Beisel, 2001). Early HIV infection is accompanied by certain micronutrient deficiencies (vitamin A and zinc) that play an important role in both the transmission of HIV and its progression (Kean et al., 2001). Improving nutrition thus strengthens the immune system against secondary infection, delays the progression of HIV/AIDS and reduces transmission from mother to child (Kean et al., 2001). Indigenous vegetables have strong nutritional and nutraceutical potential to provide a good interface between food and nutritional security and HIV/AIDS (Gari, 2003). Consumption of moringa, for example, has been demonstrated to improve the health conditions of HIV/AIDS patients by increasing the Cluster of Differentiation 4 (CD4) cells and lowering virus counts (Hirt and Lindsey, 2005).

Table C6.1 A list of the active germplasm collection of strategically important indigenous vegetables preserved and potentially used in breeding at the AVRDC genebank in Arusha, Tanzania

Vegetable Crop	Genus and species	No. of Species	No. of Accessions
Amaranth	Amaranth cruentus, A. dubius, A. graecizans, A. hybridus, A. hypochondriachus, A. retroflexus, A. shimbuya, A. thunbergii	9	546
African eggplant	Solanum aethiopicum, S. anguivi, S. macrocarpon	3	466
African nightshade	Solanum americanum, S. chenopodioides, S. cochabambense, S. eldoretianum, S. nigrum, S. nigrescens, S. nodiflorum, S. opacum, S. retroflexum, S. sarrachiodes, S. scabrum, S. villosum	12	328
Ethiopian mustard	Brassica carinata	1	154
Jute mallow	Corchorus olitorius	1	35
Hyacinth bean	Lablab purpureus	1	51
Moringa	Moringa oleifera	1	6
Mungbean	Vigna radiata	1	80
Okra	Abelmoschus caillei, A. esculentus, A. ficulneus, A. manihot	4	316
Pumpkin	Cucurbita maxima, C. moschata	2	77
Roselle	Hibiscus sabdariffa	1	297
Spider plant	Cleome gynandra	1	107
Vegetable cowpea	Vigna unguiculata	1	142
Bitter gourd	Momordica charantia	1	1
Ivy gourd	Coccinia grandis	1	1
Lagos spinach	Celosia argentea	1	1
Marigold	Tagetes erecta	1	2
Peas	Pisum sativum	1	1
Sword bean	Canavalia gladiata	1	1
Velvet beans	Mucuna pruriens	1	1
Galant soldier	Galinsoga parviflora	1	1
Sun hemp	Crotolaria spp.	2	2
Total		48	2,616

Table C6.2 Recommended nutrient intakes (RNI)[a] for women in the first trimester of pregnancy and percentage nutrient intake from 100 g of food[b]

	Protein	Vitamin A	Iron	Folate	Zinc	Calcium	Vitamin E
RNI for pregnant women (1st trimester)							
	60 g	800 µg RE[c]	30 mg	600 µg DFE[d]	11 mg	1000 mg	7.5 mg α-TE[e]
Percentage of RNI from 100 gm food							
Rice	0	0	1	2	4	0	0
Cassava (root)	2	0	1	5	3	2	0
Millet	6	0	2	14	8	0	0
Meat (chicken)	37	0	3	1	14	1	3
Mungbean	40	2	22	104	24	13	7
Vegetable soybean	18	2	13	28	13	4	78
Cabbage	3	1	1	10	2	4	2
Tomato	2	18	1	3	2	1	7
Slippery cabbage	6	106	5	30–177	11	18	58
Moringa leaves	7	146	11	49	5	10	65
Amaranth	9	160	6	31	6	32	17
Jute mallow	10	198	12	21	0	36	36
Nightshade	8	101	13	10	9	21	28
Vegetable cowpea leaves	8	193	6	27	3	54	101

a   RNI: data souce: FAO/WHO 2004. RNI for populations of pregnant women (1st trimester) and diets of low iron and zinc bioavailabilty.
b   Nutrient data sources: AVRDC nutrition laboratory and USDA nutrient database (USDA, 2010)
c   RE: retinol equivalent: 1 µg RE = 6 µg β-carotene α = 12 µg α-carotene
d   DFE: dietary folate equivalent, 1 µg DFE = 0.6 µg of folic acid supplement.
e   α-TE: α-tocopherol equivalent; 1 mg α-TE = 1 mg d-α-tocopherol = 1 mg d-α-tocopherol = 0.5 mg d-α-tocopherol.

Linking farmers to markets and marketing indigenous vegetables

Traditionally, indigenous vegetables were grown in homestead gardens for subsistence and rarely traded. However this has changed over the past decade and indigenous vegetables now contribute substantially to household incomes (Pasquini and Young, 2007). This is partly attributed to deliberate market demand creation through concerted promotion and public awareness efforts. Such efforts have been led by staff of Bioversity International allied with local non-governmental organizations (NGOs), rural communities and AVRDC (Moore and Raymond, 2006; Oniang'o et al., 2006; Irungu et al., 2007). Urban consumers now appreciate indigenous vegetables as rich sources of important nutrients as well as traditional flavours, while farmers recognize them as valuable commercial crops. Linking producer groups to market outlets in both formal and informal markets has led to a shift in production trends particularly in Tanzania, where an estimated 70 per cent of the vegetables grown and marketed in rural and peri-urban areas are indigenous vegetables, while in Kenya a 135 per cent market growth for these vegetables was realized between 2002 and 2006.

Promoting the consumption of indigenous vegetables

AVRDC employs an inclusive participatory approach to variety development that involves joint evaluation and demonstration with various stakeholders. This approach ensures the continual flow of information from farmers and consumers to researchers and back to farmers for the identification of new varieties that meet market/consumer demand. The new varieties are promoted through demonstrations, field days, seed fairs, information leaflets, distribution of seed kits for home gardens, training programmes for farmers, and workshops in collaboration with seed companies, NGOs, and National Agricultural Research and Extension Services (NARES). For example, in partnership with Farm Concern International, AVRDC and Bioversity International have introduced and promoted new lines of various indigenous vegetables in Kenya and Tanzania, successfully competing with standard vegetables in supermarkets. Currently, several supermarkets in Nairobi have attractive displays of indigenous vegetables while some restaurants, such as Ranalo Foods, now specialize in indigenous vegetables and other traditional foods (Moore and Raymond, 2006).

African eggplant as an indigenous vegetable with potential for rapid development

The genus Solanaceae comprises more than 3,000 species. Globally, it is among the most important taxon economically and is the most valuable in terms of vegetable crops (Mueller et al., 2005). These species have evolved in highly contrasting environments, and, although vegetable crops such as potato

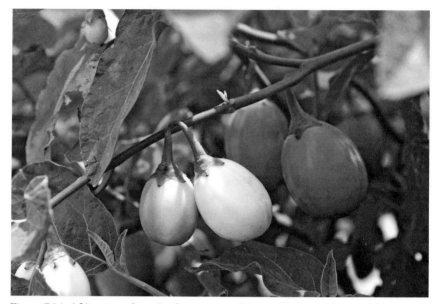

Figure C6.1 African eggplant: In the process of domestication, *Solanum aethiopicum L.* developed into four cultivated groups based on adaptation to different growing conditions and selection for either fruit or leaf consumption. The Gilo group, shown here, has edible oval or round fruit 2–12 cm long ranging in colour from white, green, red, brown to purple. The Shum group has small hairless leaves, which are consumed as a leafy green; the small, very bitter fruit is not eaten. The Kumba group produces large ridged fruit (5–10 cm in diameter) edible when green or red in colour, and has large leaves that can be consumed as a vegetable; some cultivars of this group are used for both fruit and leaf consumption, while others are mainly grown as leafy vegetables. The furrowed fruit of the Acelatum group is about 3–8 cm in diameter (Grubben and Denton, 2004; Porcher, 2010). Source: AVRDC – The World Vegetable Center

and tomato are reasonably well understood and may be regarded as 'model' species for research, the majority of the potential vegetable species within the genus remain largely under-researched, if not undiscovered. In the case of the 'aubergine' or eggplant (*Solanum melongena*), its worldwide prominence in Mediterranean agricultural environments has led to a long history of cultivation and substantive research support, mostly for purple coloured teardrop shapes or their near equivalent. This is less true for other shapes and colours of *S. melongena*. Three of its near relatives, the African eggplants (*S. aethiopicum, S. anguivi,* and *S. macrocarpon*) have received very little research attention, yet these species have potential for helping smallholder farmers grow themselves out of poverty.

African eggplant is commonly grown and consumed in the tropical areas of sub-Saharan Africa, South Asia and Southeast Asia. The fruit varies in shape from round, ovoid, or teardrop to long and thin; colours include white, yellow, green, orange, brown, and speckled. The flesh can be sweet or bitter in taste. The usual locus of production today is from smallholder growers or from kitchen garden plots, and farmer use of improved or hybrid seed is rare (Keding et al., 2007). The lack of a preferred market type and production on small farm plots provides little incentive for seed companies to invest in improved types, as each market segment is perceived to be comparatively small and ill-defined. This, in essence, is the research and development problem associated with this species. Nevertheless, African eggplant is popular and could generate much broader demand from urban populations in Africa and Asia with sufficient research and development investment.

Identification of the dimensions of the research and development problem for African eggplant

Accurate statistics on the area of land under production and the productivity of African eggplant species worldwide are essentially unavailable (FAOSTAT, 2007). This is a truism for most vegetable species not only at the global level, but also at regional and down to national levels. This is probably because such a crop is deemed by statistical collection authorities to be largely of smallholder interest only, as much of the crop is self-consumed by producer families with only the excess sold fresh in local markets. Data on vegetables are perceived as less important and more difficult to collect from smallholders or low-volume market traders than for staple crops traded internationally, such as maize and rice. Yet these species are available for sale, though in small quantities, throughout sub-Saharan Africa, South and Southeast Asian, whether it is in the Sahel, the Great Lakes, the Deccan or the Mekong regions (Chadha and Mndiga, 2007; National Research Council, 2006).

National authorities, private sector seed companies, and public sector breeders in most parts of the tropical world have shown ambivalence toward these eggplant species, with the exception of India, where many eggplant types are grown. Until recently, improved seed has not been available in most countries and only unimproved landraces have been the principal sources of seed. Research in general has been minimal, as reported by Ssekabembe and Odong (2008). In Uganda, more recently, Oluoch and Chadha (2007) have shown that of 42 lines of African eggplant, the highest five-year mean fruit yields could exceed 62 t/ha, with seed yields also above 2 t/ha. In comparison, previous yields using landraces might have been around (*Solanum scabrum*) 5–20 t/ha (Oluoch and Chadha, 2007). These authors showed that *S. aethiopicum* lines were better adapted to conditions in Arusha, Tanzania than *S. anguivi* and *S. macrocarpon*. There were considerable differences between lines, suggesting good opportunities to select superior cultivars.

In addition to good yield potential, it is evident that the eggplant, though not particularly nutritious itself, can be grown as an intercrop with nutrient-dense green leafy vegetables such as *Amaranthus* spp. Examples from Uganda suggest this is a more profitable option than sole cropping of either vegetable (Ssekabembe, 2008).

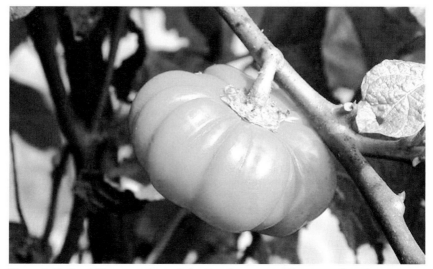

Figure C6.2 An African eggplant of the Kumba group. African eggplant fruit is eaten boiled, steamed, pickled or in stews with other vegetables and meats. Young leaves of African eggplant are high in beta-carotene and calcium. Source: AVRDC – The World Vegetable Center

The approach of AVRDC to research and advocacy for African eggplant

AVRDC – The World Vegetable Center has committed breeding and full value chain support to African eggplant. The Center seeks to provide improved varieties of different African eggplant species for release throughout sub-Saharan Africa and South and Southeast Asia. These are types deemed desirable by consumers in tropical regions for colour, shape, and taste. The Center also encourages national seed release and control authorities to make registered quality seed available to farmers. Small- and medium-scale private sector partners were encouraged to multiply seed of improved African eggplant lines and sell it directly to farmers, or to use the improved lines as parents in their own breeding or hybridization programmes.

Research and development results to date of AVRDC and its partners

Current research and development has resulted in the release of several AVRDC African eggplant varieties in Africa. In Mali, 'Soxna' produces flattened, lobed fruit turning red-orange at maturity; it has a slightly soft texture and can be eaten fresh or cooked. Variety 'L10' has slightly smaller fruit of similar characteristics. In Tanzania, variety 'DB3' has been released; it has white, medium-sized, ovoid, sweet fruits. This line is already popular with farmers, and demand for seed exceeds supply. Seed of 'DB3' will be sold by small and medium seed companies throughout Tanzania's Great Lakes Region. Other types of African eggplant will soon be available from AVRDC's breeding pipeline.

Impact on farmers and their families

Chadha and Mndiga (2007) report that several promising varieties of African eggplant were identified in Arusha, Tanzania including 'DB3', 'Tengeru White', 'AB2' and 'Manyire Green.' Seeds were distributed to 200 farmers in the Arumeru district of Tanzania (near Arusha) and an informal survey was carried out with those farmers who had collaborated in the test-growing. These farmers were generally smallholders and were able to allocate about 0.5 ha or less to growing eggplant in a single season. 'DB3' and 'Tengeru White' seemed to be the preferred types, and 'DB3' was formally released in 2011.

There was high market demand for these crops locally and incomes were said to have increased by between US$1,600 and US$2,500 per hectare per season. Farmers reported several substantial social improvements as a result of the increased income, including the ability to purchase more land, build houses, and buy improved household articles. One grower is also acting as a consolidating buyer, employing women to harvest, sort, grade and bag the crop prior to sale to local wet markets or supermarkets.

Marketing efforts to interest supermarkets in African eggplant in Tanzania and Kenya have been successful, and the fruit is now commonly seen for sale in Nairobi, Arusha and Dar es Salaam, as well as in Accra, Cotonou and other cities in West Africa (AVRDC, 2008). Most consumers in big African cities have a desire to purchase the indigenous vegetables that are more common in rural areas. This appears to be the case for African eggplant and market demand remains buoyant.

What further research is needed?

Early tests of the economic performance of improved eggplant seed have shown that African eggplant can be a profitable crop provided consumer preferences are addressed in improved varieties. However, suitable seed systems need to be developed and seed must be made available throughout countries in the tropics to adequately address the crop's potential. The complexity of ploidy relationships in intercrosses between eggplant species needs better understanding if hybrid seeds are to become more easily available. There have been some levels of success with new intra- and interspecific pipeline hybrid varieties developed by Rijk Zwaan Afrisem Co. Ltd in Arusha Tanzania (H. Peeters, pers. comm., 2010).

Little is known about the agronomy of pest resistance of the improved varieties, although evidence exists that *S. aethiopicum* has substantive resistance to bacterial wilt (*Ralstonia solanacearum*). This is seen to be of considerable value globally as *S. melongena* is generally lacking resistance to this serious and common disease (Colonnier et al., 2001). Evidence is needed to determine whether heat and drought tolerance claims can be substantiated in reality.

Lessons learned and future prospects

Indigenous vegetables were previously considered subsistence food crops as opposed to cash crops. It is now established that they attract good prices in local markets and also have potential for international trade. Among the food crops, starch crops are referred to as staple or food security crops and indigenous vegetables fall into the category of non-staple crops. Yet, indigenous vegetables often accompany staple crops in meals, and most staple crops are less palatable without associated vegetable servings. Indigenous vegetables can enhance bioavailability of micronutrients in staple crops and promote absorption (Vijayalakshi et al., 2003). In addition, some indigenous vegetables can be harvested in just 21 days, providing a rapid response to urgent needs for food and nutrition, while most of the food security crops take at least six to nine months to reach harvest. It is now recognized that food security cannot be delinked from nutritional security, to which the consumption of indigenous vegetables significantly contributes (Keatinge et al., 2011). Well-balanced diets are essential to human health and these are best achieved by greater diet diversity and increased consumption of vegetables. Continuing investment in indigenous vegetables research and development is thus a vital weapon in the continuing battle against human malnutrition worldwide.

References

AVRDC – The World Vegetable Center (2008) *Point of Impact: When putting all your eggs in one basket pays – improved indigenous vegetables have market potential*, Shanhua, Taiwan: AVRDC, p.2.

AVRDC – The World Vegetable Center (2010) *Prosperity for the Poor and Health for All: Strategic Plan 2011–2025*, Shanhua, Taiwan: AVRDC, p.41.

AVRDC – The World Vegetable Center (2011) *New variety releases expand market options for Tanzania's farmers. Fresh News from AVRDC – The World Vegetable Center*, pp.1–3.

Beisel, W.R. (2001) Nutritionally acquired immune deficiency syndromes, in: *Micronutrients and HIV Infection*. Ed. H. Friis. CRC Series in Modern Nutrition, Boca Raton, p.272.

Chadha, M.L. and Mndiga, H.H. (2007) African eggplant – from underutilized to a commercially profitable venture, *Acta Horticulturae,* vol 752, pp.521–523.

Chweya, J.A. and Eyzaguirre, P.B. (1999) Introduction, in: J.A. Chweya and P.B. Eyzaguirre (eds) *Biodiversity of Traditional Leafy Vegetables,* International Plant Genetic Resources Institute. Rome, Italy, pp.1–6.

Colonnier, C., Mulya, K., Fock, I., Mariska, I., Servaes, A., Vedel, F., Siljak-Yakovlev, S., Souvannavong, V., Ducreux, G. and Sihachakr, D. (2001) Source of resistance against *Ralstonia solanacearum* in fertile somatic hybrids of eggplant (*S. melongena* L.) with *S. aethiopicum* L., *Plant Science*, vol 160, pp.301–313.

FAO (2002) *Agrobiodiversity, Food Security and HIV/AIDS Mitigation in Sub-Saharan Africa – Strategic Issues for Agricultural Policy and Programme Responses*, Rome, Italy: FAO.

FAOSTAT (2007) FAOSTAT on-line Rome, Italy: FAO.

Gari, J.A. (2003) *Agrobiodiversity Strategies to Combat Food Insecurity and HIV/AIDS Impact in Rural Africa*, FAO (Population and Development Service), Rome, Italy; preliminary edition, p.154.

German, J.B. and Dillard, C.J. (1998) Phytochemicals and targets of chronic disease, in: W.R. Bidlack, S.T. Omaye, M.S. Meskin, and D. Jahner (eds) *Phytochemicals – A New Paradigm*, Lancaster, Pennsylvania: Technomic Publishing Company.

Grubben, G.J.H. and Denton, O.A. (2004) *Plant Resources of Tropical Africa 2. Vegetables*, PROTA Foundation, Wageningen, Netherlands. Backhuys Publishers, Leiden, Netherlands. CTA, Wageningen, Netherlands.

Hirt, H.M. and Lindsey, K. (2005) *AIDS: Artemisia annua anamed (A-3) and Moringa*, http://www.thebody.com/Forums/AIDS/SideEffects/Archive/Alternative/Q189936. html, accessed July 2012.

IFPRI (2001) Empowering Women to Achieve Food Security: Vision 2020. Focus no 6. Washington, D C: International Food Policy Research Institute.

Irungu, C., Mburu, J., Maundu, P., Grum, M. and Hoeschle-Zeledon, I. (2007) *Analysis of Markets for African Leafy vegetables within Nairobi and its Environs and Implications for On-Farm Conservation of Biodiversity*, Rome, Italy: Global Facilitation Unit for Underutilized Species, p.54.

Kean, L.G., Ntiru, M.K., and Giyose, B.D. (1999) Nutrition Briefs; Linking Multiple Sectors for Effective Planning and Programming, SARA/USAID, SANA and CRHCS Project Report.

Kean, L.G., Ntiru, M.K., and Giyose, B.D. (2001) Nutrition Briefs; Linking Multiple Sectors for Effective Planning and Programming, SARA, SANA-AED Project Report.

Keatinge, J.D.H., Yang, R.Y., Hughes, J. d'A., Easdown, W.J., and Holmer, R. (2011) The importance of vegetables in ensuring both food and nutritional security in attainment of the Millennium Development Goals, *Food Security,* vol 3, no 4.

Keding, G., Weinberger, K., Swai, I., and Mndiga, H. (2007) Diversity, Traits and Use of Traditional Vegetables in Tanzania, *AVRDC Technical Bulletin* 40, Shanhua, Taiwan: AVRDC, p.53.

Ministère de l'Agriculture (2011) *Catalogue Officiel des Especes et Varietes, Tome III. Cultures maraîchères*, Ministère de l'Agriculture, Republique du Mali, vol 38.

Moore, C. and Raymond, R.D. (2006) *Back by Popular Demand: The Benefits of Traditional Vegetables*, Rome, Italy: IPGRI, p.60.

Muchiri, S.V. (2004) Characterization and Purification of African Nightshade Accessions for Sustainable Seed Purification in Kenya, Msc Thesis in Horticulture, Jomo Kenyatta University of Agriculture and Technology, Juja, Kenya.

Mueller, L.A., Solow, T.H., Taylor, N., Skwarecki, B., Buels, R., Binns, J., Lin, C.W., Wright, M.H., Ahrens, R., Wang, Y., Herbst, E.V., Keyder, E.R., Menda, N., Zamir, D. and Tanksley, S.D. (2005) The SOL Genomics Network: A comparative resource for Solanaceae biology and beyond, *Plant Physiology*, vol 138, pp.1310–1317.

National Research Council (2006) *Lost Crops of Africa. Volume II: Vegetables*, Washington, DC: National Academies Press.

Nesamvuni, C., Steyn, N.P., and Potgieter, M.J. (2001) Nutritional value of wild leafy plants consumed by the Vhavenda, *South African Journal of Science,* vol 97, pp.52–54.

Oluoch, M.O. and Chadha, M.L. (2007) Evaluation of African eggplant for yield and quality characteristics, *Acta Horticulturae* vol 752, pp.303–306.

Oniang'o, R.K., Shiundu, K., Maunda, P. and Johns, T. (2006) Diversity, nutrition and food security: The case of African leafy vegetables, in: *Hunger and Poverty: The Role of Biodiversity*, S. Bala Ravi, I. Hoeschle-Zeledon, M.S. Swaminathan, and E. Frison, (eds) Rome, Italy: IPGRI, pp.86–100.

Pasquini, M.W. and Young, E.M. (2007) Networking to promote the sustainable production and marketing of indigenous vegetables through urban and peri-urban agriculture in sub-Saharan Africa (Indigenoveg), *Acta Hort.* (ISHS), vol 752, pp.41–48.

Porcher, M.H. (2010) Know your eggplants – Part 1. http://www.plantnames.unimelb. edu.au/new/Sorting/CATALOGUE/Pt1-African-eggplants.html.

PROTA (2004) *Plant Resources of Tropical Africa 2, Vegetables*, in: G.J.H. Grubben and O.A. Denton (eds) Leiden, The Netherlands: Backhuys Publishers, p.668.

PROTA (2009) *Vegetables of Tropical Africa, Conclusions and recommendations based on PROTA 2: 'Vegetables'*, 2nd edition. C.H. Bosch, D.J. Borus, and J.S. Siemonsma, Wageningen, (eds) Netherlands: PROTA Foundation, p.66.

Sreeramulu, N., Nodsi, G.D. and Mtotomwema, K. (1983) Effects of cooking on the nutritive value of common food plants of Tanzania: Part 1 – Vitamin C in some of the wild green leafy vegetables, *Food Chemistry*, vol 10, pp.205–210.

Ssekabembe, C.K. (2008) Effect of proportion of component species on the productivity of *S. aethiopicum* and *Amaranthus lividus* under intercropping, *African Journal of Agricultural Research,* vol 3, pp.510–519.

Ssekabembe, C.K. and Odong, T.L. (2008) Division of labour in nakati (S. aethiopicum) production in central Uganda, *African Journal of Agricultural Research*, vol 3, pp.400–406.

Vijayalakshi, P.S., Amruthavani, S., Devadas, R.P., Weinberger, K., Tsou, S.C.S., and Shanmugasundaram, S. (2003) *Enhanced Bioavailability of Iron and Mungbeans and Its Effects on Health of Schoolchildren*, Technical Bulletin 30, Shanhua, Taiwan: AVRDC.

Weinberger, K. and Msuya, J. (2004) *Indigenous Vegetables in Tanzania: Significance and Prospects*, Technical Bulletin No. 31, AVRDC – The World Vegetable Center, Shanhua, Taiwan.

Yang, R.Y. and Keding, G.B. (2009) Nutritional contribution of important African vegetables, pp.105–135, in: C.M. Shackleton, M.W. Pasquini, and A. W, Drescher (eds) *African Indigenous Vegetables in Urban Agriculture*, London, UK: Earthscan, p.29.

Case study 7

Diversifying diets: using agricultural biodiversity to improve nutrition and health in Asia

Jennifer Nielsen, Nancy Haselow, Akoto Osei and Zaman Talukder

Background

Malnutrition, including micronutrient deficiencies, is a serious public health problem among women and children throughout Asia. Underweight among preschool children in Bangladesh, Cambodia, Nepal and the Philippines is 41 per cent, 36 per cent, 39 per cent and 21 per cent respectively (NIPORT, 2009; NIS, 2011; MOHP, 2012; NSO, 2009). Anaemia and vitamin A deficiencies are also widespread, with anaemia affecting over half of children between 6 and 59 months and pregnant women in these countries (WHO, 2012). Hunger and malnutrition have consequences for survival, cognitive function, physical capacity, resistance to disease, quality of life (Victora et al., 2008) and lifetime earnings (Hoddinott et al., 2008), while low dietary diversity is associated with both poverty and stunting (Black et al., 2008).

Helen Keller International's Homestead Food Production (HFP) programme was developed in Bangladesh and later expanded to Cambodia, Nepal and the Philippines to diversify household-level agricultural production as a means to diversify dietary intake. The model introduced new varieties while preserving and promoting indigenous varieties of plants as well as poultry and livestock, emphasizing a wide range of production in order to maximize success under varying biotic, edaphic and climatic conditions; reduce the risk of loss due to pests, disease, and climate change and variability; and optimize the nutritional status of household members through consumption of a broader spectrum of macro and micronutrients and phytochemicals. Recognizing the importance of diversified agro-ecosystems, the design intentionally promotes and supports growing a variety of species year round.

The benefits of agricultural biodiversity: why, what

While the primary objective of the HFP programme is to improve food security and nutrition by promoting more diversified diets, there are clear mutually reinforcing benefits between agricultural biodiversity and human nutrition.

Helen Keller International's (HKI) first pilot home gardening programme was launched in Bangladesh in 1988 after a national blindness survey showed that households with kitchen gardens were less likely to comprise night-blind children (a clinical sign of vitamin A deficiency – VAD). The objective of the first HFP programme was thus to reduce VAD in women and children by increasing production and consumption of nutrient-rich fruits and vegetables. Within two years of the intervention, over 90 per cent of the families targeted by the pilot study were producing vegetables and fruits high in vitamin A, including carrots, spinach, amaranth and papaya year round, with vegetable consumption in the target households increasing from 5.8 to 7.5 kg per week, compared with a modest increase of 5.1 to 5.4 kg among control households. Soon after, when a study in Indonesia (de Pee et al., 1998) showed low bioavailability of beta-carotene in some plant sources, HKI integrated small animal husbandry into the model. The model has been scaled up in Bangladesh and expanded to Cambodia, Nepal, the Philippines and Indonesia. More recent surveys in the Barisal division of Bangladesh confirm the uptake findings with the practice of improved (diverse, year-round) homestead food production increasing from < 1 to 89 per cent of households between 2004 and 2009. The volume of production and the number of varieties in participating households was also found to increase, with improved home gardens producing on average 45 varieties of vegetables compared with 10 in households with traditional gardens (Talukder et al., 2010).

To diversify production systems, the HFP programme encourages the conservation of indigenous varieties of fruits and vegetables (de Pee et al., 2010), particularly underutilized species, and the introduction of micronutrient-rich species from similar agro-ecosystems to complement and improve increased intake of a wide range of nutrients. Improved local breeds of poultry are promoted as animal-source foods in addition to fish. In Asia, HKI promotes more than ten infrequently cultivated indigenous varieties of vegetables and fruits. These include varieties of mint (*Mentha* sp.), black arum (*Xanthosoma atrovirens*), kangkong (*Ipomoea aquatica*), pigeon pea (*Cajanus cajan*), drumsticks (*Moringa oleifera*), helencha (*Enhydra fluctuans*), Thankuni pata (*Centella asiatica*), neem (*Azadirachta indica*), basil (*Ocimum* sp.), country bean (*Lablab niger*), cowpea (*Vigna* sp.), taro (*Colocasia esculenta*), and coriander (*Coriandrum sativum*). Some of these are leguminous plants promoted to enhance soil nitrogen; others act as organic insect repellents. Because they are locally adapted, these plants do not require significant labour or other inputs, yet contribute to a healthy agro-ecosystem as well as nutritional diversity.

The benefits of agricultural biodiversity: how

HKI promotes the HFP model by establishing demonstration plots on local farms to showcase low-cost, low-risk cultivation practices to households interested in making the transition from traditional to more diversified vegetable, fruit and animal production. Farmers with adequate land and a demonstrated commitment to the project are selected by community leaders and trained by HKI to set up and run Village Model Farms (VMF) that provide training and demonstrations on improved agricultural techniques, technologies and poultry production activities for households participating in the programme (typically between 20–40 households per VMF). Furthermore, the VMF are used as production centres, providing targeted households with low-cost quality seeds, seedlings, saplings of locally available fruit, shade and multipurpose trees and local or improved breeds of chicks. Model farmers are trained to provide technical training on seed production and storage to ensure sustainable cultivation in subsequent planting seasons. Because of their important role in household food preparation, women are the main targets for training and technical assistance, while community support for women's leadership is carefully cultivated.

Nutrition education, based on the Essential Nutrition Actions (ENA)[1] framework, is also a fundamental component of the HFP model. Trained health staff and volunteers working at the village level lead nutrition education discussions and provide counselling to support mothers to adopt healthier practices, including the consumption of nutritious foods from the HFP during pregnancy and lactation, optimal breastfeeding and complementary feeding for infants and young children. Other elements of the behaviour change communications strategy include cooking demonstrations, engagement of fathers and grandmothers, community mobilization events and mass media messages to reinforce knowledge and support changes in community norms around nutrition. These multi-channel communication strategies reinforce awareness and adoption of improved nutrition practices.

Local community-based organizations (CBOs) are fundamental to the sustainability of the programme, as are government and non-governmental agents from agricultural, health and other sectors who are mobilized to disseminate key messages and reinforce improved practices. Group marketing strategies have helped small producers to access markets, increasing household income and livelihood options. This, in turn, helps to perpetuate the use of improved practices. Sharing, collaboration, community mobilization, mutual support and building on local organizations are also critical. Personnel from these local structures are trained to lead the initial implementation and are prepared to provide additional inputs and technical advice to help sustain the work in the communities after external support is withdrawn.

The benefits of agricultural biodiversity: health impacts

Substantive evidence exists on the role of the HFP model in contributing to improved household food security and nutrition status (Bushamuka et al. 2005). Pooled data from across the four countries in Asia, where the programme has the longest history, showed decreases in anaemia prevalence among children aged from 6 to 59 months in all programme communities, including significant differences in Bangladesh and the Philippines, and

Box C7.1 Sona Chaudhary, age 40, Nepal

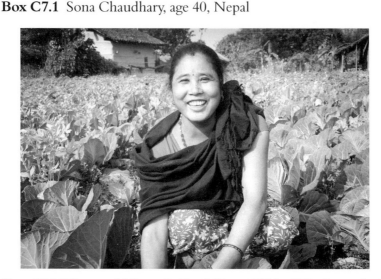

Figure C7.1 Village model farmer in Nepal. Photo: ©Helen Keller International/ George Figdor

Sona Chaudhary is a village model farmer living in a joint family made up by her husband, two brothers-in-law, two sisters-in-law, a grandson and a granddaughter. Her husband, a day labourer, is rarely home, so she has to manage many household responsibilities herself.

Sona and her family were selected to manage the village model farm as she met the minimum land requirements, was respected by the women in her village, and expressed a willingness to share knowledge and provide assistance to others. Sona received an intensive three-day training from HKI's USAID-funded AAMA project (*aama* means mother in Nepali) covering organic agriculture, planning for year-round diversified production and mentoring others in newly acquired skills.

Sona reports that prior to training received by HKI her family had very limited knowledge of vegetable production and animal husbandry, as well as of the production and application of compost manure. Her household's home garden covered an area of 65m², grew six crops – dark green leafy vegetables [DGLV] amaranth and taro; orange-fleshed pumpkin; potato, chilli and onions – and production did not meet her family's consumption needs. The family had one hen and one rooster that were allowed to graze freely with no protective coop, at high risk of predators and disease.

Through her participation in the project, Sona's garden has expanded to 1,000 m² and now produces six varieties of DGLV, including mustard leaf and spinach, carrots and mangos, in addition to pumpkin, cauliflower, cabbage, garlic, radish, green beans, broccoli and eggplant. Vegetable production is now year round. Poultry numbers have risen to 24. The fowl are well protected by a coop and are systematically vaccinated thanks to improved links with government extension services. Sona produces fertilizer from compost, pesticides using organic compounds from the garden and has been able to afford an electric pump for irrigation. Income from surplus production has also allowed her to invest in her children's education as well as in health care.

Sona is grateful for the confidence and leadership skills she gained through the training, which has enabled her to hold meetings with other women farmers, to share knowledge and techniques for improved homestead food production and nutritional practices.

greater differences in programme compared with control communities, even though intergroup differences were not statistically significant (Talukder et al., 2010). Surveys in Bangladesh also documented increases in dietary diversity (measured as consumption of at least three food groups[2] on at least three of the previous seven days) from 34 to 62 per cent among women and from 43 to 86 per cent among children aged 6–59 months. Similar outcomes were achieved in other settings, including Cambodia and Nepal. Research is currently under way in Nepal to test the impact of the intervention on child growth. At the same time, a review by the International Food Policy Research Institute of HKI's nearly 20 years of support for HFP intervention in Bangladesh recognized that the programme improved food security for nearly 5 million vulnerable people in diverse agro-ecological zones, increasing both the variety and quantity of production (Iannotti et al., 2009). Evidence from Cambodia indicates that household consumption of dark green leafy vegetables, orange vegetables and fruits, overall household dietary diversity scores and egg consumption among children increased significantly more in intervention households from baseline to end line compared with controls. Pooled analysis of data from Bangladesh and Cambodia suggests that among households with improved gardens, children consumed a mean of 13 types of vegetables compared with only four where cultivation was traditional, and the frequency of vegetable consumption was 1.6 times higher (Talukder et al., 2010).

HKI has recently begun to translate this model of biodiverse household production to sub-Saharan Africa, with an initiative under way in Burkina Faso and another planned in Tanzania. The arid climate, poor soils, and migratory labour demands on staple crop production in the Sahel pose significant challenges to the approach. Nevertheless, while year-round production may not be possible, evidence to date shows that diversified agriculture production and consumption is possible and equally critical in these settings.

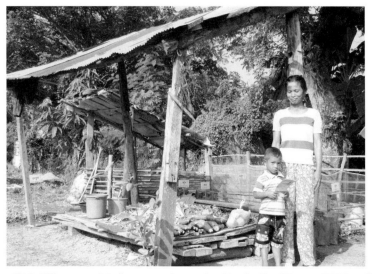

Figure C7.2 Village model farmer and son in Cambodia. Photo: ©Helen Keller International/Wendy Lee

Scale-up efforts and challenges

In Asia the positive impact of the HFP intervention on food security, dietary intake and nutritional status of household members has captured the attention of governments and development partners who have begun to scale-up efforts to other food insecure areas. In Bangladesh, where over 1 million households (approximately 5 million people) benefited from HFP interventions, the Government has provided additional funding to the programme and implemented the HFP model through government extension services. Efforts to scale-up the approach under relevant national agricultural strategies, nutritional and food security strategies, policies and programmes are also being pursued in Nepal and Cambodia. The model in Nepal was initially implemented on a small scale. In 2008, the United States Agency for International Development (USAID) supported a new phase to incorporate ENA as the nutrition education approach and to refine, replicate and evaluate the model in two districts of the Far Western Region. Based on initial promise, USAID provided further support to expand to two additional districts and also to allow the government and development partners to undertake multi-sectoral planning. More recently, an effort has begun to extend the model to food insecure areas in 20 more districts.

In Cambodia, the programme has covered 12 (out of 75) of the most food insecure districts within five provinces and is currently being replicated in an additional province, along with testing the added value of mixed pisciculture in the model. The Council of Agricultural and Rural Development under the Council of Ministers is seeking to replicate this programme in other food insecure provinces, while the Commune Councils now include the approach in their annual development plans and are directly involved in monitoring and evaluation. In the Philippines, Local Government Units have provided funding to expand the HFP practices to additional households and provinces, while in Indonesia the programme is in the pilot phase.

Current challenges to scale-up include establishing reliable input supplies; addressing soil infertility; lack of water and the need for site-specific irrigation systems; developing adequate management skills and support systems (with a multiplicity of partner NGOs); establishing on-going programme monitoring to identify and correct problems early (and transferring these tools to local partners); and promoting optimal maternal and young child nutritional intake through behaviour change communications. In addition, in Bangladesh in particular, understanding the multifactorial contributors to undernutrition and the local social and cultural constraints faced by women has been critical (Talukder et al. 2000).

Stakeholder involvement

Local government, CBO and community engagement and leadership are crucial to the success and sustainability of the HFP programme, as is collaboration involving not only the health and agriculture sectors, but also local development, education, women's development, and water and sanitation. In Bangladesh alone, HKI has forged relationships with more than 150 diverse local NGOs who co-finance activities and build community ownership. In Nepal, planning includes all relevant government sectors. Moreover health agents are included in agricultural training programmes while nutrition education is provided to agricultural extension agents to help encourage integrated approaches and build mutual appreciation of the benefits of diversification.

In all settings HKI engages local, provincial and district authorities in the planning and supervision of the programme. Local agriculture and health authorities and government representatives facilitate HFP activities at the local level, while steering/advisory committees ensure engagement at the district and provincial levels. At the national level, in some countries, coordinating councils have been successfully established. External support from bilateral donors and the private sector has also provided vital resources.

Policy impact

In Nepal, the success of the model and HKI's engagement in national policy have led to policy impact at the national level. The new phase of the programme aims to strengthen the capacity of the ministries of health, agriculture and planning to conduct coordinated, multi-sectoral planning that link agriculture to nutrition and health outcomes and implementation of programmes that strengthen small-holder agriculture, livelihoods, food security, nutrition and health. The project is working at district, regional and national levels to harmonize efforts of donors investing in agriculture and nutrition in Nepal. This broader, integrated vision

Box C7.2 Local NGO partner Prey Veng, Cambodia

One of HKI's key NGO partners in Cambodia is the Organization to Develop Our Village (ODOV), an independent, non-profit, community-based organization that has been operating in the country since 1995 and working in Prey Veng province since 2004. Criteria for partnering with HKI include at least two years on-the-ground experience in target regions, experience supporting income-generating activities, ability for modest cost-sharing in project implementation, and willingness to integrate homestead food production into the organization's core community development strategies (rather than implementing it as a free-standing activity).

Even before its partnership with HKI, ODOV's mission was to implement integrated community development programmes to improve the living standards of vulnerable households through improved food security, health and nutrition, community finance, income generation through off-farm promotion, school gardening, and commune council administration and reform activities. ODOV has collaborated with HKI since the end of 2009 to implement a homestead food production programme (HFPP) in 300 selected villages in three districts of Prey Veng, which currently reaches 3,300 households. HKI provided technical and management training to ODOV staff to strengthen their capacity to assume long-term responsibility for supporting and expanding the programme after HKI involvement, which generally ends at a day-to-day level after three years. Technical training covers homestead food production as well as nutrition education (using the Essential Nutrition Actions framework), while institutional strengthening covers financial management, programme management, monitoring and evaluation. Local partners are engaged from the very start in strategic planning, situational analysis, and baseline data collection to ensure their ownership of programmes and contributions to crafting local approaches and sustainable systems. About half of ODOV's full complement of 25 staff has supported implementation of HFP in Prey Veng.

As the project was coming to a close at the end of 2011, HKI conducted a rapid organizational assessment of ODOV. The NGO has mobilized resources from other donors to expand the HFP approach to neighbouring villages, and HFP is now an integral element of ODOV's core programme.

should support the scale-up of programmes like HFP that promote ecological approaches to production, biodiversity, dietary diversity and improved human and agricultural health. Leaders in Bangladesh, Cambodia and the Philippines have also incorporated the approach into annual development plans to improve agricultural production and nutrition. In Cambodia, the government is working with donors to mobilize additional resources for expansion of the model.

Key lessons learned

- Small-scale, diversified agriculture can be highly productive, sustainable, improve livelihoods, nutritional status and well-being in multiple ways, while promoting good stewardship of natural resources.
- Women play a necessary and key role in HFP as they translate inputs and technical training into improved household nutrition.
- Strong partnerships with a range of local community-based organizations ensure that HFP builds on and enhances local practices, is compatible with socio-cultural norms, and engages existing structures.
- A clearly defined, but flexible programme model facilitates successful replication to other food insecure areas with varying agro-ecological zones and cultural situations.
- Strong monitoring and evaluation systems and feedback loops allow effective use of data to inform and improve HFP programming.

Notes

1 http://www.hki.org/reducing-malnutrition/essential-nutrition-actions/, accessed July 2012.
2 Dark green leafy vegetables, pulses, animal-source foods, fruits, and other vegetables.

References

Black, R.E., Allen, L.H., Bhutta, Z.A., Caulfield, L.E., de Onis M., Ezzati, M., Mathers, C. and Rivera, J. (2008) 'Maternal and child undernutrition: global and regional exposures and health consequences', *Lancet*, vol 371, pp.243–260.

Bushamuka, V.N., de Pee, S., Talukder, A., Kiess, L. Panagides, D., Taher, A. and Bloem, M. (2005) 'Impact of a homestead gardening program on household food security and empowerment of women in Bangladesh', *Food and Nutrition Bulletin* vol 26 no 1 pp.17–25.

De Pee, S., Bloem, M.W., Gorstein, J., Sari, M., Satoto, Y.R., Shrimpton, R. and Muhilal (1998) 'Reappraisal of the role of vegetables in the vitamin A status of mothers in Central Java, Indonesia,' *Am J Clin Nutr,* vol 68, pp.1068–1074.

De Pee, S., Talukder, Z. and Bloem, M. (2010) 'Homestead food production for improving nutrition and health' in R.D. Semba and M. Bloem (eds) *Nutrition and Health in Developing Countries*, Humana Press, Totowa, NJ.

Hoddinott, J., Maluccio, J.A., Behrman, J.R., Flores, R. and Martorell, R. (2008) 'Effect of a nutrition intervention during early childhood on economic productivity in Guatemalan adults,' *Lancet* vol 371, pp.411–416.

Iannotti, L., Cunningham, K. and Ruel, M. (2009) 'Improving diet quality and micronutrient nutrition: homestead food production in Bangladesh', International Food Policy Research Institute Discussion Paper 00928, prepared for Millions Fed: Proven successes in agricultural development.

Ministry of Health and Population (MOHP) [Nepal], New ERA, and ICF International Inc. (2012) *Nepal Demographic and Health Survey 2011*, Kathmandu, Nepal: Ministry of Health and Population, New ERA, and ICF International, Calverton, MA.

312 Jennifer Nielsen, Nancy Haselow, Akoto Osei and Zaman Talukder

National Institute of Population Research and Training (NIPORT), Mitra and Associates, and Macro International (2009) *Bangladesh Demographic and Health Survey 2007*, Dhaka, Bangladesh and Calverton, MA: National Institute of Population Research and Training, Mitra and Associates, and Macro International.

National Institute of Statistics (NIS) Directorate General for Health, and ICF Macro (2011) *Cambodia Demographic and Health Survey 2010*, Phnom Penh, Cambodia and Calverton, MA: National Institute of Statistics, Directorate General for Health, and ICF Macro.

National Statistics Office (NSO) [Philippines] and ICF Macro (2009) *National Demographic and Health Survey 2008*, Calverton, MA: National Statistics Office and ICF Macro.

Talukder, A., Kiess, L., Huq, N., de Pee, S., Darnton-Hill, I. and Bloem, M.W. (2000) 'Increasing the production and consumption of vitamin A-rich fruits and vegetables: lessons learned in taking the Bangladesh Homestead Gardening Programme to a national scale', *Food and Nutrition Bulletin* vol 21, no 2, pp.165–172.

Talukder, A., Haselow, N.J., Osei, A.K., Villate, E., Reario, D., Kroeun, H., SokHoing, L., Uddin, A., Dhungel, S., Quinn, V. (2010) 'Homestead food production model contributes to improved household food security and nutrition status', Field Actions Science Report; available at: www.factsreports.org, accessed August 2012.

Victora, C.G., Adair, L., Fall, C., Hallal, P.C., Martorell, R., Richter, L. and Sachdev, H.S. (2008) 'Maternal and child undernutrition: consequences for adult health and human capital', *Lancet,* vol 371, pp.340–357.

World Health Organization (WHO) (2012) 'Vitamin and mineral nutrition information system' (VMNIS) [online], http://www.who.int/vmnis/database/anaemia/en/index.html, accessed July 2012.

Case study 8

Minor millets in India: a neglected crop goes mainstream

Nadia Bergamini, Stefano Padulosi, S. Bala Ravi and Nirmala Yenagi

Background

In spite of several national nutritional intervention programmes, India faces huge nutrition challenges as the prevalence of micronutrient malnutrition continues to be a major public health problem with an associated economic cost of 0.8 to 2.4 per cent of the GDP. Most vulnerable segments of the population are children, adolescents, pregnant women and lactating mothers (Arlappa et al., 2010), with estimates from the most recent National Family Health Survey (IIPS, 2007) indicating that about 46 per cent of the children under five years of age, particularly those living in rural areas (Rajaram et al., 2007), are moderately to severely underweight (thin for age), 38 per cent are moderately to severely stunted (short for age), and approximately 19 per cent are moderately to severely wasted (thin for height) (Kanjilal et al., 2010).

The overdependence on a handful of species – rice, maize, wheat and potatoes – which provide over 50 per cent of the world's caloric intake (FAO, 2010), has seen hundreds of species and varieties of food plants marginalized and becoming increasingly irrelevant in national agricultural production systems and economies. Less attention by researchers on these so-called neglected and underutilized species (NUS) (Padulosi and Hoeschle-Zeledon, 2004) translates into missed nutrition and health opportunities (Smith, 1982; Frison et al., 2006; Chadha and Oluoch, 2007; Hawtin, 2007; Smith and Longvah, 2009), since many of them offer a broader range of macro and micronutrients than those available in major staple crops.

One such group of highly promising crops is that of minor millets. They are called 'minor' because of the lack of research investment they attract, and their limited commercial importance in terms of area, production and consumption patterns (Nagarajan and Smale, 2007). By no means are they considered 'minor' in terms of their nutritional and income generation opportunities, which is what this case study will attempt to demonstrate. Once widely consumed in India and playing a key role in household food security and dietary diversity, in the last two decades these millets have been supplanted by rice as the staple grain. However, over the last 10 years, there has been increasing recognition of their favourable nutritional properties and associated benefits, also thanks to several national and international projects tackling their valorization in India and elsewhere in South Asia (Padulosi et al., 2009). Furthermore, as well as gaining credit for their role as a staple crop in marginal agricultural regions, they are increasingly being appreciated as healthy foods for urban and middle-income groups, losing the stigma of 'poor people's food' that was associated with them up until recently (Bala Ravi et al., 2010).

The benefits of agricultural biodiversity: why, what

In India, this group of small-seeded cereals is represented by six species, namely, finger millet (*Eleusine coracana* (L.) Gaertner) (Figure C8.1), kodo millet (*Paspalum scrobiculatum* (L.)), foxtail millet (*Setaria italica* (L.) Pal.), little millet (*Panicum sumatrense* Roth *ex* Roemer & Schultes), proso millet (*Panicum miliaceum* (L.)) and barnyard millet (represented by two species: *Echinochloa crusgalli* and *E. colona* (L.) Link) (Bala Ravi, 2004; Padulosi et al., 2009). Millets are hardy crops and quite resilient to a variety of agro-climatic adversities, such as poor soil fertility and limited rainfall. In view of their superior adaptability (compared for instance with rice or maize), they play an important role in supporting marginal agriculture, such as that commonly practised in the hilly and semi-arid regions of India (Bala Ravi, 2004; Padulosi et al., 2009; Bhag Mal et al., 2010).

Minor millets are nutritionally comparable or even superior to staple cereals such as rice and wheat (Gopalan et al., 2004; Geervani and Eggum, 1989). Compared with rice, 100 g of cooked grain of foxtail millet contains

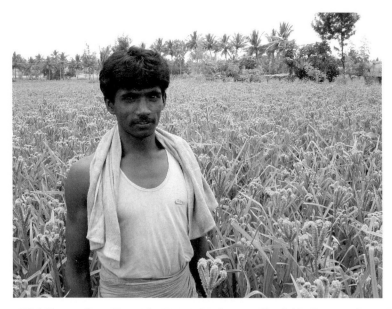

Figure C8.1 Farmer from Karnataka State in his finger millet field. Photo credit: Stefano Padulosi

almost twice the amount of protein, finger millet over 38 times the amount of calcium, and little millet more than nine times the amount of iron (Gopalan et al., 2004) (Table C8.1). Millets are rich in vitamins, minerals (calcium and iron in particular), sulphur-containing amino acids and phytochemicals, and hence are often described as 'nutritious millets' (Bala Ravi, 2004) or 'nutri-cereals' (Choudhury, 2009). They also contain high proportions of non-starchy polysaccharides and dietary fibre. Their slow release of sugar on ingestion makes them ideal food for diabetic patients, whereas the lack of gluten in their grains makes them good food for coeliac-affected people (Kang et al., 2008). Recognizing the importance of minor millets, particularly local landraces, for food and nutritional security, a 10-year project was carried out from 2001 to 2010 to promote their conservation and sustainable utilization. The project, known as the IFAD NUS project, supported by the International Fund for Agricultural Development (IFAD) and coordinated by Bioversity International, aimed at enhancing the contribution of neglected and underutilized species (NUS) – minor millets among them – in strengthening food security and incomes for the poor (Rojas et al., 2009; Bhag Mal et al., 2010).

Using highly inter-connected, community-based conservation through-use interventions, as well as participatory methods and tools, the project targeted smallholder farmers who were socio-economically disadvantaged with respect to access to food and more so to nutritious food. Implemented in 31 villages across four Indian states (Tamil Nadu, Orissa, Karnataka and Uttarakhand), the project was estimated to have influenced, directly or indirectly, some 753 households (Padulosi et al., 2009).

The benefits of agricultural biodiversity: how

The IFAD NUS project used an eight-step approach to enhance the use of minor millets in India (Figure C8.2). Project objectives, explained in detail below, were pursued by promoting the conservation, improvement and utilization of local landraces, developing enhanced cultivation practices, raising awareness on the nutritional importance and strategic role of millets in food and nutritional security, promoting innovative value addition methods and empowering local communities to become self-sustainable producers of raw and processed food products that can compete with other well-established commodity crops.

1   Provision and conservation of genetic material
    Surveys targeting the distribution of existing crop diversity were carried out to map the on-farm distribution of more common and endangered millet varieties. The establishment of village gene/seed-grain banks using culturally-acceptable approaches developed by the M.S. Swaminathan Research Foundation (MSSRF) allowed: i) the conservation of genetic diversity, ii) the creation of quality seed sources for cultivation purposes and iii) the accumulation of reasonable quantities of food grain stock to address food insecurity in most vulnerable households during lean income

Table C8.1 Nutrients in white rice and minor millets

Food (100 g)	Energy (Kcal)	Protein (g)	Fat (g)	Fiber (g)	Carbohydrate (g)	Phosphorous (mg)	Calcium (mg)	Iron (mg)
Rice (*Oryza sativa*)	346	6.4	0.4	0.2	79.0	143.0	9.0	1.0
Common millet (*Pennisetum glaucum*, "Bajra, Cambu")	361	11.6	5.0	1.2	67.5	296.0	42.0	8.0
Italian millet (*Setaria italica* "Thenai")	331	12.3	4.3	8.0	60.9	290.0	31.0	2.8
Proso millet (*Panicum miliaceum* "Pani-varagu")	341	12.5	1.1	2.2	70.4	206.0	14.0	0.8
Finger millet (*Eleusine coracana* "Ragi")	328	7.3	1.3	3.6	72.0	283.0	344.0	3.9
Little millet (*Panicum sumatrense* "Samai")	341	7.7	4.7	7.6	67.0	220.0	17.0	9.3
Kodo millet (*Paspalum scrobiculatum* "Varagu")	309	8.3	1.4	9.0	65.9	188.0	17.0	0.5

Source: Modified from Gopalan et al., 2004

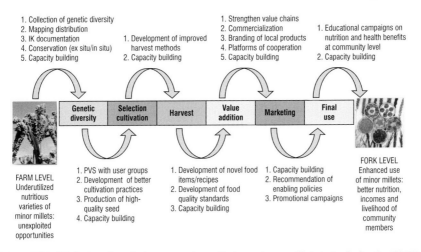

1. Collection of genetic diversity
2. Mapping distribution
3. IK documentation
4. Conservation (ex situ/in situ)
5. Capacity building

1. Development of improved harvest methods
2. Capacity building

1. Strengthen value chains
2. Commercialization
3. Branding of local products
4. Platforms of cooperation
5. Capacity building

1. Educational campaigns on nutrition and health benefits at community level
2. Capacity building

| Genetic diversity | Selection cultivation | Harvest | Value addition | Marketing | Final use |

FARM LEVEL
Underutilized nutritious varieties of minor millets: unexploited opportunities

1. PVS with user groups
2. Development of better cultivation practices
3. Production of high-quality seed
4. Capacity building

1. Development of novel food items/recipes
2. Development of food quality standards
3. Capacity building

1. Capacity building
2. Recommendation of enabling policies
3. Promotional campaigns

FORK LEVEL
Enhanced use of minor millets: better nutrition, incomes and livelihood of community members

Figure C8.2 Holistic value chain approach applied to minor millets in India by the IFAD NUS project. Text boxes list main types of interventions carried out with the close involvement of community members in target villages across the states of Uttarakhand, Tamil Nadu, Orissa and Karnataka

periods. Surveys documenting existing traditional knowledge on the health and nutritional benefits of millets were also carried out.

2   Development of better varieties to promote use

Participatory variety selections (PVS) and participatory rural appraisals (PRA) carried out in project sites led to the selection of five varieties of little millet, foxtail millet and finger millet. Selected local and improved varieties were then tested for performance in farmers' trials based on visual and quantitative assessment, such as grain and fodder yield. The agronomic potential of varieties identified from PVS and PRA was demonstrated across project villages in all four states using farmer participatory trials. Results of these demonstrations showed that the mean grain yield of varieties selected from PVS were 40 to 60 per cent higher than their local counterparts (Bhag Mal et al., 2010). Upon identification of the best varieties, farmers were then engaged in participatory seed production programmes to produce enough quality seed to be widely disseminated to farmers in target villages and elsewhere through the seed networks and Self-Help Groups (SHGs) set up by the project.

3   Development of improved cultivation practices

Improved cultivation practices were developed by blending traditional farming approaches with scientific methods. These include the use of better quality seeds; the use of density-regulated row planting instead of traditional broadcasting with high seed rate; structured intercropping of millet and other traditional crops (i.e. mung bean, chickpea, pigeon pea, lablab bean, mustard and niger) instead of their broadcasting as multi-species seed mix; use of farmyard manure; and plant density control by thinning/transplanting and weeding (Bala Ravi et al., 2010). Data gathered from 198 field demonstrations carried out in 2003 and 2004 revealed that the use of improved cultivation practices contributed to an increase of 39.8–62.8 per cent in grain yield and 34.1–47.3 per cent in fodder yield compared with traditional practices (Padulosi et al., 2009).

4   Development of more efficient processing technologies

The project successfully developed more efficient ways of grain threshing and milling, thus reducing drudgery normally associated with processing, a chore that has played a major role in the declining popularity of millets among traditional consumers (Bala Ravi et al., 2010). The provisioning of easy-to-use grain processing machines has effectively enhanced household consumption of minor millets as well as providing new livelihood options, particularly for women who are now able to complement their income by producing millet-based, locally-appropriate foods (Bala Ravi et al., 2010). Access to markets and micro-credit schemes was also supported to build long-term, economically viable and sustainable options (see also point 6).

5   Nutritional and industrial characterization of crops and products

New food-processing technologies were developed and tested to promote culturally-acceptable, millet-based products on the Indian food market. Traditional foods such as *paddu* (savoury pancakes) and novel foods such as biscuits, *laddus*, *chaklis* (popular sweet and savoury snacks), finger millet malt, finger millet flour and 'rice' of little millet and Italian millet were tested. A detailed cost-benefit analysis of product development showed that the highest benefits were associated with finger millet malt and little and Italian millet 'rice', for which a large market potential exists in India due to their importance in weaning and health foods (Bala Ravi et al., 2010). Malting of finger millet enhances the grain's energy value, making its protein, rich calcium and iron more bio-available, while enhancing the content of vitamins such as niacin and folic acid and its amino acid balance (Malleshi and Desikachar, 1986). Table C8.2 reports some of the novel foods developed by the project and their nutritive value assessed using the food composition tables of the nutritive value of Indian foods (Gopalan et al., 2004).

6   Build up of sustainable enterprises

Sustainability of activities beyond the project lifetime was achieved by establishing Self-Help Groups (SHGs) based on internal lending schemes and the creation of enterprises focusing on the cultivation, consumption, value addition and commercialization of end-products (Gruère et al., 2009). Since project inception in 2001, more than 35 SHGs were established with a total membership exceeding 386, of which 214 were women. To create market presence and promote demand for minor millet products, the MSSRF developed a branding strategy, which promoted the organic provenance and the conservation of millet genetic diversity as the products' added value. MSSRF also assisted SHGs in developing a booklet compiling traditional and novel recipes using minor millets (MSSRF, 2004), which was distributed as a part of the marketing efforts.

Table C8.2 Nutritive value of ethnic and novel foods

Parameters	Rice	Millet
Paddu – 100g		
Carbohydrates(g)	123.02	111.63
Protein(g)	19.03	20.85
Fat(g)	10.96	12.58
Ash(g)	2.02	4.75
Crude fibre(g)	0.75	12.42
Energy(kcal))	666.84	643.18
Calcium(mg)	68.86	94.08
Papad – 100g		
CHO(g)	81.82	78.51
Protein(g)	5.79	7.90
Fat(g)	3.06	4.06
Ash(g)	0.52	2.48
Crude fibre(g)	0.66	3.74
Energy(kcal)	377.98	382.18
Calcium(mg)	14.56	34.60
Biscuit – 100g		
CHO(g)	57.80	58.69
Protein(g)	4.78	4.35
Fat(g)	26.36	27.88
Ash(g)	0.28	4.55
Crude fibre(g)	0.12	0.92
Energy(kcal)	487.79	503.07
Calcium(mg)	60.40	90.16
Ladoo – 100g		
CHO(g)	64.46	63.97
Protein(g)	9.58	7.54
Fat(g)	18.91	18.39
Ash(g)	1.27	1.40
Crude fibre(g)	0.55	2.08
Energy(kcal)	500.00	483.34
Calcium(mg)	28.86	24.81
Chakli – 100g		
CHO(g)	45.48	39.13
Protein(g)	6.92	7.49
Fat(g)	32.33	32.12
Ash(g)	1.16	1.88
Crude fibre(g)	1.04	5.05
Energy(kcal)	501.33	475.58
Calcium(mg)	65.27	72.00

Source: Yenagi et al., 2010

7   Training of community members

At least 1,000 community members were trained in cultivation practices, value addition, marketing and nutrition during training efforts carried out by the IFAD NUS project in India. These training courses complemented the provision of novel technology and ranged from learning machinery operation to production of diverse value-added products suited for domestic consumption and commerce, standard codes of product quality, hygiene, packaging, labelling, marketing and account keeping. Capacity-building activities were mostly targeted at women, who are the main custodians of minor millet genetic diversity and the traditional knowledge associated with their production and consumption.

8   Raising public awareness

Numerous awareness-raising activities were organized on the nutritional importance of millets and their strategic role in providing food and nutritional security in certain agro-climatic regions. Targeting different stakeholders such as farmers (particularly women), urban housewives, government officials and rural development workers, primary and secondary school students and the wider public, activities included organizing poster sessions and millet-based product exhibitions during World Food Day, World Nutrition Day and World Diabetes Day, and during annual festivals in project villages. Similar exhibitions were organized by MSSRF during national and international conferences, as well as talks and lectures on the nutritional and health values of minor millets compared with more common cereal grains. During these events booklets and brochures were widely distributed, along with recipe books for these grains. Field demonstrations, farmers' fairs and exhibitions were also organized in project sites to promote high-yielding varieties, enhanced cultivation practices and improved processing technologies for finger millet. In addition, many TV and radio programmes promoting finger millet were organized, including a documentary in Kannada, the language of Karnataka, and English.

The benefits of agricultural biodiversity: health impacts

Investigations into the health impacts of minor millets showed promising results in a study carried out on school children from two millet-growing areas in Karnataka State. Using height and weight measurements and haemoglobin levels as measures of nutritional status, 60 school children between 11–14 years of age were monitored to assess the nutritional impact of replacing existing rice-based diets used in school feeding programmes with finger millet or foxtail millet rice. At baseline, the children, mostly from farming families, exhibited chronic energy deficiency (CED) with a BMI < 16.0, and haemoglobin levels below 12.0 g/100ml. Following a three-month intervention, research findings revealed a significant improvement with respect to weight and haemoglobin content in children fed on millets compared with the control group fed on rice (Table C8.3).

Table C8.3 Statistical analysis on the impact of millet-based food on school children

Parameter	Control				Treatment					Paired 't' test
	Initial	Final	Mean difference	't' value	Initial	Final	Mean difference	't' value		
Weight (kg)	24.58	25.25	0.67	5.12**	25.68	26.83	1.15	6.18**		2.23**
Height (cm)	133.50	134.3	0.80	9.96**	136.4	137.3	0.97	5.04**		1.51 NS
Haemoglobin (g/ml)	7.31	7.85	0.54	5.62*	7.78	10.46	2.68	14.10**		10.07**

* Significant, ** highly significant, NS not significant

Source: Annual Report 2010, MSSRF

Table C8.4 Nutrient composition of millet recipes per serving

Nutrient	Finger millet (Ragi)		Foxtail millet	
	Rice and sambar /serving	Ragi Mudde and Sambar/ serving	Rice and sambar/ serving	Millet rice
Protein (g)	15.77	16.52	17.06	25.31
Carbohydrate (g)	131.7	122.4	140.22	114.6
Fat (g)	15.0	16.2	7.18	12.88
Energy (Kcal)	691.25	773.75	696	675
Crude fibre (g)	0.67	5.77	1.1	12.8
Minerals (g)	1.77	4.92	2.18	6.23
Calcium (mg)	33.25	534.25	61.25	92.75
Phosphorous (mg)	316	500.5	358	553
Iron (mg)	1.72	6.52	2.56	5.71

Source: Yenagi et al. (not published)

In particular, haemoglobin levels of children eating millet-based school meals were significantly higher than the control group by 32.0–37.6 per cent.

Millet foods were considered very tasty and acceptable to more than 85 per cent of school children. The millet recipes developed and fed to the selected children were analysed for their nutrient composition. Results reported in Table C8.4 show that these products fulfil the nutritional standards indicated by the Supreme Court of India – which make it mandatory since 2001 to serve every child in all government schools mid-day meals containing at least 300 Kcal and 8–12 g protein a day for a minimum of 200 days (Supreme Court Order of November 28, 2001) – while providing additional amounts of micronutrients as compared with rice. Thus, millet foods represent a good source of micronutrients and have the potential to improve the nutritional status of school-going children and should therefore be recommended in the school mid-day meal programmes. These investigations were, however, limited in scale and in time and call for follow-up studies for further validation.

Policy impact

Concerted efforts to promote the nutritional and health benefits of minor millets successfully influenced public policy to include these grains in government-sponsored school feeding programmes and to subsidize public distribution systems including millets to target socio-economically and nutritionally-vulnerable populations. In 2006, Prof. M.S. Swaminathan urged the Government of India to include minor millet grains, sorghum and millet procurement and provision as part of the existing public distribution system to ensure nutritional security and sustainable production. This recommendation is now reflected in the policies of the Indian Government on 'nutri-cereals'. In his union budget speech for 2011–2012 the Finance Minister Pranab Mukherjee recognized the importance of minor millets and decreed that financial incentives would be made available to support millet farmers and 'promote higher production of these cereals, upgrade their processing technologies and create awareness regarding their health benefits'. The initiative is hoped to provide market linked production support to millet farmers in the arid and semi-arid regions of the country and to increase the nutritional security of about 25,000 villages.

Key lessons learned

The project was able to demonstrate that currently marginalized crops can be successfully used to create self-sustainable, agricultural-based enterprises that can support income generation in marginal areas of India while strengthening food and nutrition security through better use of culturally-adequate, nutritious crops. Furthermore, considering the high incidence of marginal land, poor soils and scarcity of water in many regions of India, the suitability of minor millets to grow in difficult edaphic and climatic conditions compared with other commodity crops make them ideal candidates to be used in climate change adaptation strategies in agriculture.

Barriers to their greater promotion are mostly of a policy nature, with heavy subsidies still being allocated to other commodity cereals, such as rice. Greater efforts are thus needed to convince policy makers to integrate minor millets in India's subsidized public distribution system (PDS). Such policies would not only move in the direction of enhanced food security, but would also support more resilient production systems in view of the global changes that are predicted to seriously affect the Indian continent in the coming decades (Padulosi et al., 2009).

Continued lobbying for the inclusion of minor millets in school-feeding programmes is also advocated as children could greatly benefit from the nutrients that are mobilized through a greater consumption of these crops and their products. Although the IFAD NUS project has been successful in demonstrating the value of certain interventions, more work is needed to scale-up approaches, methods and tools in wider areas of India. Greater government investment is also needed to continue developing superior varieties of minor millets as well as processing technologies that can satisfy increased demands for millet-based products across India, along with enabling policies to support their dissemination and adoption by consumers.

References

Arlappa, N., Laxmaiah, A., Balakrishna, N. and Brahmam, G.N.V. (2010) 'Consumption pattern of pulses, vegetables and nutrients among rural population in India', *African Journal of Food Science*, vol 4(10), pp.668–675.

Bhag Mal, Padulosi S. and Bala Ravi, S. (eds) (2010) *Minor Millets in South Asia: Learnings from IFAD-NUS Project in India and Nepal*, Bioversity International, Maccarese, Rome, Italy and the M.S. Swaminathan Research Foundation, Chennai, India, p.185.

Bala Ravi, S. (2004) 'Neglected millets that save the poor from starvation,' *LEISA*, India, vol 6, no 1, pp.34–36.

Bala Ravi, S., Swain, S., Sengotuvel, D. and Parida, N.R. (2010) 'Promoting nutritious millets for enhancing income and improved nutrition: A case study from Tamil Nadu and Orissa', in Bhag Mal, S. Padulosi, and S. Bala Ravi (eds) pp.19–46, *Minor millets in South Asia – Learning from the IFAD-NUS Project in India and Nepal*, Bioversity International, Maccarese, Rome, Italy and the M.S. Swaminathan Research Foundation, Chennai, India, p.185.

Chadha, M.L. and Oluoch, M.O. (2007) 'Healthy diet gardening kit for better health and income', *Acta Hort.*, vol 752, pp.581–583.

Choudhury, M. (2009) '"Konidhan" – A small millet against starvation', www.merinews. com/article/konidhan-a-small-millet-against-starvation/15772737.shtml, accessed August 2012.

FAO (2010) *Second report on the state of the world's plant genetic resources for food and agriculture*, Commission on Genetic Resources and Agriculture, FAO, Rome, Italy.

Frison, E.A., Smith, I.F., Johns, T., Cherfas, J. and Eyzaguirre, P B. (2006) 'Agricultural biodiversity, nutrition and health: Making a difference to hunger and nutrition in the developing world,' *Food Nutr. Bull.*, vol 27, pp.167–179.

Geervani, P. and Eggum, B.O. (1989) 'Nutrient composition and protein quality of minor millets', *Plant Foods for Human Nutrition*, Dordrecht, Netherlands, vol 39, issue 2, pp.201–208.

Gopalan C., Ramashastri, B.V. and Balasubramanium, S.C. (eds) (2004) *Nutritive Value of Indian Foods*, ICMR, New Delhi.

Gruère, G., Nagarajan, L., and King, O.E.D.I. (2009) 'The role of collective action in the marketing of underutilized plant species: Lessons from a case study on minor millets in South India,' *Food Policy*, vol 34, pp.39–45.

Hawtin, G. (2007) 'Underutilized plant species research and development activities – review of issues and options,' GFU/ICUC. International Plant Genetic Resources Institute, Rome, Italy.

International Institute for Population Sciences (IIPS) and Macro International (2007) *National Family Health Survey (NFHS-3), 2005–06: India: Volume I–II*. Mumbai.

Kang R.K., Jain, R. and Mridula, D. (2008) 'Impact of indigenous fiber rich premix supplementation on blood glucose levels in diabetics,' *Am. J. Food Technol.*, vol 3, no 1, pp.50–55.

Kanjilal, B., Mazumdar, P.G., Mukherjee, M. and Rahman, M.H. (2010) 'Nutritional status of children in India: household socio-economic condition as the contextual determinant,' *International Journal for Equity in Health*, pp.9–19.

Malleshi, N.G. and Desikachar, H.S.R. (1986) 'Nutritive value of malted millet flours,' *Qual. Plant, Plant Foods Hum. Nutr.*, vol 36, pp.191–196.

MSSRF (2004) *Mouth-Watering Gourmets from Traditional Foods of Kolli Hills,* published booklet from the Field station (MSSRF), Kolli Hills and Namakkal.

Nagarajan, L. and Smale, M. (2007) 'Village seed systems and the biological diversity of millet crops in marginal environments of India,' *Euphytica*, vol 155, pp.167–182.

Padulosi, S. and Hoeschle-Zeledon, I. (2004) 'Underutilized plant species: what are they?' *LEISA*, vol 20, no 1, pp.56.

Padulosi, S., Bhag Mal, Bala Ravi, S., Godwa, J., Godwa, K.T.K., Shanthakumar, G., Yenagi, N. and Dutta, M. (2009) 'Food security and climate change: role of plant genetic resources of minor millets,' *Indian Journal of Plant Genetic Resources*, vol 22, no 1, pp.1–16.

Rajaram, S., Zottarelli, L.K., and Sunil, T.S. (2007) 'Individual, household, programme and community effects on childhood malnutrition in rural India,' *Maternal & Child Nutrition*, vol 3, issue 2, pp.129–140.

Rojas, W., Valdivia, R., Padulosi S., Pinto, M., Soto, J.L., Alcócer, E., Guzmán, L., Estrada, R., Apaza, V. and Bravo, R. (2009) 'From neglect to limelight: issues, methods and approaches in enhancing sustainable conservation and use of Andean grains in Bolivia and Peru', in A. Buerkert, and J. Gebauer (eds) Agricultural biodiversity and Genetic Erosion, Contributions in Honor of Prof. Dr Karl Hammer, Supplement 92 to the *Journal of Agricultural and Rural Development in the Tropics and Subtropics*, Kassel University Press, pp.87–117.

Smith, I.F. (1982) 'Leafy vegetables as source of minerals in southern Nigerian diets,' *Nutr. Rep Intern.*, vol 26, pp.679–688.

Smith, I.F. and Longvah, T. (2009) 'Mainstreaming the use of nutrient-rich underutilized plant food resources in diets can positively impact on family food and nutrition security – data from Northeast India and West Africa,' *Acta Hort.*, vol 806, pp.375–384.

Supreme Court Order of November 28 (2001) Writ Petition (C), no 196 of 2001, http://www.righttofoodindia.org/orders/nov28.html, accessed August 2012.

Yenagi, N.B., Handigol, J.A., Bala Ravi, S., Bhag Mal, and Padulosi, S. (2010) 'Nutritional and technological advancements in the promotion of ethnic and novel foods using the genetic diversity of minor millets in India,' *Indian Journal of Plant Genetic Resources*, vol 23, no 1, pp.82–86.

Yenagi, N.B., Vijayalakshmi, D., Geeta, K., Geeta, Y., Jayarame Gowda, Dolli, S.S., Bala Ravi, S., Bhag Mal and Padulosi, S. (not published) 'Intervention studies on millets in school feeding programme and its impact on nutritional status of rural/urban school children'.

Case study 9

Local food and dietary diversity: farmers markets and community gardens in Melbourne, Australia

Kelly Donati, Christopher Taylor and Craig J. Pearson

Background

Recent policy initiatives in Australia at the metropolitan and national level have attempted to engage with ideas of food security in recognition of the threats that climate change and petrochemical dependency pose to food production as well as the barriers that socio-economic disadvantage present to accessing fresh and nutritious food. In the last five years, these threats have become more acute as agricultural production in the state of Victoria especially has been severely affected by natural disasters such as droughts, bushfires and floods. These natural disasters increase the cost of food for low-income households in Melbourne and regional areas alike (Carey et al., 2011). While the state and federal government have dedicated resources to supporting the economic sustainability of the agricultural sector and developing preventative health initiatives to encourage the consumption of fresh fruit and vegetables, Carey et al. (2011) highlight the absence of 'policy approaches that link fruit and vegetable consumption to production, either in Victoria or internationally'. This case study will focus on research carried out to explore farmers markets and community gardens as localized food systems that offer potential for improving dietary diversity and nutrition, supporting biological diversity and linking production to consumption. Data were collected using a GIS-based description of land use in Melbourne, as well as interviews carried out between 2009 and 2010 with local producers at farmers markets.

In Australia, the federal government is in the process of developing a national food plan that is likely to draw on economic measures and regulatory approaches to maintain the integrity of the country's food supply. The City of Melbourne has taken a more localized approach. Recognizing that food security is dependent on the viability of farms that surround the city, the city council is developing a food policy that addresses health and sustainability issues in Melbourne's food system. Food security is defined in this context as a stable supply of food that is available in sufficient quality and quantity, economically accessible, safe and nutritious; it also acknowledges the importance of a population that has the capacity and capability to cook and eat the food available (City of Melbourne, 2011). In 2008, the City of Melbourne endorsed the *Future Melbourne Plan*, a community visioning document that explicitly links production and consumption by setting out the ambitious target of 30 per cent of food to be either grown within the city or sourced from within 50 km of the city by 2020. This goal is to be achieved by enabling 'local residents to cultivate food for their own consumption' but also depends upon a thriving agricultural community around the city fringe (City of Melbourne, 2008). However, agricultural and urban planning policies are effectively at odds with each other in Victoria. Despite over half of the state's vegetables and approximately 17 per cent of its fruit being currently produced around Melbourne's borders (Carey et al., 2011), the council's vision for the future is challenged by state government policy that has earmarked more peri-urban agricultural land for residential development (Budge and Slade, 2009; Carey et al., 2011; Buxton et al., 2011).

Melbourne's current land allocation is shown in Figure C9.1a and Table C9.1. The map identifies large areas as public parks for conservation and as reserves (Green Wedges). The (peri-urban) area identified as farmland is relatively small (Figure C9.1b). However, in the inner city there is obviously active food production within household lots and in community gardens, and opportunities for intensification and diversification of production along transport corridors and in in-fill allotments. Further from the centre, opportunities exist for more productive land use in areas designated as low-density residential, rural conservation, and Green Wedges (the wedges being largely held as speculation for development rather than for production or conservation of, e.g., unique grasslands).

Farmers markets

Victoria's first farmers market was established in 1998 in Yarra Glen, 50 km outside of Melbourne. In 2002, a group of farmers market managers and stallholders joined to form the Victorian Farmers' Markets Association, which recently received US$2 million in state government funding to support the establishment and accreditation of more farmers markets across the state. There are now 50 accredited farmers markets in Victoria supplied by around 2,000 farmers. Twelve markets that are certified as selling locally-grown food are located within Melbourne's suburbs, eight within 125 km of the city and the rest in rural and regional areas. These are shown as white circles in Figure C9.1a.

Agricultural biodiversity

Animal genetic diversity is not recognized as a national priority in fostering food security in the National Food Plan, nor is there government support for monitoring or protecting rare breeds in Australia (Chambers, 2004). Rare breeds sold at farmers markets around Melbourne include critical, endangered or vulnerable pig breeds such as the Wessex Saddleback, Large Black and Tamworth as well as 'at risk' cattle breeds such as the Belted Galloway. Figures from the Rare Breed Trust of Australia indicate that the number of registered Tamworth and Large Black

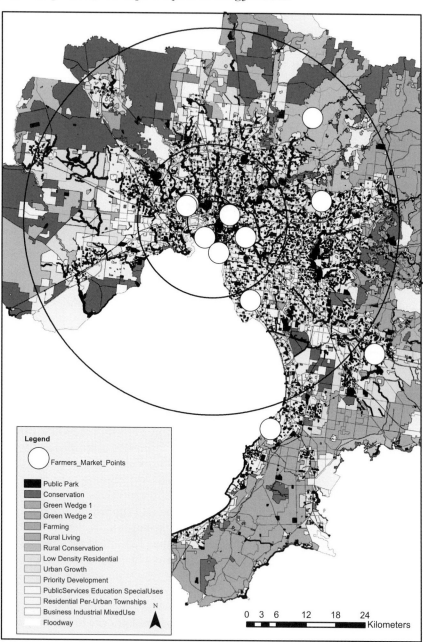

Figure C9.1a Melbourne's current land allocation by use

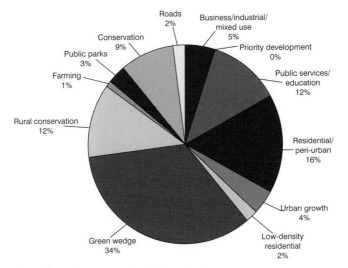

Figure C9.1b Melbourne's current land allocation by use

Table C9.1 Areas (hectares) of various Melbourne land types

Land type	0–5km	5–15km	15–40km	Total
Residential/peri-urban	2,518	31,348	66,369	123,514
Urban growth	0	0	24,245	34,414
Low density residential	0	3	8,459	16,598
Green wedge	0	0	66,054	258,711
Rural conservation	0	112	38,191	95,176
Farming	0	0	4,558	6,541
Public park	1,380	4,785	10,717	23,208
Conservation	0	719	12,941	66,061
Roads	554	2,673	7,854	16,650

pigs have more than doubled and Wessex Saddleback pig numbers have increased four-fold between 1998 and 2011 (RBTA, pers. comm., 11 December 2011). Fiona Chambers (RBTA Managing Director and Wessex Saddleback producer) believes that farmers markets provide a valuable conduit for rare breed sales to occur in small volumes and have partly contributed to the increased numbers.

Farmers markets in Victoria have a far greater diversity of plant varieties and animal breeds than is found in mainstream supply chains (see Table C9.2). The fragility of many heirloom vegetables means they are unsuited to long transport. Retail and wholesale markets also impose aesthetic and dimensional specifications which require a degree of crop uniformity that is not expected by patrons at

Table C9.2 Fruit and vegetable diversity

	Farmers Markets	Community Gardens
Aloe Vera		1
Apples	multiple (5+)★	
Amaranth		1+
Asian greens	multiple (4+)	multiple (4+)
Apricots	multiple	
Artichokes	2	1+
Asparagus	2	
Avocado	4	
Beans	multiple (7+)★	multiple (4+) ★
Beetroot	multiple (6+)★	multiple ★
Blueberries	multiple ★	
Bottle gourd		1+
Broccoli	multiple (2+)	multiple (2+)
Brussels sprouts	1+	1+
Cabbage	multiple (2+)	multiple (4+)★
Capsicum	multiple (4+)	multiple
Cauliflower	multiple (3+)	multiple (3+)
Carrots	multiple (5+)	multiple
Celeriac		
Celery	1+	Celery & Chinese celery
Cherries	1+	
Chilli	multiple (4+)	multiple
Cime di rapa	1+	
Citrus (lemons and oranges)	1+	1+
Corn/maize	multiple	multiple ★
Cucumbers	multiple (3+)	
Eggplant	multiple ★	multiple
Fennel	1+	1+
Feijoa	1+	
Garlic	multiple (3+)	1+
Grapes	1+	1+
Herbs[a]	1+	1+
Jerusalem artichokes	1+	1+
Kale (Russian, Tuscan)	1+	1+
Kohlrabi	1+	
Leeks, onions and shallots	1+	1+
Salad lettuces and greens[b]	1+	1+ (plus stem lettuce)
Melons	multiple (2+)★	multiple (3+)
Mushrooms	1+	
Nectarines	multiple	

	Farmers Markets	*Community Gardens*
Non-commercial edible plants or fruit	Mountain paw paw, nettle	multiple[c]
Nuts	almonds, pistachios (5), walnuts, chestnuts, hazelnuts	
Olives	1+	
Parsnip	1+	1+
Passionfruit	1+	1+
Peaches	multiple	
Pear	multiple (7+)★	
Peas	multiple	multiple
Pumpkin	multiple	multiple
Pepino		1+
Plums	multiple	
Potatoes	multiple (10+)★	multiple
Radish	multiple (4+)★	multiple (2+)★
Rhubarb	multiple ★	1+
Quince	1+	
Silverbeet	1+	
Strawberries	1+	1+
Sweet Potatoes	1+	1+
Tamarillo	1+	1+
Taro		1+
Tomatoes	multiple (20+)★	multiple ★
Turnip	1+	1+
Water chestnuts		1+
Watercress	1+	1+
Wild-sourced foods	Cardoons, wild watercress, mushrooms (3)	
Zucchini and squash	multiple (5+)★	multiple

★ denotes heirloom or heritage varieties
1+ denotes at least one variety identified
'Multiple' indicates unknown variety names and/or numbers
a Includes multiple basil varieties, chervil, coriander, dill, garlic chives, lemon balm, lemongrass, lemon verbena, multiple mint varieties, margoram, parsley, oregano, perilla, sage, tarragon, Vietnamese balm and Vietnamese mint.
b Includes chicory★, iceberg, watercress, butter, cos, rocket, oak, mizuna, endive, radicchio, spinach and sorrel.
c Includes arrowhead, black nightshade, canna, Chinese boxthorn, epazote, five-seasons herb, garland chrysanthemum, gotu kola (Indian pennywort), greater celandine, horehound, long-leaf coriander, mallow, luffa fruit, malabar spinach, molokhia, mugwort, orach, nettle, plantain, purple rice plant, purslane, rue, wormwood, water celery

farmers markets. In 2010, over 18 heirloom tomato varieties, ten types of potatoes and a selection of wild foods such as nettles, mushrooms, cress and cardoons were identified at the inner-city Slow Food Melbourne and Collingwood Children's farmer markets. One stallholder located 160 km from Melbourne has the largest selection of blueberry varieties in Australia and supplies the market with fresh and frozen organic blueberries year round. Another stallholder sells five types of pistachios, including a variety that the Commonwealth Scientific and Industrial Research Organisation (CSIRO) deemed unviable as a commercial crop and subsequently destroyed. An award-winning wine and olive oil producer farms a six-acre suburban property 15 km from the centre of Melbourne and, in addition to ten grape varieties, grows an astonishing array of fruits and vegetables including unusual crops such as Calabrian varieties of beans.

Dietary diversity and nutrition

Farmers markets predominantly cater and contribute to the dietary diversity of a relatively comfortable socio-economic demographic. However, they also contribute to the dietary diversity of the stallholders themselves, many of whom live in small towns in regional and rural Victoria which have been found to have limited access to fresh fruit and vegetables (Burns et al., 2004). At the end of each market, they regularly buy from or swap their remaining produce with other stallholders.

Plant variety is also likely to result in nutritional variety, although there are few data on intra-specific differences in quality among vegetables (Frison et al., 2004). However, research on Spanish greenhouse tomatoes that are bred for shelf life and uniform shape has shown that they have 'poor organoleptic and reduced nutritional qualities'. Rodríguez-Burruezo et al. (2005) who studied the internal and external qualities of North American varieties of heirloom tomatoes found that many varieties had superior nutritional and taste qualities to modern varieties sold in supermarkets.

Community gardens

Farmers markets cater largely to middle-class consumers while community gardens have stronger potential to improve access to fresh fruit and vegetables for low-income households. Melbourne has a long history of producing urban food. In 1941, almost half the population was producing its own food, more so in more affluent neighbourhoods and less so in disadvantaged areas where open land was scarce (Gaynor, 2006). Figure C9.1a illustrates opportunities for intensification of urban food production within allotments and transport corridors in the inner city and within preserved green space beyond 15 km (Table C9.1). While in Melbourne there is a resurgence of backyard and guerilla gardening – i.e. gardening on land that gardeners do not have legal right to use, often an abandoned site or area not cared for by anyone – many low-income households access land through community gardens, particularly in public housing estates.

Dietary diversity and nutrition

Community Gardens: A Celebration of the People, Recipes and Plants (Woodward and Vardy, 2005) is a valuable resource for understanding the enormous diversity of foods grown around Melbourne's public housing estates (Table C9.2) – much of which is not commonly available in retail markets – and how this food is consumed by residents for culinary and medicinal purposes. The recipes and interviews with gardeners demonstrate a clear link between garden produce and home cooking practices. This, combined with research from other urban gardens around the world, suggests that community gardens have potential for improving access to fresh fruit and vegetables by overcoming barriers to food security such as high food costs and increasing access to fresh produce that gardeners enjoy eating (Alaimo et al., 2008).

Biodiversity in community gardens

Seed saving and exchange between gardeners reduces the reliance on purchased seeds and allows them to grow and share plant varieties that are culturally relevant. Given that 75 per cent of the world's plant genetic diversity has been lost in the last century (FAO, 2004), community gardens may have broader implications for preserving agricultural biodiversity on farm and fostering food security by protecting plant varieties that have no commercial value. Galluzzi et al. (2010) describe home gardens 'as neglected hotspots of agro-biodiversity and cultural diversity'. The authors suggest that traditional crops or varieties are often 'maintained in cultivation because of personal affection and commitment of single gardeners, resulting in maintenance of a greater portion of intra-specific diversity than a market exposure permits'. Like many home and community gardens around the world, the crops grown on Melbourne's multi-cultural public housing estates are often cultivated because they have a particular relationship to a family or individual's traditions, cultural practices or culinary preferences (Baker, 2004). While community gardens may improve access to fresh fruit and vegetables, it is important not to privilege functional considerations such as nutrition or biodiversity over more affective factors such as pleasure and preference when considering the influences in production and consumption choices in community gardens.

Beyond functional understandings of farming, food and eating

A review of 16 studies on the influence of farmers markets and community gardens in the United States on dietary intake shows there is some potential for improving 'access to fruits and vegetables, especially in low-income areas that have poor access to affordable, healthful foods' (McCormack et al., 2010). However, most of these studies advocated the distribution of economic incentives, such as food coupons, to promote fruit and vegetable consumption, rather than promoting education campaigns that may ultimately prove more effective in influencing attitudes and beliefs regarding the purchase, preparation, or consumption of fruits and vegetables obtained from farmers markets or community gardens.

Drewnowski (1997) points out that most public health efforts have focused on encouraging 'consumers to replace palatable energy-dense foods with less palatable, but arguably healthier, starches and grains', with a particular emphasis on decreasing sugar and fat consumption. However, farmers market producers and gardeners alike frequently frame the motivations for their farming, gardening and consumption practices in terms of taste. One stallholder, Andrew Wood of Glenora Heritage Produce, explained that he uses non-hybrid, open pollinated, heirloom seed because, although they are more difficult to grow, he is interested in protecting biodiversity but also producing the best tasting food possible: 'I suppose you could call us gastronomic farmers... When I look at our vegetables in the field, I see the endless variety of finished dishes ready to eat' (Wood, 2010). Wood's commitment to taste is consistent with other farmers market producers who indicated that they grow particular varieties for their taste rather than yield. Similarly, many urban gardeners grow their own food not because it gives them better access to fresh fruit and vegetables, but because they have better flavour. Taste and aroma are a central part of eating and have the potential to influence moods, recall memories, serve as a warning of toxicity and more, yet the social value of the olfactory senses is frequently ignored in public health and agricultural policy and discourse (Santich, 2009).

Delind (2006) makes a case for local food systems that are more visible, convivial and sensual and that exceed the functional values represented in economic and nutritional understandings of food and farming. Focusing on functional elements of food production may overlook the primary motivation of both farmers market producers and urban gardeners. Our research indicates that consideration of the relationship between taste, cooking and eating that emerges from farmers markets and community gardens, rather than functionality, is most likely to encourage biological and dietary diversity.

References

Alaimo, K., Packnett, E., Miles, R.A., and Kruger, D.J. (2008) 'Fruit and vegetable intake among urban community gardeners,' *Journal of Nutrition Education and Behavior*, vol 40, no 2, pp.94–101.

Baker, L.E. (2004) 'Tending cultural landscapes and food citizenship in Toronto's community gardens,' *Geographical Review*, vol 94, no 3, pp.305–325.

Budge, T., and Slade, C. (2009) 'Integrating Land Use Planning and Community Food Security: A New Agenda for Government to Deliver on Sustainability, Economic Growth and Social Justice,' Prepared for the Victorian Local Governance Association and supported by VicHealth.

Burns, C., Gibbon, P., Boak, R., Baudinette, S., and Dunbar, J. (2004) 'Food cost and availability in a rural setting in Australia,' *Rural and Remote Health*, vol 4, no 311, pp.1–9.

Buxton, M., Alvarez, A., Butt, A., Farrell, S., Pelikan, M., Densley, L., and O'Neill, D. (2011) 'Scenario planning for Melbourne's peri-urban region,' RMIT University, Melbourne.

Carey, R., Krumholz, F., Duignan, K., McConell, K., Browne, J.L., Burns, C., and Lawrence, M. (2011) 'Integrating agriculture and food policy to achieve sustainable peri-urban fruit and vegetable production in Victoria, Australia,' *Journal of Agriculture, Food Systems and Community Development*, vol 1, no 3, pp.181–195.

Chambers, F. (2004) 'Status of Rare Breeds of Domestic Farm Livestock in Australia,' Compiled for the Rare Breeds Trust of Australia.

City of Melbourne (2008) 'Future Melbourne Plan,' www.futuremelbourne.com.au/wiki/view/FMPlan/WebHome, accessed June 2012.

City of Melbourne (2011) 'Food Policy Discussion Paper,' http://www.melbourne.vic.gov.au/CommunityServices/Health/FoodPolicy/Documents/Food_Policy_Discussion_Paper.pdf, accessed June 2012.

Delind, L. (2006) 'Of bodies, place, and culture: re-situating local food,' *Journal of Agricultural and Environmental Ethics*, vol 19, pp.121–146.

Drewnowski, A. (1997) 'Taste preferences and food intake,' *Annual Review of Nutrition*, vol 17, pp.237–253.

Food and Agriculture Organization of the United Nations (2004) 'Fact Sheet: What is happening to agrobiodiversity?' http://www.fao.org/docrep/007/y5609e/y5609e02.htm, accessed June 2012.

Frison, E.A., Cherfas, J., Eyzaguirre, P.B., Johns, T. (2004) 'Biodiversity, nutrition and health: making a difference to hunger and conservation in the developing world,' Keynote Address to the Seventh Meeting of the Conference of the Parties to the Convention on Biological Diversity (COP 7), 9–20 February 2004, Kuala Lumpur, Malaysia, available at: www.cbd.int/doc/speech/2004/sp-2004-02-09-cop-02-en.pdf, accessed June 2012.

Galluzzi, G., Eyzaguirre, P., and Negri, V. (2010) 'Home gardens: neglected hotspots of agro-biodiversity and cultural diversity,' *Biodiversity and Conservation*, vol 19, no 13, pp.3635–3654.

Gaynor, A. (2006) *Harvest of the Suburbs: an Environmental History of Growing Food in Australian Cities*, University of Western Australia Press, Crawley WA.

McCormack, L.A., Laska, M.N., Larson, N.I., and Story, M. (2010) 'Review of the nutritional implications of farmers' markets and community gardens: a call for evaluation and research efforts,' *Journal of the American Dietetic Association*, vol 110, no 3, pp.399–408.

Rodríguez-Burruezo, A., Prohens, J., Roselló, S., and Nuez F. (2005) 'Heirloom varieties as sources of variation for the improvement of fruit quality in greenhouse-grown tomatoes,' *Journal of Horticultural Science and Biotechnology*, vol 80, no 4, pp.453–460.

Santich, B. (2009) *Looking for Flavour*, Wakefield Press, Adelaide SA.

Wood, A. (2010) 'A matter of taste,' *Langton's Magazine* http://www.langtons.com.au/Magazine/Wood.aspx?MagazineId=316, accessed June 2012.

Woodward, P., and Vardy, P. (2005) *Community Gardens: A Celebration of the People, Recipes and Plants*, Hyland House, Flemington Vic.

Case study 10

'Please pick me': how Incredible Edible Todmorden is repurposing the commons for open source food and agricultural biodiversity

John Paull

Background

Perhaps it is the recipes, the climate, or the Manchester School of free trade advocacy. Whatever the reasons, food has not been one of Britain's great gifts to the world. Apparently, British school children generally do not wonder where their next meal is coming from beyond the supermarket freezer. In a survey, 36 per cent of school children did not know that the main ingredient of chips was potato, and 37 per cent were unaware that cheese is made from milk (Homeyard, 2005); and while 99 per cent could use a DVD player, only 58 per cent could use a vegetable peeler and only 43 per cent could boil an egg (Slattery, 2006).

The English town of Todmorden in West Yorkshire (North West England), with a population of about 17,000, was once a thriving hub of activity supporting the rapacious textile industry of a Great Britain in the midst of an Industrial Revolution that oversaw the near-extinction of non-industrial textile production. Now the region has one of Britain's highest unemployment rates. Houses in Todmorden are modest even by English standards. Front yards are non-existent or tablecloth size; and ditto backyards.

In the past, food production was off-shored with cheaper land and labour under foreign skies to 'better' climates, and, with British ships 'ruling the waves', feeding Britain cheaply took priority over feeding Britain locally or seasonally.

The wisdom of scouring the world for the cheapest foodstuffs while neglecting British agriculture and local food production came adrift during WWII when German U-boats were doing their darnedest to torpedo supply. At the Economic Reform Club, Lord Northbourne raised the question: could Britain feed itself? (Northbourne, 1940). The campaign 'Dig for Victory' and food rationing and shortages, which extended into the 1950s for Britain, brought home to the British their lack of food security and sovereignty.

Thus, when the Incredible Edible Todmorden (IET) project raises the question of food self-sufficiency for Todmorden – and by extension the rest of Britain – it is treading on historical carcasses and the skeletons of British

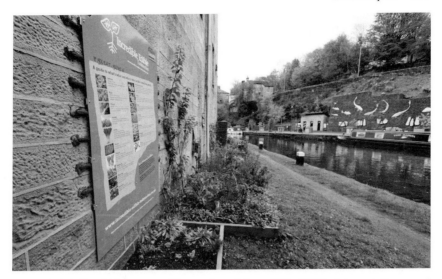

Figure C10.1 Canalside – vegetable patch and Incredible Edible interpretative panel along the canal tow path at Todmorden. Photo credit: John Paull

imperialism, the dogmas of free trade, and the faded 'greatness' and arrogance of an empire well past its use-by-date.

On a daily basis, newspapers report dysfunctional eating and the obesity epidemic engulfing Britain. The National Health Service (NHS) is funding lap-band surgery for obese Britons as young as 16 years old (Bond, 2011). British women are the fattest in Europe and a quarter are obese (Bates and Hope, 2011), while national facilities are expended on repurposing resources. For one morbidly obese Briton: 'On one occasion firefighters had to be called out to demolish the front wall of his former home so they could drive a fork lift truck inside to lift him out and put him into an ambulance … Two female carers take up to four hours to wash (him) because his size makes it impossible for him to clean himself' (Whitelocks and Bates, 2011).

The benefits of agricultural biodiversity: why, what

In March 2008 a public meeting was held in Todmorden. The topic was food – and the premise was 'we need to talk'. The meeting attracted about 60 attendees and was a local response to the growing awareness that Britain needs to have a conversation about food. In many ways it was a meeting against the tide of the Americanization of the British diet, of the Tesco-ization[1] of food retailing, of the dissociation of food from its agricultural and geographic provenance, as well as of a centuries-late response to the off-shoring of British agricultural biodiversity and of food production generally.

From that meeting, *Incredible Edible Todmorden* (IET) was born. The town was scoured for land and space that could be repurposed for food growing.

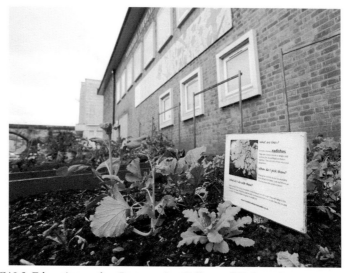

Figure C10.2 Education – the Community College of Todmorden tempts passers-by with open access radishes growing in a pavement plot. Photo credit: John Paull

Permission gardens and guerilla gardens[2] appeared around town planted out with cabbage and carrots, rhubarb and radishes, chard and chives, becoming 'propaganda gardens' – their very presence, designed to precipitate public and private discourse on the subject of food. They serve as 'Trojan horses' to smuggle food issues into public awareness.

A herb garden planted out beside a footpath and planter pots outside the Hippodrome Theatre added edibility to the streetscape of Todmorden. One senior school and six primary schools in the town all now grow food and the local cemetery has had an Incredible Edible make-over tended by school children. The local medical centre features an apothecary garden, and planter boxes in the adjacent car park have been shared out between IET and Blooming Todmorden, a practical compromise between the contesting ideologies of prettification versus edibility.

The novelty of IET's produce is that this is help-yourself food where passers-by are invited and encouraged to pick this fresh local produce. A message on IET boards is: 'Go on, take some. It's all free.' Signage presents pictures and names of planted produce, and suggests when it is ready to pick and how it may be cooked. Against an image of kale, consumers are advised: 'Harvest: June–February. Use in any recipes that are suited to cabbage or Brussels sprouts.' Of lovage (*Levisticum officinale*) we read: 'Harvest: All year. A lesser-known and underrated herb. Tastes a little like celery, so great in soups and stocks'. Adjacent to an image of chard: 'Harvest: All year. Great as a side dish. Just cook and add olive oil and salt. Mmmmm.'

Many are now familiar with open-source journals where the content is free to the end user, but the concept of open-source food, of picking and eating something that someone else had planted and nurtured, took some time to catch on, and represents a cultural change in Todmorden.

Plots are mixed – there is no monoculture for IET – which is visually more interesting and attractive, and encourages mixed picking as well as sampling of the unfamiliar.

The benefits of agricultural biodiversity: how

IET has created 40 public fruit and vegetable gardens. The gardens and orchards in 'the commons' are the public face of IET and they are its most visible, tangible and immediate community benefit. They are a constant reminder that 'food doesn't grow on supermarket shelves, you know'. They deliver visual interest, opportunities for participation and engagement, gastronomic novelty and amenity, as well as fresh seasonal local nourishment.

IET has also created a variety of communication, educative and celebratory events in the town. Such events have included street cook-offs, 'Tod Talks', targeted campaigns such as 'Every Egg Matters' which maps local egg production, cooking courses, the field to plate lunch, and seed swaps. Regular newsletters, an active website (www.incredible-edible-todmorden.co.uk, accessed August 2012), presentations beyond the local district, and veggie tourism, all serve to maintain the momentum of IET.

A celebrity visit, such as by Prince Charles, to IET adds endorsement and gains media exposure beyond what free carrots in an obscure West Yorkshire town may otherwise attract. It can add Todmorden to the celebrity-circuit and, as an online commentator offered: 'Congratulations to the folk of Todmorden for being so innovative that the Prince of Wales just had to come to see it for himself' (wrinkles, in Moseley, 2010).

The benefits of agricultural biodiversity: impacts

The local and immediate outcome of IET is the transformation of the commons with edible townscaping. IET has raised the profile of food in general and local food in particular. Residents and food vendors have a raised awareness of localness. A survey of Todmorden shoppers reported that 64 per cent 'buy locally produced food regularly', with the leading reasons for doing so being to 'support the local economy' followed by 'quality and freshness' (Lee-Woolf, 2009).

The Todmorden local market has survived and even prospered with a banner declaring: 'Your Local Market. Great people, great value, great service. Local food on sale here. Put markets back into market towns.' Of the fresh produce on offer in the market, many items are prominently labelled as 'local'. This creates a motivation for producers to grow such differentiated produce and shoppers to preference it.

The movement against the Tesco-ization of small-town Britain is active in Todmorden. Decals reading 'Save our markets. No more supermarkets'

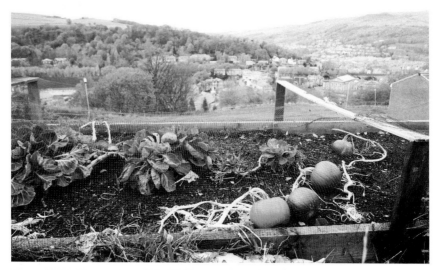

Figure C10.3 Views – Incredible Edible pumpkins planted with a view over Todmorden, West Yorkshire, UK. Photo credit: John Paull

are on prominent display throughout the town and a recent application for a further supermarket has been declined by the local council. The *Todmorden News* carried the comment endorsing that decision: 'This should now send Sainsbury's a clear signal, should they appeal, that they are not welcome in Tod. This message could also be extended to any other supermarket chain wishing to build another supermarket in the town. Three is enough thank you!' (Sutcliffe, 2011).

The first Todmorden cheese was launched on the market in August 2009. The new Pextenement Cheese Company restored a seventeenth-century dairy, and its East Lee branded cheese is made from local organic milk (Pextenement, 2010). It is perhaps at the forefront of a new wave of niche, boutique and artisan local food products.

A survey in Todmorden had 47 per cent of respondents reporting that they 'have grown food at home this year' while 35 per cent reported that they are 'fairly new to food growing'. Seventy-nine per cent stated that they 'would like more food growing around town' (Lee-Woolf, 2009).

A local mother stated: 'I'd never grown a vegetable in my life and I had absolutely no idea how to do it, but when I heard about Incredible Edible from another mum ... I knew it made sense. I started in my own garden by growing vegetables. It was far easier than I'd expected it to be. This year we've had potatoes, leeks, carrots, cabbage, strawberries, onions, garlic, peas, parsnips and sprouts, and I don't spend more than two hours a week in the garden' (Pauline Mullarkey, quoted in Moorhead, 2009).

Scale up efforts and challenges

IET has used a strategy of 'find what works', and duplicate it. The Todmorden core activities of creating propaganda gardens and propaganda orchards using local and heritages varieties have been successfully replicated across the town. Sites continue to be identified, and the corpus of such gardens and orchards continues to grow.

Residents of at least sixteen towns and villages[3] have adopted the Incredible Edible model and moniker and are in various stages of reproducing the Todmorden project for themselves. These copy-cats are generally villages and small towns. It remains to be tested if Incredible Edible is a small-town phenomenon that can readily be scaled up to larger conurbations, cities, and perhaps even mega-cities. Scaling down is plausibly a less problematic enterprise.

A different species of 'scale-up' is about to be tested in Todmorden. Following a successful application to the Lottery Fund, IET has been awarded £500,000 to expand its vision of local food with plans for an ambitious demonstration project including aquaponics, with integrated orchards, bees, and an 'edible learning landscape'. Just how will this major injection of funds with its attendant commitments, demands, promises, staffing, infrastructure, management, and reporting requirements impact on what has been a volunteer enterprise? Stories of lottery winners squandering their winnings are by now a cliché. Just how will IET articulate its own change of fortunes, and perhaps even negotiate with a potential 'saving Nemo' backlash? What is certain is that half a million pounds will change the dynamics of IET and, when the cash runs out, IET will have a fascinating narrative to share – about scalability (and fish).

Stakeholder involvement

'If you eat, you're in' is a tag of IET. It identifies that we are all stakeholders in the enterprise of food, and thereby all potential constituents of the Incredible Edible project.

Pam Warhurst, one of the IET founders, characterizes 'The Model' of IET as 'Three plates spinning' where she says 'One is boring, two is clever, three's a show!' According to Warhurst these 'plates' are the 'Community – Everyone', the 'Business sector including farmers' and 'Learning/education – cradle to cradle' (Warhurst, 2010). IET has successfully recruited these three plates into the IET vision.

IET began without funding and it was the sweat-equity of community members that was initially invested in the enterprise. An early engagement with food businesses was to give them each blackboards where they could advertise what was 'local'. Businesses have reciprocated and their support has generally been in kind – timber, plants, seeds, planter boxes, signage, and the space for planting.

All schools in Todmorden participate. The catering manager of Todmorden High School, Tony Mulgrew, reported that the school started growing food in

February 2009. By the summer of that year the school was serving soup in their dining room made with their own school-grown tomatoes, potatoes, courgettes, beans, endive and chard (Moorhead, 2009).

Policy impact

IET is a vehicle to argue for systemic change, and its proponents are not blind to the wider context of their small-town project, perhaps even to the global context. The emphasis has been on direct action, and as Pam Warhurst says: 'We're bored to death and cynical about strategies and policies and rhetoric' (quoted in Paull, 2011). Nevertheless the IET people are not silent about the bigger picture, and the opportunities for engineering systemic change at the policy level. Ten proposals have been generated that, if implemented at a government policy level, would inject, by fiat, food growing into urban planning (Table C10.1).

IET's success to date has been the success of a grass-roots idea that has taken hold in its hometown and has spread to other towns and villages. Just how this success might port to government is unclear as well as contested. A recent newspaper report about Todmorden and its Incredible Edible project attracted favourable feedback from readers as well as tapping a vein of cynicism about government intervention (Graff, 2011). One correspondent commented: 'This is one light at the end of the tunnel that is not an oncoming train' (mkb, in Graff, 2011). Another expressed optimism that others would take up the idea: 'Wonderful inspiring ladies, with a beautiful vision. I dearly hope more towns,

Table C10.1 Proposals from Incredible Edible Todmorden for edible townscaping (Warhurst, 2010)

1. Build schools for the future that have the living edible world at their heart
2. Transform health buildings with edible plants and trees as an integral part of the design and workplace
3. All public bodies to release land for food growing
4. Plan for food - Support local food production through the planning system with local plans identifying places for growing
5. Tick all the boxes - Make growing a performance indicator for 'wellbeing' for all Public Services
6. Insist all new homes have ready-to-grow spaces
7. All social landlords to allocate space for growing
8. Charter for truly local markets - support local food producers and farmers and campaign for the reallocation of subsidies
9. Make sure public bodies like schools and health authorities have as a priority to procure local food
10. Invest in food skills for the future. We need incredible degrees and diplomas, cooks and technologists, farmers and fabulous food producers

cities and villages think the same and take part in this fantastic scheme' (Kroger, in Graff, 2011). A positive role for government was envisaged by one reporter: 'Perfect! The way it should be. I don't want to knock the beautiful flower beds around town but increased fruit and vegetable planting (instead of flowers to some extent) should be a national policy' (PrivateSi, in Graff, 2011), while others raised a note of caution regarding its involvement. One correspondent pleaded: 'Please do not involve government, ministers or councillors – that is instant death to anything. People feel they are being pushed and so rebel or are disinterested. It would instantly be loaded with health and safety rules as well. Keep councillors out' (Flora, in Graff, 2011). Another wrote: 'I agree that it's a brilliant idea but like an earlier comment "don't get the politicians involved, local or national" they'll find a way to tax it and throw the "elf and safety" book at it' (Get it right eh, in Graff, 2011).

Whether IET could successfully make the transition from 'grass-roots' and citizen activism to local government or national government policy, remains uncharted territory. While some draw from a deeply sceptical vein, what is clear is that the IET group are themselves optimistic and more than optimistic since they are actively advocating a governmental uptake of Incredible Edible precepts.

Key lessons learned

There are at least seven lessons that can be drawn from the successes of the IET project. These lessons can be characterized as: champions; actions; visibility; engagement; media and message; replication; and contagion.

Firstly, the success of IET has been driven by local champions who have imaginatively, enthusiastically and articulately taken up the challenge of localizing food. The initial public meeting moved the project past the idea stage, and taking action is the important second lesson of IET. Thirdly, those actions, whether permission gardens or guerilla gardens, shared the common element of visibility. IET gardens are highly visible. They are labelled with IET logos and interpretational text ranging from handwritten, for example 'Food to Share – Please do not pull veg. then leave to die – this is sad and wasteful. Enjoy it!' through to the professionally illustrated signage, in full-colour and sponsored.

The fourth lesson of IET has been engagement. IET actively recruited from the outset its 'three spinning plates' – community, business and the education sector. This engagement leveraged commonalities, resources, skill sets, and interests. The success of IET has been accompanied by regular coverage in the *Todmorden News* which has provided frequent refreshment of the message in the local weekly newspaper. The fifth lesson is the constructing of regular stories, photo opportunities, fresh angles, the framing of messages (e.g. 'If you eat, you're in').

A sixth lesson from IET is replication. Find out what works and do that, again and again. Some activities, such as street gardens and verge orchards, can proliferate to occupy the available niches. Rituals that work, for example street cook-offs and seed swaps can become regular or annual fixtures. The seventh lesson of IET is to foster contagion – keep it simple, open, replicable, non-proprietorial, and continually refresh the momentum.

IET is successfully reinvigorating food discourse, 'one stick of rhubarb at a time'. Food is increasingly being acknowledged as the issue of our times. Incredible Edible has created a vehicle to inject food issues into the public domain and to project them well beyond its hometown of Todmorden.

Acknowledgements

Warm thanks are extended to the University of Oxford and the team of Incredible Edible Todmorden.

Notes

1　Tesco is a British multinational grocery and general merchandise retailer.
2　Gardening on land that the gardeners do not have legal right to use, often an abandoned site or area not cared for by anyone.
3　Todmorden as well as: Accrington; Cloughmills; Glossop; Holmes Chapel; Hoylake; Huddersfield; Lambeth; Llandrindod; Prestwich; Ramsbottom; Rossendale; Totnes; Wakefield; Wight; and Wilmslow.

References

Bates, C. and Hope, J. (2011) British women are the fattest in Europe with a quarter so overweight their health's at risk, *The Daily Mail*, 25 November.

Bond, A. (2011) Schoolgirl who became Britain's youngest gastric bypass patient loses ten stone in just one year, *The Daily Mail*, 12 December.

Graff, V. (2011) Carrots in the car park, radishes on the roundabout. The deliciously eccentric story of the town growing all its own veg., *The Daily Mail*, 10 December.

Homeyard, S. (2005) Food 4 thought: Online Kids 5th–12th October, report prepared by TNS, London, for British Heart Foundation (BHF).

Lee-Woolf, C. (2009) A critical evaluation of the contribution that community-based action makes to sustainable development in the UK food system, MSc thesis, Imperial College London.

Moorhead, J. (2009) Todmorden's good life: introducing Britain's greenest town – 'Grow your own' fever has gripped the Pennines community, which is aiming for self-sufficiency, *The Independent*, 29 November.

Moseley, T. (2010) Prince Charles visits Todmorden, *The Lancashire Telegraph*, 8 September.

Northbourne, Lord (1940) Where is the food to come from? In *Three Addresses on Food Production in Relation to Economic Reform* (pp.3–9), London: The Economic Reform Club and Institute.

Paull, J. (2011) Incredible Edible Todmorden: Eating the Street, *Farming Matters*, vol 27, no 3, pp.28–29.

Pextenement (2010) Pextenement Cheese Company, Specialty Cheese made from Todmorden Organic Milk. Retrieved 14 December 2011, www.pextenement.co.uk, accessed August 2012.

Slattery, L. (2006) Techno whizz kids who can't boil an egg or peel a potato, British Heart Foundation, press release, 2 November.

Sutcliffe, P. (2011) Delighted with decision – three supermarkets is enough, thanks, *Todmorden News*, 30 August.

Warhurst, P. (2010) Incredible Edible Todmorden. Incredible Edible Todmorden London Conference in Peckham, John Donne School, Peckham, 9 October.

Whitelocks, S. and Bates, C. (2011) Former world's fattest man begs for NHS operation to remove folds of skin after losing 40 stone, *The Daily Mail*, 25 November.

Case study 11

Cultivating health with leafy vegetables in coastal Tanzania

Petra Bakewell-Stone

Background

Levels of food insecurity are persistently high in Tanzania, with 34 per cent (13.9 million) of the population undernourished (FAO, 2011). The main nutritional disorders affecting Tanzanians include protein-energy malnutrition and deficiencies in iron, vitamin A and iodine (Lorri, 1996; Kinabo, 2008).

Underlying causes of malnutrition are complex and multi-faceted, but have in part been attributed to declining consumption of nutrient-rich traditional and leafy vegetables (Pendaeli et al., 2010; Oniang'o et al., 2006; Ogoye-Ndegwa and Aagaard-Hansen, 2006). Low-income households typically have unbalanced diets consisting mainly of carbohydrates complemented by a small quantity of low-end protein. When consumed, leafy vegetables are often exotic (including cabbage and collard greens) and purchased at a high price from local markets. Even in relatively wealthy urban households, children consume low amounts of leafy vegetables due to lack of availability and knowledge. Other reasons for the declining consumption of traditional vegetables include Westernisation, negative perceptions associated with these foods, lack of awareness about their benefits, shortage of land on which to grow or collect them, as well as the time needed to gather and prepare them (RESEWO, 2009).

Local groups in many different countries are now taking action to reverse the negative effects of the 'nutrition transition' (which refers to 'changes in diet and activity patterns' – Popkin, 2001: 871), including declining dietary diversity and associated nutritional disorders such as obesity, high blood pressure, cholesterol and diabetes (Turner and Ommer, 2003).

In 2006, over cups of *Bidens pilosa* (Blackjack) tea, a group of senior women citizens – siblings, neighbours and old school friends – living on the Regent Estate in Dar es Salaam, Tanzania, decided to start the Regent Estate Senior Women's Organisation (RESEWO). Their aim was to promote the identification, cultivation and use of traditional foods and vegetables. RESEWO's original membership of 12 grew to 22 by 2006, and in 2011 counted over 60 members. Most are retired professionals over 60 years of age, and all but two are women. Reasons for membership include: maintaining heritage species, conserving agricultural biodiversity, teaching others about forgotten or underutilised foods

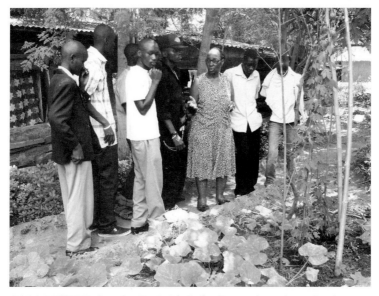

Figure C11.1 RESEWO founder, Freda Chale, leading students through a demonstration garden in the Village Museum in Dar es Salaam. Photo credit: P. Bakewell-Stone

and the value of traditional vegetables, and improving the health of vulnerable groups as well as their own.

This case study reports on the findings of an ethnobotanical study conducted with RESEWO members in Kinondoni district and their counterparts, mature homegardeners, in Bagamoyo district (Dar es Salaam and Pwani regions, respectively). Research focused on documenting the use of traditional plant species by communities for health and food security, as well as factors promoting and influencing leafy vegetable cultivation.

Kinondoni district covers an area of 531 km² and in 2002 housed a population of over one million (Mbonile and Kivelia, 2008); the contiguous Bagamoyo district covers 9847 km² and has an estimated population of 277,673 (MoAFC, 2010). The region is characterised by a tropical climate with an average temperature of 28°C and average annual rainfall ranging between 800–1500 mm. Climatic changes, including a decrease in rainfall and increase in temperature (Mbonile and Kivelia, 2008), are affecting planting seasons, as well as yields and types of vegetables grown.

Whereas in Bagamoyo, agriculture, livestock-keeping and fishing are the population's main livelihood strategies, in Kinondoni most households depend on informal businesses such as selling agricultural commodities.

In addition to drought and pest epidemics, major challenges faced by the agricultural sector include low levels of education and a lack of extension services. This results in low access to improved technology and farm inputs, weak irrigation, limited processing, storage and marketing infrastructure, lack of credit and low investment. Rural–urban migration, particularly among the younger generations, and the prevalence of HIV/AIDS and other diseases put pressure on the availability of farm labour. In addition, due to unsustainable land management practices, deforestation and over-grazing, soils are being heavily degraded and becoming more susceptible to erosion.

The benefits of agricultural biodiversity: why, what

The cultivation and use of micronutrient-rich leafy vegetables with medicinal properties has been promoted as a means to improve health and food security (Turner and Ommer, 2003), their use underlining the 'multiple roles of botanicals as constituents of both an indigenous diet and herbal pharmacopoeia' (Etkin and Ross, 1983: 232). High in antioxidants, folic acid, protein per calorie and omega-3, leafy greens are an important component of diets in many places in the world (Nabhan, 2004) and contribute significant amounts of vitamins A and C to the diets of resource-poor households in sub-Saharan Africa (van Rensburg et al., 2004). The nutritional quality of these vegetables is characterised by biologically-active plant metabolites including carbohydrates, vitamins, hormones, organic and amino acids, phenolics, flavonoids and glucosinolates. Essential for plant growth, development and defence, metabolites determine plant colour, taste and smell along with the plant's medicinal and nutritional properties (Hounsome et al., 2008: 48). This explains the sustained use of leafy greens throughout history as essential ingredients for relishes, herbal preparations and other traditional forms of phytotherapy amongst communities and traditional healers in Tanzania, as well as the supplementary role they play in diets by adding variety and improving palatability and taste of staple foods (Lyimo et al., 2003). Research carried out by Marshall (2001) on the use of wild and weedy greens by a community in Kenya demonstrated that patterns of harvesting and using these plants results in greater dietary diversity while maximising the plants' nutritional benefits. In Marshall's study group wild greens were gathered and cooked with between one and four other taxa of weedy greens, and combinations of greens eaten varied from day to day, providing different sources of nutrients, vitamins and minerals.

Across East Africa the domain of leafy vegetables is both large and diverse, encompassing a wide variety of edible plants (over 50 different species reportedly used in Tanzania). Many are cultivated, although there is a large amount of variation in management intensity from wild gathered to fully domesticated. A number of species of wild and weedy leafy vegetables traditionally consumed in East Africa show potential for domestication. These include *Talinum portulacifolium*, *Cleome gynandra*, *Solanum nigrum*, *Bidens pilosa*, *Basella alba* and *Portulaca oleracea*. They are often preferred due to their environmental suitability and contribution to 'climate proofing' by resisting drought. Growing leafy vegetables is amongst a portfolio of livelihood strategies used by smallholders to adapt to climate change, improve nutritional security and become more self-sufficient.

For the present study, besides management status, leafy vegetables were differentiated on the basis of leaf shape, life cycle, abundance, propagation

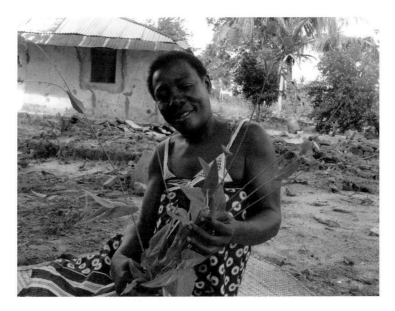

Figure C11.2 Fatuma Shariff, Chairwoman of a community-based organisation in Kiromo village, Bagamoyo district, showing *kilemba cha bwana* (*Emilia javanica*) a wild leafy vegetable used traditionally in the coastal region of Tanzania. Photo credit: P. Bakewell-Stone

technique, perceived status, use, preparation method and taste. Whilst the great majority of plants described as leafy vegetables were herbaceous, some tree species were also included such as Guava (*Psidium guajava*), Baobab (*Adansonia digitata*) and Moringa (*Moringa oleifera*). This variation can be explained by the biocultural diversity existing across Tanzania's 120 tribes and nine agro-ecological zones.

During the documentation phase of this study, the most commonly nominated leafy vegetables were *Launaea cornuta* and *Bidens pilosa*. Their frequency of mention indicates the underlying criteria for their utilisation in coastal Tanzania including bitter-tasting, weedy, use reliant on traditional knowledge and medicinal. Both are used in traditional healthcare as anti-malarials and are good candidates for improving micronutrient status. *Bidens pilosa* is valued as a nutritious vegetable, tea-substitute and home remedy for a number of ailments.

The benefits of agricultural biodiversity: how

In order to promote the use of these plants and raise awareness of their nutritional properties, the founders of RESEWO transferred traditional vegetable seeds from their native areas to homegardens. The organisation now grows and promotes a range of different traditional leafy vegetables on their demonstration plots at the Village Museum in Dar es Salaam and in their own homegardens. They also distribute seeds, vegetables and information materials, such as recipe books (Pendaeli et al., 2010), as well as helping establish school gardens and developing a community seed bank. Members of RESEWO adopt such approaches because they attribute protein–energy deficiency not only to poverty but also to lack of education and awareness, particularly with regards to nutritious foods.

The benefits of agricultural biodiversity: health impacts

Whether used as foods or for their medicinal properties, the consumption of leafy vegetables and the ingestion of the phytochemicals they contain 'can explain diverse cultural food behaviours and health outcomes' (Johns et al., 1996). Growing leafy vegetables is providing homegardeners in the coastal region of Tanzania with daily access to safe and nutritious food and medicine. This is important, for example, in reducing iron and vitamin A deficiencies in vulnerable groups such as the elderly and in pregnant women, and for improving maternal health and reducing child illness and mortality (Lyimo et al., 2003). Cowpea (*Vigna unguiculata*) and sweet potato (*Ipomoea batatas*), both known to have high iron contents, are being recommended for pregnant women and for treating anaemia. Other nutrient-rich leaves include those of squash (*Cucurbita maxima*) that provide vitamin A and *Cleome gynandra* containing high levels of vitamin C, iron and calcium.

A wide range of leaves are used traditionally for the treatment of diarrhoea and other stomach complaints. The increasing incidence of HIV/AIDS and diabetes has seen a rise of people turning to traditional plants to treat disease-related problems, e.g. lemongrass for lesions and ulcers. Leafy vegetables and plants in general are considered a safer alternative to (often counterfeit) store-bought medication. They are often associated with longevity and increased immunity – as is the case for baobab (*Adansonia digitata*) – and sometimes also increased appetite (*Caylusea abyssinica*).

During the documentation phase of the study, many people were keen to testify to the efficacy of leafy vegetables in preventing, alleviating or treating different ailments. *Bidens pilosa*, for instance, has been successfully used to treat high blood pressure and anaemia as well as preventing malaria; one couple reported not suffering from malaria since 1965 as a result of drinking one to two cups of *Bidens pilosa* tea on a daily basis. Therapeutic claims made about its use are well supported by the literature (Moshi et al., 2010), with a number of studies reporting similar ethnomedical uses in other countries and providing evidence of its phytochemical and curative properties (Boily and van Puyvelde, 1986; Chhabra and Mahunnah, 1994; Rivera and Obon, 1995).

Scale up efforts and challenges

In and around Dar es Salaam leafy vegetable cultivation is reportedly increasing, in part due to the efforts of RESEWO to promote them. These include strategies being developed with the Slow Food movement including cookery demonstrations and disseminating traditional food cookbooks, alongside nutritional education and education on preserving agricultural biodiversity through utilisation.

In addition, the World Vegetable Centre in Arusha is distributing nutritional seed kits containing germplasm of improved varieties of *Amaranthus* spp., *Corchorus olitorius*, *Brassica carinata*, *Crotalaria* spp., *Solanum scabrum*, *Cleome gynandra*, *Moringa oleifera* and *Vigna unguiculata*.

When asked to envision their ideal future, RESEWO members said that they wanted to see more Tanzanians eating traditional foods and Tanzania 'a healthier nation in which malnutrition and poverty have been alleviated and food security and incomes improved by the increased cultivation and use of traditional foods and vegetables' (RESEWO, 2011: 8).

To achieve this vision, it is recommended that RESEWO continues to advise people on establishing and maintaining traditional food and medicine homegardens. The organisation provides a valuable service to surrounding communities by offering nutritional advice and informal health counselling. Intergenerational transfer of knowledge between older members of the community and school children or students is particularly important.

There is a need for strengthened awareness raising, publicity, training, outreach, extension, practical cooking demonstrations and taste education to promote appropriate preparation of foods that maximise their nutrient value. Increased human and financial resources are required for this mission. The need for more sites for cultivation, marketing and demonstration was also highlighted. These focal points could be centres for learning, networking and advocacy around traditional foods, as well as loci for seed-saving and seed bank establishment, natural pest control and post harvest management. Other priorities include establishing rainwater harvesting and irrigation facilities, as well as heightened investment in solar drying, for a simple technique that can be widely applied to most types of leafy vegetables using easily constructed and efficient solar dryers (Martin et al., 1998).

Stakeholder involvement

Rather than acting in isolation, individuals cultivating leafy vegetables are part of social networks. RESEWO, Slow Food and other local groups and networks are tightly linked, allowing for the effective exchange of knowledge and planting materials between homegardeners and women's groups across the country.

RESEWO also seeks institutional involvement by carrying out extensive consultations with local government actors and district agricultural authorities through meetings, workshops, community trainings, conferences and seminars, as well as informal networking. This is facilitated by the fact that the *Chagga* community, which is mostly involved in RESEWO's work, tend of have large and well-connected families, with a high representation in government institutions.

Policy impact

Global agricultural policies emphasise common food crops such as cassava, maize, pigeon peas and beans, meaning that other traditional vegetables have received less attention. In addition, the introduction of imported vegetables, often considered more highly than local varieties by extension services, has undermined the use of indigenous and traditional vegetables (Eyzaguirre and Linares, 2004).

Although rarely promoted in policy, there is great scope for traditional leafy vegetables to be incorporated into national health and nutrition programmes. One good example is the campaign promoted by the Tanzania Food and Nutrition Centre that encourages the cultivation of nutrient-rich vegetables (particularly those rich in iron and vitamin C, which enhances iron availability) at the household level (Lorri, 1996). Further suggestions to promote the use of traditional leafy vegetables in diets as a way of improving dietary diversity and micronutrient status of vulnerable groups – including orphans and people living with HIV/AIDS and kwashiorkor – include: i) engaging district hospitals to carry out awareness-raising campaigns targeting pregnant women and lactating mothers; ii) working with district agricultural projects to monitor food security; iii) carry out research on improved varieties of traditional leafy greens; and iv) provide training on nutrition, food preservation and improved growing practices.

Key lessons learned

Leafy vegetable diversity is an important part of Tanzania's biocultural heritage, particularly in the context of changing dietary patterns, food security, nutrition and health. Supported by the background literature, RESEWO firmly believes that traditional leafy greens can provide a substantial contribution to poverty reduction, as well as increasing food security and improving health in vulnerable communities, showing great promise to reliably and cost-effectively provide food, medicine and, potentially, cash income.

The reasons for growing leafy vegetables not only relate to the plants' phytochemical characteristics, but also to the traditional knowledge and cultural beliefs associated with these species, along with the way they shape the communities' livelihood strategies. In particular, traditional leafy vegetables are grown because of their environmental suitability, ease of cultivation and preparation, and culinary and medicinal uses. Integrating promising taxa into existing crop systems is an affordable means of mitigating malnutrition.

Acknowledgements

I am very grateful to all members of the Regent Estate Senior Women's Organisation and the coastal communities of Tanzania for their participation, academic supervisors (Professor Roy Ellen and Dr Julia Wright) and partners for their critical review, and the UK's Economic and Social Research Council for funding the research via the University of Kent.

References

Boily, Y. and van Puyvelde, L. (1986) 'Screening of medicinal plants of Rwanda (Central Africa) for antimicrobial activity,' *Journal of Ethnopharmacology*, vol 16, pp.1–13.

Chhabra, S.C. and Mahunnah, R.L.A. (1994) 'Plants used in traditional medicine by Hayas of the Kagera region, Tanzania'. *Economic Botany*, vol 48, pp.121–129.

Etkin, N.L. and Ross, P.J. (1983) 'Malaria, Medicine, and Meals: Plant Use among the Hausa and Its Impact on Disease,' in L. Romanucci-Ross, D.E. Moerman, and L.R. Tancredi, (eds) *The Anthropology of Medicine: From Culture to Method*. New York: Praeger.

Eyzaguirre, P.B. and Linares, O.F. (2004) *Homegardens and agrobiodiversity*, Washington: Smithsonian Books.

Food and Agriculture Organization of the United Nations (FAO) (2011) FAOSTAT Online Statistical Service, Rome: FAO, http://faostat.fao.org, accessed June 2012.

Hounsome, N., Hounsome, B., Tomos, D. and Edwards-Jones, G. (2008) 'Plant metabolites and nutritional quality of vegetables,' *Journal of Food Science*, vol 73, no. 4, pp.48–65.

Johns, T., Mhoro, E.B., and Uiso, F.C. (1996) 'Edible plants of Mara region, Tanzania,' *Ecology of Food and Nutrition*, vol 35, pp.71–80.

Kinabo, J. (2008) Tanzania Nutrition Profile, Nutrition and Consumer Protection Division, Rome: FAO, ftp.fao.org/ag/agn/nutrition/ncp/tza.pdf, accessed June 2012 .

Lorri, W. (1996) Editorial, *Nutrition Newsletter*, Tanzania Food and Nutrition Centre, December, no 005.

Lyimo, M., Temu, R.P.C. and Mugula, J.K. (2003) 'Identification and nutrient composition of indigenous vegetables of Tanzania,' *Plant Foods for Human Nutrition*, vol 58, pp.85–92.

Marshall, F. (2001) 'Agriculture and use of wild and weedy greens by the Piik AP Oom okiek of Kenya,' *Economic Botany*, vol 55, no.1, pp.32–46.

Martin, F.W., Ruberté, R.M., and Meitzner, L.S. (1998) *Edible Leaves of the Tropics*, third Edition. ECHO, North Fort Myers, FL.

Mbonile, M.J., and Kivelia, J. (2008) 'Population, environment and development in Kinondoni district, Dar es Salaam,' *Geographical Journal*, vol 174, no. 2, pp.169–175.

MoAFC (2010) Kilimo Kwanza Bagamoyo, Inawezekana timiza wajibu wako. Agricultural Sector Development Programme/District Agricultural Development Plans, Ministry of Agriculture, Food and Cooperatives.

Moshi, M., Otieno, D., Mbabazi, P. and Weisheit, A. (2010) 'Ethnomedicine of the Kagera Region, north western Tanzania, Part 2: The medicinal plants used in Katoro Ward, Bukoba District,' *Journal of Ethnobiology and Ethnomedicine*, vol 6, no 19, doi:10.1186/1746-4269-6-19.

Nabhan, G.P. (2004) *Why some like it hot; Food, Genes and Cultural Diversity*, Washington: Island Press.

Ogoye-Ndegwa, C. and Aagaard-Hansen, J. (2006) 'Dietary and Medicinal Use of Traditional Herbs Among the Luo of Western Kenya,' in A. Pieroni, and L.L. Price (eds) *Eating and Healing; Traditional Food as Medicine*, Oxford: Haworth Press, pp.323–343.

Oniang'o, R.K., Shiundu, K., Maundu, P. and Johns, T. (2006) 'Diversity, nutrition and food security: the case of African leafy vegetables,' in S. Bala Ravi, I. Hoeschle-Zeledon, M.S. Swaminathan and E. Frison (eds) *Hunger and poverty: the role of biodiversity – Report of an International Consultation on The Role of Biodiversity in Achieving the UN Millennium Development Goal of Freedom from Hunger and Poverty*, International Plant Genetic Resources Institute, Rome, Italy, pp.83–100.

Pendaeli, E., Chale, F., Mwasha, I. and Shao, S. (eds) (2010) *Cooking with traditional leafy vegetables; Indigenous plants in Tanzania's kitchen*, Slow Food Foundation for Biodiversity, Dar es Salaam: RESEWO.

Popkin, B.M. (2001) 'The Nutrition Transition and Obesity in the Developing World,' *Journal of Nutrition*, vol 131, no 3, pp.871–873.

RESEWO (2009) *Ripoti utafiti juu ya ufahamu, hisia na mazoea ya jamii kuhusu mboga na vyakula asilia: wilaya za mkuranga na kinondoni*, Regent Estate Senior Women's Organisation.

RESEWO (2011) *Five Year Strategic Plan* (2011–2016), Regent Estate Senior Women's Organisation.

Rivera, D. and Obon, C. (1995) 'The ethnopharmacology of Madeira and Porto Santo islands; A review,' *Journal of Ethnopharmacology*, vol 46, pp.73–93.

Turner, N.J. and Ommer, R. (2003) *'Our Food is Our Medicine': Traditional Plant Foods, Traditional Ecological Knowledge and Health in a Changing Environment*. Proceedings of the First Nations Nutrition and Health Conference.

van Rensburg, J.W.,S., de Ronde, J.A., Venter, S.L., Netshiluvhi, T.R., van den Heever, E. and Vorster, H.J. (2004) 'Role of indigenous leafy vegetables in combating hunger and malnutrition,' *South African Journal of Botany*, vol 70, no 1, pp.52–59.

Case study 12

The Food Acquisition Programme in Brazil: contributions to biodiversity, food security and nutrition

Catia Grisa and Claudia Job Schmitt

The Food Acquisition Programme[1] (PAA)

Former Brazilian President Lula da Silva's first term was marked by the incorporation of hunger, food security and nutrition as key themes in the policy agenda, particularly after the launch of the *Zero Hunger Programme*. This programme provided a set of structural and emergency actions aimed at ensuring human right to food and at eradicating the structural causes of poverty. The creation of the PAA, which encompassed in the same policy instrument consumption subsidies to people suffering from food insecurity and support to family farming,[2] was an innovative measure, and part of the contemporary structuring of an integrated food security policy framework in Brazil (Delgado et al., 2005; Schmitt, 2005).

The programme acquires family farm products and forwards them to public programmes and social organizations supporting people with limited access to food or suffering from food insecurity, thus enabling the establishment of different production–consumption patterns. The PAA operates using different purchasing schemes that enable: i) the setting up of local food networks that support the distribution of family farm products to food insecure populations through a number of social programmes; ii) price regulation of specific products destined to form public security food stocks; iii) the acquisition of food during the growing season to be stored and subsequently sold through farmer organizations (i.e. associations and cooperatives) that can, thereby, position themselves on the market under more favourable terms and; iv) the purchase and donation of milk to socially vulnerable families via a public distribution circuit. The implementation of these mechanisms involves a range of actors, including the federal and state governments, municipalities, as well as farmer and social service organizations. The different buying modalities that operate at different scales, can be used as a toolbox of sorts, and adapted to fit the different local contexts.

From 2003 to 2010, more than US\$2.03 billion (3.5 billion reais) were spent on the purchase of approximately 3.1 million tonnes of food (Brasil, 2011); and between 2008 and 2010, the number of farming families involved in the PAA reached 160,000 per year – only a small percentage (3.7 per cent) considering the total number of family farms existing in Brazil (4.3 million, according to

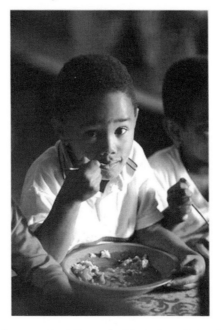

Figure C12.1 A child eating food from the Food Acquisition Programme. Source: CONAB

the Agricultural Census of 2006). The PAA is currently being implemented in approximately 40 per cent of Brazilian municipalities, reaching more than 25,000 governmental and non-governmental organizations per year, including schools, child care organizations, nursing homes and community kitchens among others, with 15 million people benefiting from food distribution every year (Brasil, 2011).

Promoting diversification and the sustainable management of biodiversity for food and nutrition: PAA's contribution

In many contexts, the PAA has promoted changes in the productive matrix of family farming as well as in the links between farm units and markets. Public procurement schemes are helping to strengthen polyculture, historically a traditional feature of a "farmer's way of life" in Brazil (Wanderley, 1999). This is happening because in many regions of Brazil, the "modernization of agriculture" has led farmers to specialize in the production of a limited number of commodity crops and to adopt unsustainable agricultural practices based on the intensive use of pesticides and other chemical inputs, which, in turn, has exposed these families to economic, social and health vulnerability. Furthermore, the PAA has encouraged the diversification of production, thus connecting agricultural supply to a diversified demand. For example, in a survey conducted in the state of Paraná (southern region of Brazil), Ghizelini (2010) noted that products that farmers were unaccustomed to selling on the market, or that had little commercial value, were included in a wide range of "marketable" products. Prior to implementation of the PAA only 4 per cent of family farms included in the survey used to market their vegetables; after accessing the programme, 98 per cent of the surveyed households included these crops in their social reproduction strategies.

In addition to providing incentives for diversification, the PAA is also rescuing, recovering and commercially promoting forgotten regional and local products, some of which had never been marketed before. The result of this work is the revitalization and preservation of traditional knowledge, food customs and local cultures associated with these foods that had been lost over generations because of the negative perceptions associated with them; foods that were considered "old-fashioned" or had been eroded by the mercantilization of agriculture (Ploeg, 2008; 2003). Within the state of Rio Grande do Sul (Southern Brazil), which was partly colonized by European settlers, the PAA helped revitalize colonial mills. According to Pandolfo (2008), these mills carry the historical legacy of generations of family farmers and have an important role in preserving the culture and the food habits of rural households. This example illustrates a broader process of recovery of regional food practices that is being carried out in different regions of Brazil. Foods such as hominy (dried maize), babassu palm (*Attalea speciosa*) flour, pine nuts, coconut oil, baru nut (*Dipteryx alata*) flour, cupuaçu (*Theobroma grandiflora*), palm hearts, umbu (*Spondias* sp.), maxixe (*Cucumis anguria*) and jambú (*Syzygium* sp.), among others, are being served more frequently in schools and social care organizations.

Some of these regional foods purchased by the PAA derive from sustainable extractivist practices. In 2008, the PAA acquired 28 types of extractivist products, benefiting over 8,000 extractivist families, especially women who are often the main collectors of these products. Furthermore, the acquisition of extractivist products – such as those derived from the babassu palm (oil and flour) – has multiple benefits: on the one hand, it promotes the conservation and sustainable use of this palm tree; on the other, it grants children, the elderly and socially vulnerable groups access to food with high nutritional value. In the state of Acre, in the Amazon, before the PAA programme was established, Brazil nut extractivists depended entirely on the market opportunities provided by brokers, who would mostly buy the nuts below their market value. Under the PAA programme, extractivists are guaranteed the sale of their production and have seen the price of the nuts almost double (Cordeiro, 2007). The above-mentioned examples demonstrate that positive interactions between social and ecological processes can be achieved while conserving and sustainably managing biodiversity for food and nutrition.

In order to provide healthy, pesticide-free food to socially vulnerable groups, the PAA also promotes the commercialization of agro-ecological or organic food by supporting production systems that embrace sustainable and biodiversity conservation practices, while emphasizing the use of local resources. To this end, the programme provides a price premium of 30 per cent for environmentally-

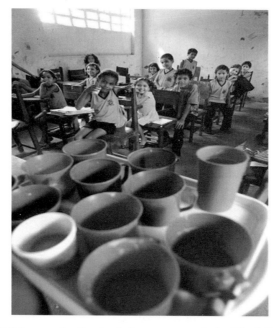

Figure C12.2 Children at school eating babassu coconut derived food. Source: CONAB

sound food products. However, the main challenge for policy makers and farm organizations remains the provision of incentives for the expansion of these agro-ecological practices and the development of mechanisms of conformity assessment that can be easily accessed by family farmers and adapted to different local contexts.

It is also worth mentioning that the PAA allows the purchase, donation and exchange of traditional and local seed varieties, as well as commercial non-hybrid seeds. The aim is to rescue and preserve biodiversity, stimulate the production and exchange of such seeds and promote the autonomy and sustainability of farming practices. These seeds carry with them the history of generations, connecting ecological processes, agricultural practices, knowledge and culture, while enabling farmers to become less dependent on external inputs and more empowered in their relations with technical experts and traders (Londres and Almeida, 2009). Several family farming organizations and technical advising non-governmental organizations (NGOs) are relying on institutional markets as an effective support mechanism for initiatives focusing on biodiversity conservation and management.

Changing the menus: PAA's contribution to food security and nutrition

The PAA contributes to enhancing food and nutritional security on both sides of the food chain by improving diets at the farm level, while ensuring that vulnerable groups have access to good quality food. Evidence of the nutritional impacts of the PAA is still limited; however, a number of surveys indicate important changes in dietary diversity and health status of families benefiting from the PAA programme.

In families producing food for the PAA, research has shown increases in dietary diversity, as well as in quantity and quality of food for self-consumption (Becker, 2010; Costa, 2010; Delgado et al., 2005). In general, products marketed through the programme are those normally consumed by households, and promoting the commercialization of these food stuffs seems to positively affect production for self-consumption. As pointed out by Zimmermann and Ferreira (2008), the PAA has been responsible for including fresh fruit and vegetables in the diets of family farmers. Before the programme, many farmers had no fruit trees in their farms and did not value native fruits. Similarly, Costa (2010) noted that families who took part in the PAA scheme were changing eating habits, incorporating vegetables into their diets and expanding their knowledge about healthy eating. Research carried out on organizations involved in the PAA distribution scheme showed an increase in the quality and diversity of food offered to scheme recipients (Triches, 2010; Costa, 2010; Zimmermann and Ferreira, 2008).

Despite the fact that PAA provides only a portion of the food needs of these social programmes, savings resulting from donations have helped expand the food supply capacity of social service organizations and helped them invest in dietary diversification. In schools, for instance, the PAA now ensures that fresh, locally-produced, often organic food is made available in the canteens, as opposed to the processed meals that were previously served and that were incompatible with regional food cultures. Preliminary observations seem to confirm that the initiative is contributing to the attendance, performance and well-being of school children (Zimmermann and Ferreira, 2008; Ortega, Jesus and Só, 2006).

Lessons learned

As discussed above, the implementation of the PAA has demonstrated that public policy can simultaneously support family farming while addressing food security and nutrition as well as biodiversity conservation. The knowledge and experience accumulated and the positive results of the PAA have inspired other initiatives dealing with institutional markets. In 2009, for example, the Brazilian National School Meals Programme (PNAE) decreed that at least 30 per cent of the food purchased through its programme should be acquired directly from family farmers through simplified acquisition procedures.

Despite this success, the Brazilian government has faced a number of challenges during the design and implementation of the PAA. The inclusion of underprivileged farmers, in general, and specific groups of farmers (such as agrarian reform settlers, indigenous groups, *quilombolas*,[3] babassu and coconut harvesters, etc.), is still limited due to their fragile organizational structure.

In many cases, information gaps and limited access to public institutions – an expression of the social inequalities that still prevail in Brazilian society – prevent farmers from fully benefiting from the programme. However, it should be highlighted that the PAA has demonstrated in a wide variety of settings its worth as a powerful tool to promote market access by family farmers while supporting ecologically-friendly agriculture and extractivist activities.

Notes

1 In Portuguese, *Programa de Aquisição de Alimentos* (PAA).
2 Within Brazilian public policy, the term family farming designates a heterogeneous universe composed by rural farmers, modernized family farmers, agrarian reform settlers, quilombolas, extractivists and indigenous peoples, among others.
3 The Associação Brasileira de Antropologia (Brazilian Anthropology Association) defines *quilombola* communities as "groups who resist changing their traditional way of life". Living in temporary settlements, most *quilombolas* descend from the African slaves who were shipped to Brazil at the beginning of the 16th century to work on plantations until the abolition of slavery in 1888.

References

Becker, C. (2010) 'A eficácia de uma política pública: análise do Programa de Aquisição de Alimentos (PAA) em municípios do território Zona Sul do Rio Grande do Sul', Dissertação de Mestrado, Universidade Federal de Pelotas, RS/Brasil.

Brasil (2011) 'Programa de Aquisição de Alimentos – PAA' (Caderno Base III Seminário Nacional PAA), Brasília, MDA.

Cordeiro, A. (2007) 'Resultados do programa de aquisição de alimentos – PAA: a perspectiva dos beneficiários', Brasília, CONAB.

Costa, I.B. (2010) 'Nesta terra, em se plantando tudo dá? Política de Soberania e Segurança Alimentar e Nutricional no meio rural paranaense, o caso do PAA,' Tese de Doutorado, Universidade Federal do Rio Grande do Norte, RG/Brasil.

Delgado, G.C., Conceição, J.C.P.R. and Oliveira, J.J. (2005) 'Avaliação do programa de aquisição de alimentos da agricultura familiar,' Brasília, IPEA.

Ghizelini, A.A.M. (2010) 'Atores sociais, agricultura familiar camponesa e o espaço local: uma análise a partir do Programa de Aquisição de Alimentos,' Tese de Doutorado, Universidade Federal do Paraná, PR/Brasil.

Londres, F., Almeida, P. (2009) 'Impacto do controle corporativo no setor de sementes sobre agricultores familiares e sistemas alternativos de distribuição: estudo de caso do Brasil,' Rio de Janeiro, ASPTA.

Ortega, A. C., Jesus, C.M., Só, L.L.S. (2006) 'O PAA-leite na Bahia e em Minas Gerais: uma avaliação preliminar de seus modelos de implementação', *Cadernos do CEAM*, ano V, no 24, pp.57–89.

Pandolfo, M.C. (2008) 'O programa de aquisição de alimentos como instrumento revitalizador dos mercados regionais,' *Agriculturas*, vol 5, no 2, pp.14–17.

Ploeg, J.D. Van der (2003) *The virtual farmer: past, present and future of the Dutch peasantry*, Royal Van Gorcum, Assen.

Ploeg, J.D. Van der (2008) 'Camponeses e impérios alimentares: lutas por autonomia e susutentabilidade na era da globalização,' Porto Alegre, UFRGS.

Schmitt, C.J. (2005) 'Aquisição de alimentos da agricultura familiar: integração entre política agrícola e segurança alimentar e nutricional,' *Revista de Política Agrícola*, ano XIV, no 2, pp.78–88.

Triches, R.M. (2010) 'Reconectando a produção ao consumo: a aquisição de gêneros alimentícios da agricultura familiar no Programa de Alimentação Escolar,' Tese de Doutorado, Universidade Federal do Rio Grande do Sul, RS/Brasil.

Wanderley, M.N.B. (1999) 'Raízes históricas do campesinato brasileiro,' in J.C. Tedesco (Org.) *Agricultura Familiar: realidades e perspectivas*, Passo Fundo, Editora UPF, pp.23–56.

Zimmermann, S.A., Ferreira, A.P. (2008) 'El programa de adquisición de alimentos de la agricultura familiar en Mirandiba-PE,' in G. Scotto, *Aun hay tiempo para el sol: pobrezas rurales y programas sociales*, Rio de Janeiro, Actionaid.

Index